HEALTH AND HUMAN DEVELOPMENT

PAIN MANAGEMENT YEARBOOK 2015

HEALTH AND HUMAN DEVELOPMENT

JOAV MERRICK - SERIES EDITOR –

MEDICAL DIRECTOR,
MINISTRY OF SOCIAL AFFAIRS, JERUSALEM, ISRAEL

Adolescent Behavior Research: International Perspectives
Joav Merrick and Hatim A Omar (Editors)
2007. ISBN: 1-60021-649-8

Complementary Medicine Systems: Comparison and Integration
Karl W Kratky
2008. ISBN: 978-1-60456-475-4

Pain in Children and Youth
P Schofield and J Merrick (Editors)
2008. ISBN: 978-1-60456-951-3

Alcohol-Related Cognitive Disorders: Research and Clinical Perspectives
Leo Sher, Isack Kandel and Joav Merrick (Editors)
2009. ISBN: 978-1-60741-730-9

Challenges in Adolescent Health: An Australian Perspective
David Bennett, Susan Towns and Elizabeth Elliott and Joav Merrick (Editors)
2009. ISBN: 978-1-60741-616-6

Children and Pain
P Schofield and J Merrick (Editors)
2009. ISBN: 978-1-60876-020-6

Living on the Edge: The Mythical, Spiritual, and Philosophical Roots of Social Marginality
Joseph Goodbread
2009. ISBN: 978-1-60741-162-8 (Hardcover)
2011. ISBN: 978-1-61470-192-7 (E-book)
2013. ISBN: 978-1-61122-986-8 (Softcover)

Obesity and Adolescence: A Public Health Concern
Hatim A Omar, Donald E Greydanus, Dilip R Patel and Joav Merrick (Editors)
2009. ISBN: 978-1-60692-821-9

Poverty and Children: A Public Health Concern
Alexis Lieberman and Joav Merrick (Editors)
2009. ISBN: 978-1-60741-140-6

Bone and Brain Metastases: Advances in Research and Treatment
Arjun Sahgal, Edward Chow and Joav Merrick (Editors)
2010. ISBN: 978-1-61668-365-8

Chance Action and Therapy: The Playful Way of Changing
Uri Wernik
2010. ISBN: 978-1-60876-393-1

International Aspects of Child Abuse and Neglect
Howard Dubowitz and Joav Merrick (Editors)
2010. ISBN: 978-1-61122-049-0

Advanced Cancer, Pain and Quality of Life
Edward Chow and Joav Merrick (Editors)
2011. ISBN: 978-1-61668-207-1

Advances in Environmental Health Effects of Toxigenic Mold and Mycotoxins
Ebere Cyril Anyanwu
2011. ISBN: 978-1-60741-953-2

Alternative Medicine Yearbook 2009
Joav Merrick (Editor)
2011. ISBN: 978-1-61668-910-0

Behavioral Pediatrics, 3rd Edition
Donald E Greydanus, Dilip R Patel, Helen D Pratt and Joseph L Calles Jr. (Editors)
2011. ISBN: 978-1-60692-702-1

Chance Action and Therapy: The Playful Way of Changing
Uri Wernik
2011. ISBN: 978-1-61122-987-5

Child Health and Human Development Yearbook 2009
Joav Merrick (Editor)
2011. ISBN: 978-1-61668-912-4

Climate Change and Rural Child Health
Erica Bell, Bastian M Seidel and Joav Merrick (Editors)
2011. ISBN: 978-1-61122-640-9

Clinical Aspects of Psychopharmacology in Childhood and Adolescence
DE Greydanus, JL Calles Jr., DP Patel, A Nazeer and J Merrick (Editors)
2011. ISBN: 978-1-61122-135-0

Drug Abuse in Hong Kong: Development and Evaluation of a Prevention Program
Daniel TL Shek, Rachel CF Sun and Joav Merrick (Editors)
2011. ISBN: 978-1-61324-491-3

Environment, Mood Disorders and Suicide
Teodor T Postolache and Joav Merrick (Editors)
2011. ISBN: 978-1-61668-505-8

International Aspects of Child Abuse and Neglect
Howard Dubowitz and Joav Merrick (Editors)
2011. ISBN: 978-1-60876-703-8

Narratives and Meanings of Migration
Julia Mirsky
2011. ISBN: 978-1-61761-103-2

Positive Youth Development: Evaluation and Future Directions in a Chinese Context
Daniel TL Shek, Hing Keung Ma and Joav Merrick (Editors)
2011. ISBN: 978-1-60876-830-1 (Hardcover)
2011. ISBN: 978-1-62100-175-1 (Softcover)

Positive Youth Development: Implementation of a Youth Program in a Chinese Context
Daniel TL Shek, Hing Keung Ma and Joav Merrick (Editors)
2011. ISBN: 978-1-61668-230-9

Principles of Holistic Psychiatry: A Textbook on Holistic Medicine for Mental Disorders
Soren Ventegodt and Joav Merrick
2011. ISBN: 978-1-61761-940-3

Public Health Yearbook 2009
Joav Merrick (Editor)
2011. ISBN: 978-1-61668-911-7

Randomized Clinical Trials and Placebo: Can You Trust the Drugs Are Working and Safe?
Søren Ventegodt and Joav Merrick
2011. ISBN: 978-1-61470-151-4 (E-book)
2012. ISBN: 978-1-61470-067-8 (Hardcover)

Rural Child Health: International Aspects
Erica Bell and Joav Merrick (Editors)
2011. ISBN: 978-1-60876-357-3

Rural Medical Education: Practical Strategies
Erica Bell and Craig Zimitat and Joav Merrick (Editors)
2011. ISBN: 978-1-61122-649-2

Self-Management and the Health Care Consumer
Peter William Harvey
2011. ISBN: 978-1-61761-796-6

Sexology from a Holistic Point of View
Soren Ventegodt and Joav Merrick
2011. ISBN: 978-1-61761-859-8

Social and Cultural Psychiatry Experience from the Caribbean Region
Hari D Maharajh and Joav Merrick (Editors)
2011. ISBN: 978-1-61668-506-5

The Dance of Sleeping and Eating among Adolescents: Normal and Pathological Perspectives
Yael Latzer and Orna Tzischinsky (Editors)
2011. ISBN: 978-1-61209-710-7

Understanding Eating Disorders: Integrating Culture, Psychology and Biology
Yael Latzer, Joav Merrick and Daniel Stein (Editors)
2011. ISBN: 978-1-61728-298-0 (Hardcover)
2011. ISBN: 978-1-61470-976-3 (Softcover)

Adolescence and Chronic Illness. A Public Health Concern
Hatim Omar, Donald E Greydanus, Dilip R Patel and Joav Merrick (Editors)
2012. ISBN: 978-1-60876-628-4

AIDS and Tuberculosis: Public Health Aspects
Daniel Chemtob and Joav Merrick (Editors)
2012. ISBN: 978-1-62081-382-9

Alternative Medicine Yearbook 2010
Joav Merrick (Editor)
2012. ISBN: 978-1-62100-132-4

Alternative Medicine Research Yearbook 2011
Joav Merrick (Editor)
2012. ISBN: 978-1-62081-476-5

Applied Public Health: Examining Multifaceted Social or Ecological Problems and Child Maltreatment
John R Lutzker and Joav Merrick (Editors)
2012. ISBN: 978-1-62081-356-0

Building Community Capacity: Minority and Immigrant Populations
Rosemary M Caron and Joav Merrick (Editors)
2012. ISBN: 978-1-62081-022-4

Building Community Capacity: Skills and Principles
Rosemary M Caron and Joav Merrick (Editors)
2012. ISBN 978-1-61209-331-4

Child and Adolescent Health Yearbook 2009
Joav Merrick (Editor)
2012. ISBN: 978-1-61668-913-1

Child and Adolescent Health Yearbook 2010
Joav Merrick (Editor)
2012. ISBN: 978-1-61209-788-6

Child Health and Human Development Yearbook 2010
Joav Merrick (Editor)
2012. ISBN: 8-1-61209-789-3

Conceptualizing Behavior in Health and Social Research: A Practical Guide to Data Analysis
Said Shahtahmasebi and Damon Berridge
2013. ISBN: 978-1-60876-383-2

Human Immunodeficiency Virus (HIV) Research: Social Science Aspects
Hugh Klein and Joav Merrick (Editors)
2012. ISBN: 978-1-62081-293-8

Our Search for Meaning in Life: Quality of Life Philosophy
Soren Ventegodt and Joav Merrick
2012. ISBN: 978-1-61470-494-2

Public Health Yearbook 2010
Joav Merrick (Editor)
2012. ISBN: 978-1-61209-971-2

Public Health Yearbook 2011
Joav Merrick (Editor)
2012. ISBN: 978-1-62081-433-8

Textbook on Evidence-Based Holistic Mind-Body Medicine: Basic Philosophy and Ethics of Traditional Hippocratic Medicine
Søren Ventegodt and Joav Merrick
ISBN: 978-1-62257-052-2

Textbook on Evidence-Based Holistic Mind-Body Medicine: Basic Principles of Healing in Traditional Hippocratic Medicine
Søren Ventegodt and Joav Merrick
2012. ISBN: 978-1-62257-094-2

Textbook on Evidence-Based Holistic Mind-Body Medicine: Healing the Mind in Traditional Hippocratic Medicine
Søren Ventegodt and Joav Merrick
2012. ISBN: 978-1-62257-112-3

Textbook on Evidence-Based Holistic Mind-Body Medicine: Holistic Practice of Traditional Hippocratic Medicine
Søren Ventegodt and Joav Merrick
2012. ISBN: 978-1-62257-105-5

Textbook on Evidence-Based Holistic Mind-Body Medicine: Research, Philosophy, Economy and Politics of Traditional Hippocratic Medicine
Søren Ventegodt and Joav Merrick
2012. ISBN: 978-1-62257-140-6

Textbook on Evidence-Based Holistic Mind-Body Medicine: Sexology and Traditional Hippocratic Medicine
Søren Ventegodt and Joav Merrick
2012. ISBN: 978-1-62257-130-7

The Astonishing Brain and Holistic Consciousness: Neuroscience and Vedanta Perspectives
Vinod D Deshmukh
2012. ISBN: 978-1-61324-295-7

Translational Research for Primary Healthcare
Erica Bell, Gert P Westert and Joav Merrick (Editors)
2012. ISBN: 978-1-61324-647-4

Treatment and Recovery of Eating Disorders
Daniel Stein and Yael Latzer (Editors)
2012. ISBN: 978-1-61470-259-7 (Hardcover)
2013. ISBN: 978-1-62808-248-7 (Softcover)

Adolescence and Sports
Dilip R Patel, Donald E Greydanus, Hatim Omar and Joav Merrick (Editors)
2013. ISBN: 978-1-60876-702-1

Advanced Cancer: Managing Symptoms and Quality of Life
Natalie Pulenzas, Breanne Lechner, Nemica Thavarajah, Edward Chow and Joav Merrick (Editors)
2013. ISBN: 978-1-62808-239-5

Alternative Medicine Research Yearbook 2012
Søren Ventegodt and Joav Merrick (Editors)
2013. ISBN: 978-1-62808-080-3

Building Community Capacity: Case Examples from Around the World
Rosemary M Caron and Joav Merrick (Editors)
2013. ISBN: 978-1-62417-175-8

Bullying: A Public Health Concern
Jorge C Srabstein and Joav Merrick (Editors)
2013. ISBN: 978-1-62618-564-7

Food, Nutrition and Eating Behavior
Joav Merrick and Sigal Israeli
2013. ISBN: 978-1-62948-233-0

Health and Happiness from Meaningful Work: Research in Quality of Working Life
Soren Ventegodt and Joav Merrick (Editors)
2013. ISBN: 978-1-60692-820-2

Health Promotion: Community Singing as a Vehicle to Promote Health
Joav Merrick (Editors)
2013. ISBN: 978-1-62618-908-9

Health Promotion: Strengthening Positive Health and Preventing Disease
Jing Sun, Nicholas Buys and Joav Merrick (Editors)
2013. ISBN: 978-1-62257-870-2

Health Risk Communication
Marijke Lemal and Joav Merrick(Editors)
2013. ISBN: 978-1-62257-544-2

Human Development: Biology from a Holistic Point of View
Søren Ventegodt, Tyge Dahl Hermansen and Joav Merrick (Editors)
2013. ISBN: 978-1-61470-441-6

Managed Care in a Public Setting
Richard Evan Steele
2013. ISBN: 978-1-62417-970-9

Mental Health from an International Perspective
Joav Merrick, Shoshana Aspler and Mohammed Morad (Editors)
2013. ISBN: 978-1-62948-519-5

Pain Management Yearbook 2011
Joav Merrick (Editor)
2013. ISBN: 978-1-62808-970-7

Pain Management Yearbook 2012
Joav Merrick (Editor)
2013. ISBN: 978-1-62808-973-8

Pediatric and Adolescent Sexuality and Gynecology: Principles for the Primary Care Clinician
Hatim A Omar, Donald E Greydanus, Artemis K Tsitsika, Dilip R Patel and Joav Merrick (Editors)
2013. ISBN: 978-1-60876-735-9

Public Health Concern: Smoking, Alcohol and Substance Use
Joav Merrick and Ariel Tenenbaum (Editors)
2013. ISBN: 978-1-62948-424-2

Public Health Yearbook 2012
Joav Merrick (Editor)
2013. ISBN: 978-1-62808-078-0

Alternative Medicine Research Yearbook 2013
Joav Merrick (Editor)
2014. ISBN: 978-1-63321-094-3

India: Health and Human Development Aspects
Joav Merrick (Editor)
2014. ISBN: 978-1-62948-784-7

Public Health: Improving Health via Inter-Professional Collaborations
Rosemary M. Caron and Joav Merrick (Editors)
2014. ISBN: 978-1-63321-569-6

Public Health Yearbook 2013
Joav Merrick (Editor)
2014. ISBN: 978-1-63321-095-0

Suicide from a Public Health Perspective
Said Shahtahmasebi and Joav Merrick
2014. ISBN: 978-1-62948-536-2

Alternative Medicine Research Yearbook 2014
Joav Merrick (Editor)
2015. ISBN: 978-1-63482-161-2

Cancer: Bone Metastases, CNS Metastases and Pathological Fractures
Breanne Lechner, Ronald Chow, Natalie Pulenzas, Marko Popovic, Na Zhang, Xiaojing Zhang, Edward Chow and Joav Merrick (Editors)
2015. ISBN: 978-1-63483-949-5

Cancer: Pain and Symptom Management
Breanne Lechner, Ronald Chow, Natalie Pulenzas, Marko Popovic, Na Zhang, Xiaojing Zhang, Edward Chow and Joav Merrick (Editors)
2015. ISBN: 978-1-63483-864-1

Cancer: Spinal Cord, Lung, Breast, Cervical, Prostate, Head and Neck Cancer
Breanne Lechner, Ronald Chow, Natalie Pulenzas, Marko Popovic, Na Zhang, Xiaojing Zhang, Edward Chow and Joav Merrick (Editors)
2015. ISBN: 978-1-63483-904-4

Cancer: Survival, Quality of Life and Ethical Implications
Breanne Lechner, Ronald Chow, Natalie Pulenzas, Marko Popovic, Na Zhang, Xiaojing Zhang, Edward Chow and Joav Merrick (Editors)
2015. ISBN: 978-1-63483-905-1

Cancer: Treatment, Decision Making and Quality of Life
Breanne Lechner, Ronald Chow, Natalie Pulenzas, Marko Popovic, Na Zhang, Xiaojing Zhang, Edward Chow and Joav Merrick (Editors)
2015. ISBN: 978-1-63483-863-4

Forensic Psychiatry: A Public Health Perspective
Leo Sher and Joav Merrick (Editors)
2015. ISBN: 978-1-63483-339-4

Leadership and Service Learning Education: Holistic Development for Chinese University Students
Daniel TL Shek, Florence KY Wu and Joav Merrick (Editors)
2015. ISBN: 978-1-63483-340-0

Mental and Holistic Health: Some International Perspectives
Joseph L. Calles Jr., Donald E Greydanus and Joav Merrick (Editors)
2015. ISBN: 978-1-63483-589-3

Pain Management Yearbook 2014
Joav Merrick (Editor)
2015. ISBN: 978-1-63482-164-3

Public Health Yearbook 2014
Joav Merrick (Editor)
2015. ISBN: 978-1-63482-165-0

Public Health Yearbook 2015
Joav Merrick (Editor)
2016. ISBN: 978-1-63484-514-4

Alternative Medicine Research Yearbook 2015
Joav Merrick (Editor)
2016. ISBN: 978-1-63484-511-3

Pain Management Yearbook 2015
Joav Merrick (Editor)
2016. ISBN: 978-1-63484-515-1

HEALTH AND HUMAN DEVELOPMENT

PAIN MANAGEMENT YEARBOOK 2015

JOAV MERRICK
EDITOR

New York

Additional color graphics may be available in the e-book version of this book.

Library of Congress Cataloging-in-Publication Data

ISBN: 978-1-63484-515-1

ISSN: 2163-7504

Published by Nova Science Publishers, Inc. † New York

CONTENTS

INTRODUCTION

Cancer Pain, Cannabis and Cannabinoids

***Michael C Tjong, MD(C)*[1]*, Joav Merrick, MD, MMedSc, DMSc*[2-6] *and Luluel Khan, MD*[1,*]**

[1]Sunnybrook Health Sciences Centre, Odette Cancer Centre, Department of Radiation Oncology, Toronto, Ontario, Canada

[2]National Institute of Child Health and Human Development, Jerusalem, Israel

[3]Office of the Medical Director, Health Services, Division for Intellectual and Developmental Disabilities, Ministry of Social Affairs and Social Services, Jerusalem, Israel

[4]Division of Pediatrics, Hadassah Hebrew University Medical Center, Mt Scopus Campus, Jerusalem, Israel

[5]Kentucky Children's Hospital, University of Kentucky College of Medicine, Lexington, Kentucky, US

[6]Center for Healthy Development, School of Public Health, Georgia State University, Atlanta, US

Introduction

Pain is one major symptom of cancer patients, and many patients receive inadequate management of their cancer pain (1). Various medications are used to manage cancer pain such as NSAIDs and opioids. For patients whose cancer symptoms are not relieved by commonly available medications, cannabis and cannabinoids emerged as alternative options (2, 3). Many patients with terminal cancer considering the use of cannabis and cannabinoids to provide pain relief. It is important to objectively appraise cannabinoids efficacy and safety profile in relieving cancer pain before regularly prescribing them to patients.

Oral cannabinoids and smoked cannabis efficacy has been demonstrated with acceptable safety in nociceptive and neuropathic non-cancer chronic pain (4, 5). A study by Ellis et al. (6, 7) demonstrated that the active substance in cannabis, Δ^9-tetrahydrocannabinol (Δ^9-THC)

* Correspondence: Luluel Khan, MD, Sunnybrook Health Sciences Centre, Odette Cancer Centre (T2-136a), Department of Radiation Oncology, 2075 Bayview Avenue, Toronto, ON M4N 3M5, Canada. E-mail: luluel.khan@gmail.com.

is both efficacious and well-tolerated for neuropathic pain in HIV patients. However, the current literature available about the use of cannabinoids in cancer pain provided mixed results (8). Early trial indicated that oral Δ^9-THC in sufficient dose to alleviate cancer pain comes with adverse effects of sedation, dizziness, and confusion (9). In recent systematic review by Campbell (10), it was concluded that Δ^9-THC is no more effective than codeine in alleviating cancer pain with significant side effects. These studies may discourage the use of Δ^9-THC as a monotherapy in cancer care palliation. Nonetheless, cannabinoids may have a role in refractory cancer pain unresolved by opioids (2). Sativex, a mixture of Δ^9-THC and cannabidiol (CBD) is shown to be efficacious in relieving cancer pain intractable by opioids alone (3).

Similarly, the potential use of cannabinoids in alleviating other cancer symptoms such as nausea and anorexia have yielded mixed results. In 1975, Sallen et al. (11) reported the anti-emetic effect of Δ^9-THC on patient receiving chemotherapy. A systematic review of 30 randomized trials showed better response with cannabinoids compared to placebo and conventional anti-emetics including chlorpromazine, prochlorperazine, and metoclopramide in acute, but not chronic setting (8, 12). Nonetheless, new anti-emetic 5-hydroxytryptamine (5-HT) receptor 3 has been developed since the review and shown to be highly efficacious in alleviating chemotherapy induced nausea and vomiting (CINV) (8, 13). In a randomized trial with 243 patients, cannabis extract and Δ^9-THC were shown to be no better than placebo in improving quality of life and appetite of patients with cancer-related anorexia-cachexia (CRAC) syndrome (14).

Based on current evidence, the use of cannabinoids in treating cancer pain may be limited to intractable pain, which is not fully resolved by opioids. While cannabinoid monotherapy was shown to be efficacious in treating cancer pain, the effective dose is associated with significant adverse effects (9). Considering the safety profile of cannabis products and availability of effective alternatives, more evidence is needed to justify more widespread use of cannabinoids in treating chemotherapy induced emesis, and cancer-related anorexia and cachexia (8, 13). Lastly, no study has been conducted on the use of smoked cannabis in cancer pain. With the legalization of medical marijuana in Canada, United States and some other countries, information from such studies would assist physicians in ensuring proper prescription of medical marijuana for cancer pain.

REFERENCES

[1] Deandrea S, Montanari M, Moja L, Apolone G. Prevalence of undertreatment in cancer pain. A review of published literature. Ann Oncol 2008;19(12):1985-91.

[2] Farquhar-Smith WP. Do cannabinoids have a role in cancer pain management? Curr Opin Support Palliat Care 2009;3(1):7-13.

[3] Johnson JR, Burnell-Nugent M, Lossignol D, Ganae-Motan ED, Potts R, Fallon MT. Multicenter, double-blind, randomized, placebo-controlled, parallel-group study of the ef?cacy, safety, and tolerability of THC:CBD extract and THC extract in patients with intractable cancer-related pain. J Pain Symptom Manage 2010;39(2):167-79.

[4] Ware MA, Wang T, Shapiro S, Robinson A, Ducruet T, Huynh T, et al. Smoked cannabis for chronic neuropathic pain: A randomized controlled trial. CMAJ 2010;182(14):E694-701.

[5] Lynch ME, Campbell F. Cannabinoids for treatment of chronic non-cancer pain; a systematic review of randomized trials. Br J Clin Pharmacol 2011;72(5):735-44.

[6] Ellis RJ, Toperoff W, Vaida F, van den Brande G, Gonzales J, Gouaux B, et al. Smoked edicinal cannabis for neuropathic pain in HIV: a randomized, crossover clinical trial. Neuropsychopharmacology 2009;34(3):672-80.

[7] Abrams DI, Guzman M. Cannabis in cancer care. Clin Pharmacol Ther 2015 Mar 16. [Epub ahead of print]

[8] Bowles DW, O'Bryant CL, Camidge DR, Jimeno A. The intersection between cannabis and cancer in the United States. Crit Rev Oncol Hematol 2012;83(1):1-10.

[9] Noyes R Jr, Brunk SF, Avery DA, Canter AC. The analgesic properties of delta-9-tetrahydrocannabinol and codeine. Clin Pharmacol Ther 1975;18(1):84-9.

[10] Campbell FA, Tram?r MR, Carroll D, Reynolds DJ, Moore RA, McQuay HJ. Are cannabinoids an effective and safe treatment option in the management of pain? A qualitative systematic review. BMJ 2001;323(7303):13-6.

[11] Sallen SE, Zinberg NE, Frei E. Antiemetic effect of delta-9-THC in patients receiving cancer chemotherapy. New Engl J Med 1975;293:795-797.

[12] Tramer MR, Carroll D, Campbell FA, Reynolds DJ, Moore RA, McQuay HJ. Cannabinoids for control of chemotherapy induced nausea and vomiting: quantitative systematic eview. BMJ 2001;323(7303):16-21.

[13] Hall W1, Christie M, Currow D. Cannabinoids and cancer: causation, remediation, and palliation. Lancet Oncol 2005;6(1):35-42.

[14] Strasser F, Luftner D, Possinger K, Ernst G, Ruhstaller T, Meissner W, et al. Comparison of orally administered cannabis extract and delta-9-tetrahydrocannabinol in treating patients with cancer-related anorexia-cachexia syndrome: a multicenter, phase III, randomized, double-blind, placebo-controlled clinical trial from the Cannabis-In-Cachexia-Study-Group. J Clin Oncol 2006;24(21):3394-400.

SECTION ONE:
CANCER, INTELLECTUAL DISABILITY AND PAIN

In: Pain Management Yearbook 2015
Editor: Joav Merrick

ISBN: 978-1-63484-515-1

Chapter 1

REVIEW OF FENTANYL FORMULATIONS IN THE MANAGEMENT OF BREAKTHROUGH CANCER PAIN

Michelle Zhou[1], BSc, Marissa Slaven[2], MD, Andrea Forgione[1], BSc, Mark Pasetka[1], PharmD, Liang Zeng[1], MD(C), Henry Lam[1], MLS, Lori Holden[1], MRT(T), Natalie Pulenzas[1], BSc(C), Nicholas Lao[1], BMSc(C), Edward Chow[1], MBBS, and Carlo DeAngelis[1*], PharmD

[1]Sunnybrook Health Sciences Centre, University of Toronto, Toronto, Ontario, Canada

[2]McMaster University, Hamilton, Ontario, Canada

Breakthrough pain (BTP) has been commonly described as a transient exacerbation of pain that breaks through well-controlled persistent pain either spontaneously or in relation to a predictable trigger. The purpose was to summarize the evidence for dosing, frequency, definition of tolerance, and dose conversions between opioids in cancer patients administered various fentanyl ROO preparations. A literature search was conducted and 16 studies identified. Each definition varied but the majority classified BTP as a transient flare. The lowest OTFC starting dose of 200 mcg was used in all but two studies, 100 mcg for both sublingual and buccal preparations and 50mg for intranasal fentanyl. Six of the nine OTFC studies as well as the intranasal study also noted that patients should not receive more than four doses in a 24-hour period. The maximum number of doses of sublingual per day varied in each study. The most common symptoms regardless of the formulation were nausea, vomiting and constipation. BTP is a severe transitory pain that is sudden in onset and has a short duration. Many forms of fentanyl have been utilized in management of BTP. An entry dose of 60 mg of oral morphine was required in a majority of the studies and adverse events were as expected in patients medicated with opioids. The majority of patients required more than the minimum dose. Beginning treatment with larger doses would reduce the time to onset of pain relief. Future studies should investigate using larger doses in the prospective setting.

---

* Correspondence: Carlo DeAngelis, PharmD, Department of Pharmacy, Odette Cancer Centre, Sunnybrook Health Sciences Centre, 2075 Bayview Avenue, Toronto, Ontario M4N 3M5, Canada. E-mail: carlo.deangelis@sunnybrook.ca.

Keywords: breakthrough cancer pain, oral transmucosal fentanyl citrate, dose, frequency, tolerance

Introduction

Breakthrough pain (BTP) has commonly been described as a transient exacerbation of pain that breaks through well-controlled persistent pain spontaneously, to a predictable trigger, or to end-dose failure (1-2). Recent reviews however, do not include pain due to end-of-dose failure as a cause of breakthrough pain (3). Episodes of spontaneous pain occur without warning and are thus not related to an identifiable trigger, whereas pain associated with an identifiable cause is classified as incidental pain. Incidental pain is further divided into volitional (brought on by a voluntary act such as walking), non-volitional (brought on by an involuntary act such as sneezing) or procedural (brought on by therapeutic interventions) (4).

Clinical features of breakthrough pain also vary among individuals in frequency of occurrence, onset, duration, and intensity. One prospective study found that upon evaluating the type of cancer BTP in 159 patients, 26% experienced spontaneous pain while more than half (54%) related their cancer pain to a particular activity (5). A more recent study by Davies et al. also evaluated the type of cancer BTP in 320 patients across four Northern European countries (Denmark, Germany, Sweden, and United Kingdom) (6). One hundred and forty-one (44%) cancer patients reported incidental BTP, 124 (39%) noted spontaneous BTP, and 54 (17%) a combination of the two. Of the 141 cancer patients with incidental BTP, 106 were identified as volitional, 19 were non-volitional and 11 were procedural in nature (6).

Davies et al. further classified the intensity of BTP as mild, moderate, and severe and discovered a median of 3 episodes per day, each lasting 60 minutes in duration and peaking at 15 minutes (6). Generally, BTP is relatively rapid in onset, moderate to severe in intensity, is less than one-hour in duration, and may occur up to four times a day (2, 7-10).

BTP is a negative prognostic factor that interferes with various daily activities along with mood, waking ability, work, sleep, enjoyment of life, and relationships (6). The interference with daily activities is usually assessed on a numerical scale from 0 to 10, where 0 indicates no interference due to pain, and 10 represents complete interference. Median scores for daily activities, mood, waking ability, work, sleep, enjoyment of life, and relationships were 7, 5.5, 5, 7, 4, 5.5, and 6 respectively. In total, 90% of cancer patients find BTP to interfere with daily activities (6).

Although, cancer BTP is highly prevalent, the term is not well understood since no single definition has been widely accepted; and a lack of consistency in medical literature and clinical practice has been noted (2, 6, 11). Only 55% of physicians stated the correct opioid dose for cancer BTP, that being defined as 10% of a patient's total daily dose and administered every one to two hours as needed (12). This suggests that when alternative opioids are needed, physicians are not calculating the correct doses for cancer BTP management (12). As a result, this pain is often under-diagnosed and undertreated (2).

For over 20 years, the World Health Organization (WHO) has recommended managing cancer pain using a three-step approach: starting with NSAIDS, then gradually increasing from a weak opioid to stronger opioids if the pain persists (13). This approach has been shown to control 80% of pain, although opioid tolerance has been an ongoing concern in 50%

of cancer patients (14-17). Traditionally, morphine, a strong opioid, has been recommended to manage BTP (13, 17-18). A survey of European clinicians showed morphine to be preferred (50%) over fentanyl (14%), oxycodone (4%), methadone (2%), and hydromorphone (1%), but its use was based on availability and cost rather than efficacy or tolerability (19-20). Until recently, fentanyl has only been available in limited formulations (injection or as a transdermal delivery system) in Canada. In the past few years, new preparations have been created to deliver fentanyl to patients. With its rapid-onset (RO), fast elimination, and greater degree of pain relief, fentanyl offers an alternative to morphine (21-23).

Several fentanyl products (buccal, sublingual and intranasal) are available with slight differences in their pharmacokinetic profiles. Oral transmucosal fentanyl citrate (OTFC) is a fentanyl lozenge available in six dosage strengths (200, 400, 600, 800, 1200 and 1600 mcg) and reach their peak effect in 20-40 minutes (24). Fentanyl buccal and sublingual tablets (FBTs, FSTs) have also been approved for use in cancer BTP. These tablets reach mean peak plasma concentrations within 35-90 minutes (25). Yet another formulation is the fentanyl buccal soluble film (FBSF). These contain a muco-adhesive layer that adheres to the moist mucosal membrane and dissolves in only a minimum of saliva within 15-30 min after application (26). There are now two sublingual products available for use; one a spray and the other a fentanyl ethypharm, of which the former has been reported to significantly reduce pain 5 minutes after administration (27). Fentanyl ethyharm is a new sublingual formulation of fentanyl citrate in tablet form. An alkalinizing layer surrounds the fentanyl citrate to increase the solubility as well as provide an optimal environment for dissolution and absorption (28). The onset of action for this preparation has been reported to be 6 minutes following administration (28). The intranasal fentanyl spray (INFS) is an alternative formulation with the benefit of fast systemic penetration. Since this formulation bypasses the oral/gastrointestinal route, it is quickly absorbed through the nasal mucosa, attaining peak plasma concentrations within 12-15 minutes for all the dosage strengths (50-200 mcg) (25). Fentanyl pectin nasal spray (FPNS) is another intranasal preparation and is available in 100 or 400 mcg doses (29). Previous studies have demonstrated significant reductions in pain 5 minutes after a dose, reaching a maximum plasma concentration at a median time of 19.8 minutes (30).

The purpose of this study is to review the definition of breakthrough pain as well as the various formulations of fentanyl, including starting doses, frequency of use, equianalgesic dosing, tolerance and side-effects for the treatment of cancer pain.

METHODS

A systematic literature review was conducted using the OvidSP platform on Medline (1946 to 2014) and Embase (1980 to 2014). A combination of MeSH or EMTREE subject headings and free text keywords including "transmucosal," "buccal," "sublingual," "intranasal," and "mucosal administration" were coupled with "fentanyl." Articles were limited to those published in English.

The selection of studies in the systematic search is illustrated in Figure 1.

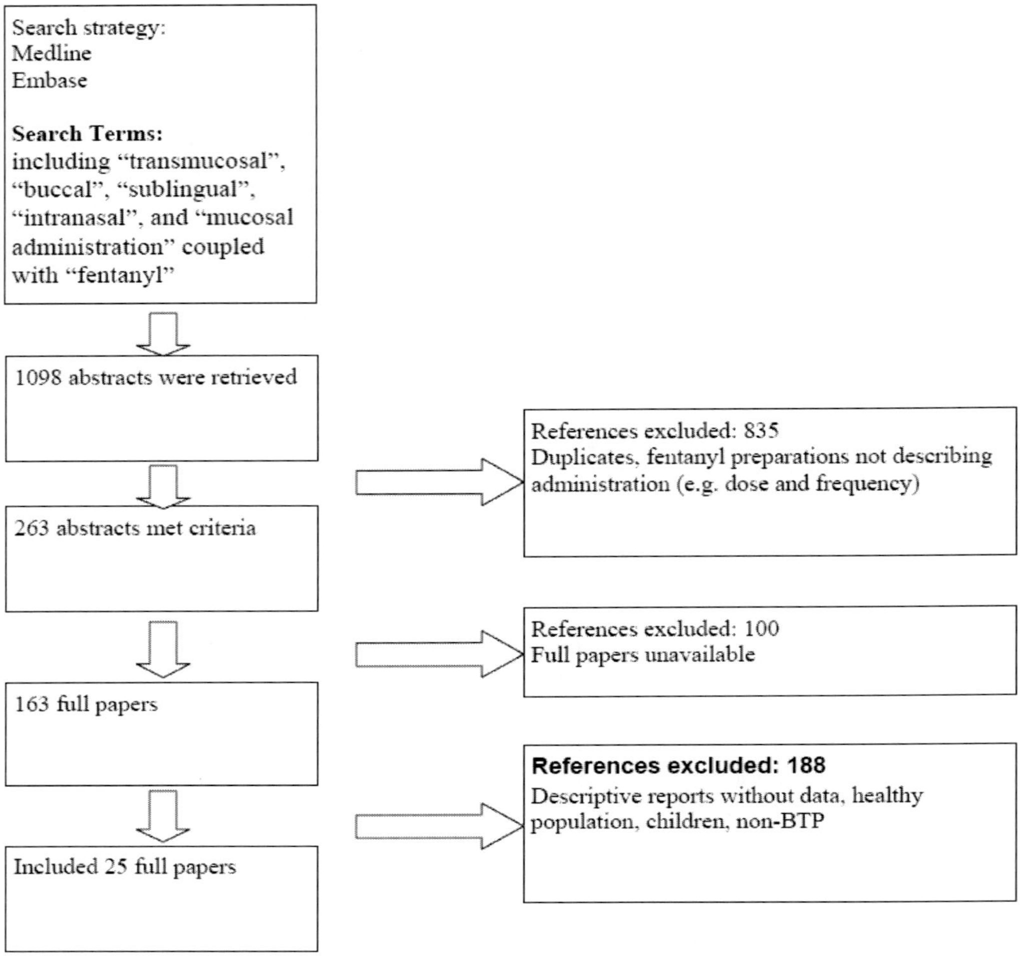

BTP= breakthrough pain.
RCTs= randomized controlled trials.

Figure 1. Flow chart of included studies.

Titles and abstracts detailing the administration of transmucosal fentanyl products in adult cancer patients with BTP were extracted for review. Previous reviews on this topic were also extracted and their reference lists were cross-checked. Descriptive reports without data were excluded. Full articles fulfilling the aforementioned criteria were obtained. Primary outcomes of interest were starting doses, frequency of use, tolerance, and guidelines for dose conversions between opioids. Other information extracted included BTP definitions, and side-effects. MZ, AF and LZ independently identified articles through this process, and consensus was sought if discrepancies occurred.

RESULTS

A total of 1,098 articles were identified for potential inclusion. After titles and abstracts were reviewed, 753 abstracts were excluded. One hundred twenty six full-length articles were obtained of which nine studied oral, seven sublingual, six buccal, and three intranasal study fulfilled the aforementioned criteria respectively (see tables 1a-d and 2a-d).

Table 1a. Summary of Study Design and Patient Population Characteristics for Administration of OTFC

References	Study Design	Population (sample size)	Mean Age (years)
Portenoy et al., 1999(8)	Randomized, double-blinded multi-center study	Ambulatory outpatient cancer patients (n=65)	53
Farrar et al., 1998 (21)	Randomized, open-labeled double-blinded multi-center placebo study	Cancer outpatients (n=130)	54
Coluzzi et al., 2001 (22)	Randomized double-blinded study	Cancer outpatients (n=134)	55
Payne et al., 2001(31)	Open-labeled study	Cancer outpatients (n=155)	54
Hanks et al., 2004 (32)	Open-labeled study	Cancer outpatients (n=57)	59
Mercadante et al., 2007 (33)	Randomized crossover control study	Cancer outpatients (n=25)	59
Mercadante et al., 2009 (34)	Randomized open-labeled cross-over study	Cancer outpatients (n=139)	62
Fine et al., 1991 (35)	Open-labeled study	Advanced in patients with cancer (n=10)	61
Burton et al., 2004 (36)	Case report	Cancer outpatients (n=39)	55

Table 1b. Summary of Study Design and Patient Population Characteristics for Administration of Sublingual Fentanyl Formulations

References	Study Design	Population (sample size)	Mean Age (years)
Sublingual Fentanyl (SLF)			
Velazquez Rivera et al., 2014 (3)	Prospective, double-blind controlled study	Cancer outpatients (n=20)	65.25
Rauck RL et al., 2009(37)	Placebo-controlled multi-center Phase III trial	Cancer outpatients (n=78)	55
Nalamachu S et al., 2011(38)	Open-label multicenter phase III trial	Cancer outpatients (n=139)	57

Table 1b. (Continued).

References	Study Design	Population (sample size)	Mean Age (years)
Mercadante S et al., 2013 (39)	Open-label study	Cancer patients admitted to acute palliative care unit (n=70)	61.7
Lennernas B et al., 2010 (40)	Phase II multicenter cross over study	Opioid tolerant locally advanced or metastatic cancer outpatients (n=23)	63
Fentanyl Sublingual Spray			
Rauck RL et al., 2012 (27)	Open-label dose titration followed by Randomized double-blind placebo-controlled phase III trial	Cancer patients (n=130)	55.6
Fentanyl Ethypharm			
Novotna S et al., 2014 (28)	Open-label dose titration followed by Randomized placebo-controlled multicenter study	Cancer outpatient (n= 91)	64.5

Table 1c. Summary of Study Design and Patient Population Characteristics for Administration of Buccal Fentanyl Formulations

References	Study Design	Population (sample size)	Mean Age (years)
Fentanyl Buccal Tablets			
Zeppetella G et al., 2010 (41)	Randomized double blind placebo control study	Cancer outpatients (n=248)	>18
Mercadante S et al., 2011 (42)	Prospective study	Cancer outpatients (n=12)	58.9
Mercadante S et al., 2012 (43)	Randomized multicenter unblinded study	Cancer outpatients (n=80)	1)61.3 2)65.4
Mercadante S et al., 2013 (44)	Open-label study	Cancer outpatients (n=30)	68.9
Kosugi T et al., 2014 (45)	Randomized double blinded placebo-controlled study	Cancer outpatients (n=101*)	62.0*
Fentanyl Buccal Soluble Film			
Rauck RL et al., 2010 (26)	Multicenter crossover study	Cancer outpatients (n=151)	57

*Baseline demographics included those that were later excluded from the remainder of the study.

Table 1d. Summary of Study Design and Patient Population Characteristics for Administration of Nasal Fentanyl Formulations

References	Study Design	Population (sample size)	Mean Age (years)
Intranasal Fentanyl Spray			
Kongsgaard et al., 2014 (11)	Observation, prospective cohort study	Cancer patients (n=309)	60
Mercadante et al., 2009 (34)	Randomized open label crossover study	Cancer outpatients (n=139)	62
Fentanyl Pectin Nasal Spray			
Radbruch et al., 2012 (30)	Multicentre, open-label study	Cancer patients (n=403)	53.8

Definition of breakthrough pain

Of the nine included OTFC studies, seven provided a definition of BTP (8, 21, 22, 31-34). On the other hand, all seven studies describing sublingual fentanyl preparations defined BTP in cancer patients as did the six fentanyl buccal studies. Likewise, all three intranasal fentanyl studies have also defined BTP. Definitions provided varied in description with five of the OTFC studies classified BTP as a transient flare (8, 21, 32-34). The remaining studies defined BTP as intermittent and acute in duration (22, 31). The seven sublingual studies also classified BTP as transient with 6 of the studies defining BTP as a rapid onset (27, 28, 37-40). Similarly, all buccal and intranasal studies defined BTP as transient pain occurring in a patient with otherwise well-controlled persistent pain (11, 26, 30, 34, 41-45). Additionally, one buccal and one intranasal study specified that the episodes were of rapid onset (30, 41).

Minimum starting dose and frequency of use

The lowest OTFC starting dose of 200mcg was used in all but two studies (see table 2a). Fine et al. dosed OTFC by weight (10-15mcg/kg), while Payne et al. started at 400mcg (31, 35). Regardless of these starting doses, all patients required titrated doses for adequate pain relief. Frequency of use ranged from one dose every 30 minutes to two hours (8, 21, 22, 31, 34-36). six of the nine studies recommended no more than four doses per day however, three remaining studies did not specify a maximum per day (21, 33, 36).

Three formulations of sublingual fentanyl were studied among the reviews: sublingual fentanyl tablets, fentanyl sublingual spray and fentanyl ethypharm. Of the 5 studies regarding sublingual fentanyl tablets, 3 required dose titrations for effective pain relief (see table 2b) (3, 37, 38). Of these studies utilizing dose titrations, two of them used 100mcg as a starting dose (see table 2b) (37, 38). Lennernas et al. compared various doses of 100, 200 and 400mcg rather than dose titration (40). This group also stated that a maximum of 4 doses could be taken per day, while other studies did not specify. Another study that did not require dose titration examined doses proportional to basal opioid regimens (39). The dose given to patients was calculated according to previous publications and local policies: 100 mcg to those who received 60 mg of oral morphine equivalents (OMEs), 200 mcg to those with 120 mg of OMEs, and so on. Of the sublingual tablet studies, only two groups specified a 2 hour time period before a dose could be repeated (37, 39). Rauck et al. conducted a dose titration study for fentanyl sublingual spray for which the starting dose used was 100 mcg (27). This group also stated that a second dose could not be administered within 2 hours following the initial dose, and a maximum of two doses being used per day (29). Novotna et al. studied a new formulation of known as fentanyl ethypharm (28). This group titrated doses starting at 133 mcg and increasing to a maximum of 800 mcg. Similar to the other sublingual formulations, doses can be repeated after 2 hours; however, up to four doses can be taken daily, as opposed to two (28).

Table 2a. Dosage and Administration for OTFC

References	Starting Dose	Frequency of Use	Max # of Doses per Day	Morphine Equivalent Dose	Duration of Previous Opioid Exposure
Portenoy PK et al., 1999 (8)	200mcg	Every 30 minutes	4	60-1000mg of oral morphine/day	Not specified
Farrar JT et al., 1998 (21)	200mcg	Every 2 hours	Not specified	At least 60mg/day of oral morphine or at least 50mcg/hour transdermal fentanyl	Not specified
Coluzzi PH et al., 2001 (22)	200mcg	Every 30 minutes	4	60-1000mg of oral morphine/day or transdermal fentanyl therapy (50-300mcg/hr)	Not specified
Payne R et al., 2001 (31)	200 or 400mcg	Every 30 minutes	4	60-1000mg of oral morphine/day or transdermal fentanyl therapy (50-300mcg/hr)	Not specified
Hanks GW et al., 2004 (32)	200mcg	Not specified	4	60-1000mg of oral morphine/day	3 days
Mercadante S et al., 2007 (33)	200mcg	Not specified	Not specified	60mg of oral morphine/day	Not specified
Mercadante S et al., 2009 (34)	200mcg	Every 30 minutes	4	60-500mg of oral morphine/day	≥1 month
Fine PG et al., 1991 (35)	10-15mcg/kg	Every 2 hours	4	Not specified	Not specified
Burton AW et al., 2004 (36)	200-600mcg	Every 30 minutes	Not specified	At least 40mg of oral morphine/day	Not specified

Studies examining buccal administration of fentanyl were divided into FBTs and FBSFs. Of the five buccal fentanyl tablet studies, three compared starting doses to the local policy, whereby patients receiving 600 mg of oral morphine were administered 1000 mcg of FBT (seec table 2c) (42-44). In the remaining studies, Zeppetella et al. titrated from an initial starting dose of 100 mcg; and Kosugi et al. used an initial dose of 50 mcg for patients receiving less than 60 mg per day of opioid taken around the clock (ATC), and 100 mcg for those receiving 60-1000 mg ATC daily (41-45). Mercadante et al. were the only group to specify a minimum time period before the next dose (44). This group required a two hour interval before subsequent doses. The single fentanyl buccal soluble film study used a starting dose of 200 mcg, and found doses greater than 400 mcg to be optimal (26). The investigators did not allow a subsequent dose to be taken within 4 hours of the initial administration, nor was a maximum dose specified.

Trials investigating the intranasal route of administration were grouped into the type of formulations: Instanyl® (an INFS) and fentanyl pectin nasal spray (FPNS). Of the three studies included in our analysis, two looked at INFS and one examined FPNS (see table 2d). For Instanyl®, both Mercadante et al. and Kongsgaard et al. utilized starting doses of 50 mcg, titrated to a max of 200 mcg (11, 34). The former of the two studies indicated a minimum time limit of 30 minutes was required before a dose could be repeated for pain, up to a maximum of four doses per day (34). In a trial conducted by Radbruch et al. FPNS was administered to patients at a starting dose of 100 mcg and titrated an additional dose per episode to a maximum of 800 mcg (30). A maximum of four doses per day could be administered to patients, although no minimum dosing interval was specified (30).

Table 2b. Dosage and Administration for Sublingual Fentanyl Formulations

References	Starting Dose	Frequency of Use	Max # of Doses per Day	Morphine Equivalent Dose	Duration of Previous Opioid Exposure
Sublingual Fentanyl (SLF)					
Velazquez Rivera et al., 2014 (3)	Not specified	Not specified	Not specified	Not specified	1 day
Rauck RL et al., 2009 (37)	100mcg	Every 2 hours	Not specified	60-1000mg/day oral morphine or 50-300mcg/h of transdermal fentanyl	Not specified
Nalamachu S et al., 2011 (38)	100mcg	Not specified	Not specified	60-1000mg/day or transdermal fentanyl 50-300ug/h	Not specified
Mercadante S et al., 2013 (39)	Varied based on basal opioid regimen	Every 2 hours	Not specified	At least 60 mg/day of oral morphine equivalents	2 days
Lennernas B et al., 2010 (40)	100,200, or 400mcg	Not specified	4	30-1000mg/d oral morphine or 25-300ug/h transdermal fentanyl	Not specified

Table 2b. (Continued).

References	Starting Dose	Frequency of Use	Max # of Doses per Day	Morphine Equivalent Dose	Duration of Previous Opioid Exposure
Fentanyl Sublingual Spray					
Rauck RL et al., 2012 (27)	100mcg	Every 2 hours	2	At least 60mg oral morphine, 30mg oxycodone, or 8 mg oral hydromorphone per day, 25 mcg transdermal fentanyl per hour, or equianalgesic doses of other opioids	At least 1 week
Fentanyl Ethypharm					
Novotna S et al., 2014 (28)	133 mcg	Every 2 hours	4	60-1000 mg/day of oral morphine or at least 25 mcg/h of transdermal fentanyl or at least 30 mg/day of oxycodone or 8mg/day of oral hydromorphone or equianalgesic dose of an alternative opioid	At least 1 week

Table 2c. Dosage and Administration for Buccal Fentanyl Formulations

References	Starting Dose	Frequency of Use	Max # of Doses per Day	Morphine Equivalent Dose	Duration of Previous Opioid Exposure
Fentanyl Buccal Tablets					
Zeppetella G et al., 2010 (41)	100-800mcg	Not specified	Not specified	oral morphine [≥60 mg/day], transdermal fentanyl [≥25 mg/h], or an equivalent dose of an alternative opioid	At least 1 week

References	Starting Dose	Frequency of Use	Max # of Doses per Day	Morphine Equivalent Dose	Duration of Previous Opioid Exposure
Mercadante S et al. 2011 (42)	Not specified	Not specified	Not specified	>500mg of oral morphine	Not specified
Mercadante S et al., 2012 (43)	100mcg or doses proportional to basal opioid regimen	Not specified	Not specified	At least 60mg of oral morphine	Not specified
Mercadante S et al., 2013 (44)	Doses proportional to basal opioid	Every 2 hours	Not specified	At least 60mg of oral morphine	Not specified
Kosugi T et al., 2014 (45)	50mcg for 30-<60mg/day ATC or 100mcg for 60-1000mg/day mg ATC	Not specified	Not specified	At least 30mg (low ATC group) or at least 60mg (high ATC group)	At least one week
Fentanyl Buccal Soluble Films					
Rauck RL et al., 201026	200mcg	Every 4 hours	Not specified	60-1000mg/day morphine or 50-300mcg/h of transdermal fentanyl	Not specified

Table 2d. Dosage and Administration for Nasal Fentanyl Formulations

References	Starting Dose	Frequency of Use	Max # of Doses per Day	Morphine Equivalent Dose	Duration of Previous Opioid Exposure
Intranasal Fentanyl Spray					
Kongsgaard et al., 2014 (11)	50 mcg	Not specified	Not specified	Not specified	Not specified
Mercadante et al., 2009 (34)	50, 100, 200mg	Every 30 minutes	4	60–500 mg/day of oral morphine	>1 month
Fentanyl Pectin Nasal Spray					
Radbruch et al., 2012 (30)	100 mcg	Not specified	4	At least 60 mg/day of oral morphine	Not specified

Table 3. Guidelines for Converting between Opioids

References	Dose Conversion
Portenoy PK et al., 199 (98)	Standard relative potency table*
Mercadante S et al., 2007 (33)	60mg of oral morphine = 400mcg of OTFC

* Jacox et al., 1994.

Conversion between opioids

Only two OTFC studies made reference to equianalgesic dose ratios between opioids (Table 3). Portenoy et al. determined morphine equivalent doses for patients receiving an opioid other than morphine from a standard potency table published by *Jacox et al. 1994*; however, this table did not specify a ratio for fentanyl use (8). The study by *Mercadante et al.* did indicate a conversion ratio for daily morphine to fentanyl of 150 (60 mg of morphine daily is equivalent to 400 mcg of OTFC) (33).

Tolerance and entry requirement

Patients using oral transmucosal fentanyl should be opioid tolerant to avoid the risk of life-threatening respiratory depression. By definition, opioid tolerance is achieved in patients taking a minimum of 60 mg per day of oral morphine equivalents or 25 mcg per hour of transdermal fentanyl for a minimum duration of one week. Of the nine OTFC studies in this review, seven fulfilled this requirement using at least 60 mg of oral morphine per day; however, only one study described patients taking opioids for the required duration of one week or greater (see table 2a). Interestingly, three studies specified using at least 50 mcg per hour of transdermal fentanyl (21, 22, 31). Four sublingual studies fulfilled the requirement of using at least 60 mg of oral morphine per day or 25 mcg per hour of transdermal fentanyl, but again, only one study specified the required duration of one week or greater (see table 2b). Two studies defined opioid tolerance as 30 mg or greater of oxycodone or 8mg of oral hydromorphone daily (27, 28).

For the buccal preparation, five studies fulfilled the requirement using at least 60 mg of oral morphine per day or 25 mcg per hour of transdermal fentanyl (see table 2c). Of these, one trial considered patients using 30 mg of oral morphine as a low ATC opioid group (45).

The rationale regarding accepting of the lower ATC administration was that this group compared efficacy and safety in Japanese patients who generally weight less than western patients as well as receive lower than 60 mg morphine equivalents per day (45). Another study specified 50-300 mcg per hour of transdermal fentanyl as opioid tolerant (26). Another group considered patients with greater than 500 mg of oral morphine (42). The rationale behind this group was that the purpose of the study was to assess the safety and efficacy of fentanyl buccal tablets in patients receiving high doses of opiods as background medications (42). Only two studies described patients taking opioids for the required duration of one week or greater (41, 45). For patients receiving intranasal administration of fentanyl, two studies specified patients were receiving a minimum of 60 mg per day of oral morphine (see table

2d). Of the two, only one fulfilled the required one week duration of basal opioid administration (34).

Side-effects

The three most frequently reported side-effects for all included studies are reported in table 4. All of these side-effects are comparable to those commonly observed with opioid therapy; however, whether the incidence or severity of these side-effects depended on the doses administered was not specified. The majority of patients reported nausea, somnolence and dizziness regardless of the type of fentanyl product. Additionally, for the 118 patients classified as opioid-tolerant by Mercadante et al. the incidences of nausea, vomiting, and constipation were also reported to be 7.6%, 3.4%, and 3.4%, respectively (34). Mercadante et al. reported that although patients experienced nausea and dizziness with FBT use, these symptoms were already present from the basal opioid regimen (34).

Discussion

BTP may be associated with or without a precipitating cause. When considering the former, the pain is referred to as incident, while the latter is termed spontaneous. Some researchers define BTP as a transient flare whereas others classify BTP based on precipitating factors. Results from an international survey have also shown that the definition for BTP varies from country to country because there is no literal translation (46).

Fentanyl has been reported to be effective for moderate to severe BTP; however, controversy remains in terms of its administration in opioid-tolerant patients. The present review evaluates starting doses of fentanyl preparations for opioid-tolerant, as well as the frequency of use, dose conversions, and side-effects.

Various clinical trials have shown that OTFC in doses ranging from 200-1600 mcg are effective for patients receiving maintenance opioid therapy. Low-dose (200 mcg) is to be started and titrated upward until pain is relieved or intolerable side effects are experienced (47). OTFC doses should not exceed 20% of a patient's twenty four hour opioid dose consumption (33).

An initial dosage of 200 mcg is usually recommended in the elderly, for patients who are sensitive to the side effects of opioids, or patients with coexisting pulmonary disease (47).

Table 4. Incidence of Side-Effects after Fentanyl Use for Cancer-Related BTP

References	Side-Effects	Incidence	Percentage
OTFC			
Portenoy PK et al., 1999 (8)	Somnolence	18/65 patients	28%
	Dizziness	9/65 patients	14%
	Nausea	7/65 patients	10%
Farrar JT et al., 1998 (21)	Dizziness	22/130 patients	17%
	Nausea	18/130 patients	14%
	Somnolence	11/130 patients	8%

Table 4. (Continued).

References	Side-Effects	Incidence	Percentage
Coluzzi PH et al., 2001 (22)	Somnolence Nausea Constipation	20/134 patients 18/134 patients 14/134 patients	15% 13% 10%
Payne R et al., 2001 (31)	Somnolence Constipation Nausea	14/155 patients 13/155 patients 12/155 patients	9% 8% 8%
Hanks GW et al., 2004 (32)	Nausea Vomiting Dizziness	8/57 patients 4/57 patients 4/57 patients	14% 7% 7%
Mercadante S et al., 2007 (33)	Nausea Drowsiness Confusion	4/12 episodes 7/12 episodes 1/12 episode	7.5% 13.2% 1.8%
Mercadante S et al., 2009 (34)	Nausea Vomiting Constipation	9/118 patients 4/118 patients 4/118patients	7.6% 3.4% 3.4%
Fine PG et al., 1991 (35)	None reported		
Burton AW et al., 2004 (36)	None reported		
Sublingual Fentanyl Formulations			
Velazquez Rivera et al., 2014 (3)	Nausea, Constipation Somnolence Vomiting	Each 3/20 patients 2/20 patients 1/20 patients	Each 15% 10% 5%
Rauck RL et al., 2009 (37)	Nausea Vomiting Somnolence		12.2% 5.3% 4.6%
Nalamachu S et al., 2011 (38)	Nausea Vomiting Dehydration	12/139 patients 8/139 patients 5/139 patients	8.6% 5.8% 3.6%
Mercadante S et al., 2013 (39)	Nausea Drowsiness	Not specified	Not specified
Lennernas B et al., 2010 (40)	Pain Vomiting Nausea	4 episodes 2 episodes 1 episode	26.7% 13.3% 6.7%
Rauck RL et al., 2012 (27)	Nausea Somnolence Vomiting	17/130 patients 11/130 patients 10/130 patients	13.1% 8.5% 7.7%
Novotna S et al., 2014 (28)	Vomiting Nausea diarrhea	77 treatment emergent AEs reported by 25/91 patients	5.5% 4.4% 3.3%
Buccal Fentanyl Formulations			
Zeppetella G et al., 2010 (41)	Nausea Dizziness Headache	43/248 patients 41/248 patients 26/248 patients	17.3% 16.5% 10.5%

References	Side-Effects	Incidence	Percentage
Mercadante S et al., 2011 (42)	Not specified		
Mercadante S et al., 2012 (43)	Not specified		
Mercadante et al., 2013 (44)	Nausea Dizziness		
Kosugi et al., 2014 (45)	Somnolence Anemia Vomiting	28/103 patients 15/103 patients 14/103 patients	27.2% 14.6% 13.6%
Rauck RL et al., 2010 (26)	Somnolence Nausea Dizziness	9/151 patients 8/151 patients 7/151 patients	6.0% 5.3% 4.6%
Intranasal Fentanyl Formulations			
Intranasal Fentanyl Spray			
Mercadante S et al., 2009 (11)	Nausea Vomiting Constipation	9/118 patients 4/118 patients 4/118patients	7.6% 3.4% 3.4%
Kongsgaard et al., 2014 (34)	Not specified		
Fentanyl Pectin Nasal Spray			
Radbruch et al. 2012 (30)	Dizziness Vomiting Constipation, somnolence	Not specified	5.2% 3.7% each 3.5%

On the other hand, a reasonable OTFC starting dose for most opioid-tolerant patients (taking at least 60 mg of oral morphine per day, 25 mcg of transdermal fentanyl per hour, or an equianalgesic dose of another opioid for one week or longer) was found to be 400 mcg (40, 47). Streisand et al. also agreed that opioid-tolerant patients require higher OTFC starting doses (48). Subsequently, the need for rescue medications and titration was lower for patients receiving 400 mcg of OTFC compared to 200 mcg (40, 19).

Mercadante et al. examined the use of sublingual and buccal fentanyl preparations in doses proportional to basal regimen (39, 44). Proportional doses were effective and safe in managing BTP while titration was thought to prolong suffering due to dose failures (39, 44). Therefore, beginning titrations with larger starting doses may also reduce the time to onset of pain relief and reduce suffering. In many of the trials included, the initial dose of OTFC was insufficient to manage BTP. Many patients required larger doses for OTFC to be effective. This suggests that a starting dose of 200 mcg may not be optimal in an adult population, and beginning treatment of BTP with larger doses of OTFC or other transmucosal fentanyl preparations may be warranted. For example, studies found sublingual fentanyl doses of 400 mcg to be effective, greater than 400 mcg for FBT, and 200 mg for Instanyl. Conversely, Kongsgaard et al. noted that a majority of patients using Instanyl had a maintenance dose of 50 mcg (11). However, a study found that INFS formulations could achieve up to 89% bioavailability within patients' systems (49). Thus, any discrepancy in terms of maintenance doses for the same formulation may be the result of inter-patient differences, such as lifestyle, or the type of cancer with which they are afflicted. However, different formulations also have differing bioavailability, which ultimately affects the maintenance dose as well (49). Future studies should determine factors that cause a discrepancy between maintenance doses of patients given the same medication. Also future studies should determine factors where initial doses are not sufficient, thus larger doses are required and explore the doses in a prospective setting.

Frequency of use also varies by patient and response, and as a result, management of BTP may require additional doses of fentanyl. Various clinical trials have found it beneficial to repeat OTFC use in 30 minutes if pain is still present (8, 22, 31, 34, 36). Others suggest using another OTFC unit after 2 hours (21, 35). On the other hand, Cleary showed that the use of OTFC every 4 to 6 hours is sufficient since such a dose is adequate in managing persistent pain, but patients are advised not to consume more than four doses in a 24-hour period (51). If more than four OTFC units are consistently used per day dose, adjustments are made to around-the-clock opioids (47). For sublingual preparations, doses were repeated after 2 hours. However, the duration between doses varied for buccal preparation. For the INFS study, doses were given every 30 minutes and up to 4 doses daily (34).

Opioid tolerance, a reduction in response to a drug after repeated administration, can cause difficulties when determining the dose of alternate opioids for some patients. Numerous studies have classified opioid-tolerant patients as taking at least 60mg of oral morphine per day, 25mcg of transdermal fentanyl per hour, or an equianalgesic dose of another opioid for one week or longer. This review evaluated fentanyl starting doses and administration in opioid-tolerant patients.

The most challenging aspect of opioid switching is deciding on the starting dose. Despite the availability of equianalgesic dose ratios, these ratios fail to consider individual patient factors such as previous opioid therapy, opioid tolerance or underlying disease (52, 53). In addition to the guidelines available in this review, relative potency ratios of OTFC to IV morphine have been evaluated by Lichtor et al. and Lu et al. (54, 55). Similarly, these studies indicate that the opioid effect of 200mcg of OTFC is equivalent to 2-4 mg of IV morphine (30 mg per day of oral morphine) and 400 mcg of OTFC is equivalent to 4-8 mg of IV morphine (60 mg per day of oral morphine) (10-20:1). This means that 90 mg, 120 mg, 180 mg, and 240 mg of oral morphine per day is equivalent to 600 mcg, 800 mcg, 1200 mcg and 1600 mcg of OTFC, respectively (54, 55). Studies examining sublingual, buccal and intranasal fentanyl preparations did not provide dose conversion guidelines. As a result, the entry dose of 60 mg of oral morphine equivalents required in the included studies is not based on data presented in the literature. Lowering this criterion would allow for the treatment of a greater number of patients.

Overall, fentanyl appears well-tolerated based on the studies in this review. The side-effects reported are typical of those associated with opioid analgesics, and recent study by Mercadante et al. also confirmed that incidence and severity of these side-effects are independent of the doses administered (56).

In conclusion, BTP is a severe transitory pain that is sudden in onset and has a short duration. Currently, patients beginning at the lowest available dose often require a greater number of administrations or a greater dose to effectively manage BTP. Low doses of OTFC are effective in opioid-naïve or elderly patients with cancer pain; however, to reduce the use of rescue medications and titration in opioid-tolerant patients, a starting dose of 400 mcg is warranted. Similarly, fentanyl sublingual has been effective at 400 mcg or greater than 400 mcg for buccal preparations. This suggests that introduction of larger starting doses of transmucosal fentanyl preparations may be required. Adverse events were consistent and similar to those reported in patients taking oral morphine. Also, the entry dose of 60 mg of oral morphine equivalents required in the included studies is not based on data presented in the literature.

Future studies should explore the factors that influence different maintenance doses of patients administered the same preparation. Also, factors that cause the need for titration to a higher dose and /or the use of a higher dose in a prospective setting should be explored.

ACKNOWLEDGMENTS

We thank the generous support of the Bratty Family Fund, Michael and Karyn Goldstein Cancer Research Fund, Pulenzas Cancer Research Fund, Joseph and Silvana Melara Cancer Research Fund, and the Ofelia Cancer Research Fund.

REFERENCES

[1] Haugen DF, Hjermstad MJ, Hagen N, Caraceni A, Kaasa S, European Palliative Care Research Collaborative. Assessment and classification of cancer breakthrough pain: a systematic literature review. Pain 2010;149(3):476-82.

[2] Rhiner MI, von Gunten CF. Cancer breakthrough pain in the presence of cancer-related chronic pain: fact versus perceptions of health care providers and patients. J Support Oncol 2010;8(6):232-8.

[3] Velázquez Rivera I, Muñoz Garrido JC, García Velasco P, Espana Ximenez de Encico I, Velazquez Clavarana L. Efficacy of sublingual fentanyl vs. oral morphine for cancer-related breakthrough pain. Adv Ther 2014;31(1):107-17.

[4] Davies A, Buchanan A, Zeppetella G, Porta-Sales J, Likar R, Weismayr W, et al. Breakthrough cancer pain: an observational study of 1000 European oncology patients. J Pain Symptom Manage 2013;46(5):619-28.

[5] Gutgsell T, Walsh D, Zhukovsky DS, Gonzales F, Lagman R. A prospective study of the pathophysiology and clinical characteristics of pain in a palliative medicine population. Am J Hosp Palliat Care 2003;20(2):140-8.

[6] Davies A, Zeppetella G, Andersen S, Damkier A, Vejlgaard T, Nauck F, et al. Multi-centre European study of breakthrough cancer pain: Pain characteristics and patient perceptions of current and potential management strategies. Eur J Pain 2011;15(7):756-63.

[7] Portenoy RK, Hagen NA. Breakthrough pain: definition, prevalence and characteristics. Pain 1990;41:273–81.

[8] Portenoy RK, Payne R, Coluzzi P, Raschko JW, Lyss A, Busch MA, et al. Oral trans-mucosal fentanyl citrate (OTFC®) for the treatment of breakthrough pain in cancer patients: A controlled dose titration study. Pain 1999;79:303–12.

[9] Goudas LC, Bloch R, Gialeli-Goudas LLM, Lau J, Carr DB. The epidemiology of cancer pain. Cancer Invest 2005;23:182-90.

[10] Svendsen KB, Andersen S, Arnason S. Breakthrough pain in malignant and non-malignant diseases: a review of prevalence, characteristics and mechanisms. Eur J Pain 2005;9(2):195-206.

[11] Kongsgaard UE, Eeg M, Greisen H. The use of Instanyl® in the treatment of breakthrough pain in cancer patients: a 3-month observational prospective, cohort study. Support Care Cancer 2014;22(6):1655-62.

[12] Gallagher R, Hawley P, Yeomans W. A survey of cancer pain management knowledge and attitude of British Columbian physicians. Pain Res Manag 2004;9(4):188-94.

[13] World Health Organization. Cancer Pain Relief, 2nd ed. Geneva: World Health Organization, 1996.

[14] Zech DF, Grond S, Lynch J, Hertel D, Lehmann K. Validation of World Health Organization Guidelines for cancer pain relief: a 10-year prospective study. Pain 1995;63(1):65–76.

[15] Meuser T, Pietruck C, Radbruch L. Symptoms during cancer pain treatment following WHO-guidelines: a longitudinal follow-up study of symptom prevalence, severity and etiology. Pain 2001;93(3):247–57.

[16] Collett BJ. Opioid tolerance: the clinical perspective. Br J Anaesth 1998;81:58-68.

[17] Hanks GW, Conno F, Cherny N, Hanna M, Kalso E, McQuay HJ, et al. Morphine and alternative opioids in cancer pain: the EAPC recommendations. Br J Cancer 2001;84(5):587–93.

[18] Kuip EJM, Zandvliet ML, Mathijessen RHJ, Van der Rijt CCD. Pharmacological and clinical aspects of immediate release fentanyl preparations: a criterion for selection. Eur J Hosp Pharm 2012;19:38-40.

[19] Klepstad P, Kaasa S, Cherny N, Hanks G, de Conno F. Pain and pain treatments in European palliative care units. A cross sectional survey from the European Association for Palliative Care Research Network. Palliat Med 2005;19(6):477–84.

[20] Droney J, Riley J. Recent advances in the use of opioids for cancer pain. J Pain Res 2009;2:135-55.

[21] Farrar JT, Cleary J, Rauck R, Busch M, Nordbrock E. Oral transmucosal fentanyl citrate: Randomized, double-blinded, placebo-controlled trial for treatment of breakthrough pain in cancer patients. J Natl Cancer Inst 1998;90:611–6.

[22] Coluzzi PH, Schwartzberg L, Conroy JD, Charapata S, Gay M, Busch MA, et al. Breakthrough cancer pain: A randomized trial com- paring oral transmucosal fentanyl citrate (OTFC) and morphine sulfate immediate release (MSIR) Pain 2001;91:123–30.

[23] Christie JM, Simmonds M, Patt R, Coluzzi P, Busch MA, Nordbrock E, et al. Dose- titration, multicenter study of oral transmucosal fentanyl citrate for the treatment of breakthrough pain in cancer patients using transdermal fentanyl for persistent pain. J Clin Oncol 1998;16:3238–45.

[24] Mystakidou K, Katsouda E, Parpa E, Tsiatas ML, Vlahos L. Oral transmucosal fentanyl citrate: overview of pharmacological and clinical characteristics. Drug Deliv 2006;13:269-76.

[25] Mercadante S. The use of rapid onset opiods for breakthrough cancer pain: the challenge of its dosing. Crit Rev Oncol Hematol 2011;80(3):460-5.

[26] Rauck R, North J, Gever LN, Tagarro I, Finn AL. Fentanyl buccal soluble film (FBSF) for breakthrough pain in patients with cancer: a randomized, double-blind, placebo-controlled study. Ann Oncol 2010;21(6):1308-14.

[27] Rauck R, Reynolds L, Geach J, Bull J, Stearns L, Scherlis M, et al. Efficacy and safety of fentanyl sublingual spray for the treatment of breakthrough cancer pain: a randomized, double-blind, placebo-controlled study. Curr Med Res Opin 2012;28(5):859-70.

[28] Novotna S, Valentova K, Fricova J, Richterova E, Harabisova S, Bullier F, et al. A Randomized, placebo-controlled study of a new sublingual formulation of fentanyl citrate (fentanyl ethypharm) for breakthrough pain in opioid-treated patients with cancer. Clin Ther 2014;36(3):357-67.

[29] Bulloch MN, Hutchison AM. Fentanyl pectin nasal spray: a novel intranasal delivery method for the treatment of breakthrough cancer pain. Expert Rev Clin Pharmacol 2013;6(1):9-22.

[30] Radbruch L, Torres LM, Ellershaw JE. Long-term tolerability, efficacy and acceptability of fentanyl pectin nasal spray for breakthrough cancer pain. Support Care Cancer 2012;20(3):565-73.

[31] Payne R, Coluzzi P, Hart L, Simmonds M, Lyss A, Rauck R, et al. Long-term safety of oral transmucosal fentanyl citrate for breakthrough cancer pain. J Pain 2001;22(1):575-83.

[32] Hanks GW, Nugent M, Higgs CM, Busch MA, OTFC Multicentre Study Group. Oral transmucosal fentanyl citrate in the management of breakthrough pain in cancer: an open, multicenter dose-titration and long-term use study. J Palliat Med 2004;18:698-704.

[33] Mercadante S, Villari P, Ferrera P, Casuccio A, Mangione S, Intravaia G. Transmucosal fentanyl vs. intravenous morphine in doses proportional to basal opioid regimen for episodic-breakthrough pain. Br J Cancer 2007;96:1828-33.

[34] Mercadante S, Radbruch L, Davies A, Poulain P, Sitte T, Perkins P, et al. A comparison of intranasal fentanyl spray with oral transmucosal fentanyl citrate for the treatment of breakthrough cancer pain: an open-label, randomized, crossover trial. Curr Med Res Opin 2009;25:2805-15.

[35] Fine PG, Marcus M, De Boer, AJ. An open label study of oral transmucosal fentanyl citrate (OTFC) for the treatment of breakthrough cancer pain. Pain 1991;45:149–55.

[36] Burton AW, Driver LC, Mendoza TR, Syed G. Oral transmucosal fentanyl citrate in the outpatient management of severe cancer pain crises: a retrospective case series. Clin J Pain 2004;20(3):195-7.

[37] Rauck RL, Tark M, Reyes E, Hayes TG, Bartkowiak AJ, Hassman D, et al. Efficacy and long-term tolerability of sublingual fentanyl orally disintegrating tablet in the treatment of breakthrough cancer pain. Curr Med Res Opin 2009;25(12):2877-85.

[38] Nalamachu S., Hassman D, Wallace MS, Dumble S, Derrick R, Howell J. Long-term effectiveness and tolerability of sublingual fentanyl orally disintegrating tablet for the treatment of breakthrough cancer pain. Curr Med Res Opin 2011;21(3):519-30.

[39] Mercadante S, Prestia G, Casuccio A. The use of sublingual fentanyl for breakthrough pain by using doses proportional to opioid basal regimen. Curr Med Res Opin 2013;29(11):1527-32.

[40] Lennernäs B, Frank-Lissbrant I, Lennernäs H, Kälkner KM, Derrick R, Howell J. Sublingual administration of fentanyl to cancer patients is an effective treatment for breakthrough pain: results from a randomized phase II study. J Palliat Med 2010;24:286-93.

[41] Zeppetella G, Messina J, Xie F, Slatkin NE. Consistent and clinically relevant effects with fentanyl buccal tablet in the treatment of patients receiving maintenance opioid therapy and experiencing cancer-related breakthrough pain. Pain Pract 2010;19(4):287-93.

[42] Mercadante S, Ferrera P, Adile C, Casuccio A. Fentanyl buccal tablets for breakthrough pain in highly tolerant cancer patients: preliminary data on the proportionality between breakthrough pain dose and background dose. J Pain Symptom Manage 2011;42(3):464-9.

[43] Mercadante S, Gatti A, Porzio G, Lo Presti C, Aielli F, Adile C, et al. Dosing fentanyl buccal tablet for breakthrough cancer pain: dose titration versus proportional doses. Curr Med Res Opin 2012;28(6):963-8.

[44] Mercadante S, Porzio G, Aielli F, Averna L, Ficorella C, Casuccio A. The use of fentanyl buccal tablets for breakthrough pain by using doses proportional to opioid basal regimen in a home care setting. Support Care Cancer 2013;21(8):2335-9.

[45] Kosugi T, Hamada S, Takigawa C, Shinozaki K, Kunikane H, Goto F, et al. A randomized, double-blind, placebo-controlled study of fentanyl buccal tablets for breakthrough pain: efficacy and safety in Japanese cancer patients. J Pain Symptom Manage 2014;47(6):990-1000.

[46] Hwang SS, Chang VT, Kasimis B. Cancer breakthrough pain characteristics and responses to treatment at a VA medical center. Pain 2003;101:55-64.

[47] Aronoff GM, Brennan MJ, Pritchard DD, Ginsberg B. Evidence-based oral transmucosal fentanyl citrate (OTFC®) dosing guidelines. Pain Medicine 2005;6(4):305-14.

[48] Streisand JB, Busch MA, Egan TD, Smith BG, Gay M, Pace NL. Dose proportionality and pharmacokinetics of oral transmucosal fentanyl citrate. Anesthesiology 1998;88:305-9.

[49] Lötsch J, Walter C, Parnham MJ, Oertel BG, Geisslinger G. Pharmacokinetics of non-intravenous formulations of fentanyl. Clin Pharmacokinet 2013;52(1):23-36.

[50] Chwieduk CM, McKeage K. Fentanyl sublingual: in breakthrough pain in opioid-tolerant adults with cancer. Drugs 2010;70(17):2281-8.

[51] Cleary JF. Use of oral transmucosal fentanyl citrate as around-the-clock medication in patients with cancer [Abstract 606]. In: 16th Annual Scientific Meeting of the American Pain Society, New Orleans, LA, 1997.

[52] Anderson R, Saiers JH, Abram S, Schlicht C. Accuracy in equianalgesic dosing. Conversion dilemmas. J Pain Symptom Manage 2001;21(5):397-406.

[53] Gammaitoni AR, Fine P, Alvarez N, McPherson ML, Bergmark S. Clinical application of opioid equianalgesic data. Clin J Pain 2003;19(5):286-97.

[54] Lichtor JL, Sevarino FB, Joshi GP, Busch MA, Nordbrock E, Ginsberg B. The relative potency of oral transmucosal fentanyl citrate compared with intravenous morphine in the treatment of moderate to severe postoperative pain. Anesth Analg 1999;89:732-8.

[55] Lu JK, Bailey PL. Dose-related respiratory pharmacology of oral transmucosal fentanyl citrate (OTFC®) versus intravenous morphine: A randomized, double-blind, double-dummy study [Abstract]. Anesthesiology 2003;99:A967.

[56] Mercadante S. Managing breakthrough pain. Curr Pain Headache Rep 2011;15:244-9.

Submitted: November 11, 2014. *Revised:* December 15, 2014. *Accepted:* January 08, 2015.

In: Pain Management Yearbook 2015
Editor: Joav Merrick

ISBN: 978-1-63484-515-1

Chapter 2

THE INTERNAL GATEWAY TO HEALING TRAUMA-SPECTRUM MANIFESTATIONS (TSM): A SHIP® PERSPECTIVE ON SPONTANEOUS HEALING REACTIONS (SHRS)

Johan O Steenkamp*, BA, BA Hons, MAPsych, DLitt et Phil
Private Practice, Brooklyn, South Africa

Innate autonomic self-regulation towards people's natural healthy blueprint disposition reflects the SHIP® (Spontaneous Healing Intra-systemic Process) point of reference. SHIP® proposes that spontaneous healing reactions (SHRs) are subcortical somatic flashbacks in the service of autonomic self-regulation and the gateway to healing trauma-spectrum manifestations. Mapping through the integration of experiential research on SHRs and literature on brain specificity is documented in support of this assumption.

Keywords: autonomic self-regulation, individual specific field, psychology, SHIP®, spontaneous healing reactions (SHRs), trauma, trauma-spectrum manifestation (TSM)

INTRODUCTION

Unresolved neurological changes in the brain induced by trauma, especially developmental trauma, are an initiating complement for trauma-spectrum manifestations (TSM), an integrated SHIP® diagnosis for trauma-related dis-eases (1). ("The trauma spectrum" was introduced by Van der Kolk in 1988 (2)). TSM diagnosis incorporates the doctrine that chronic dis-eases are part of people's internal natural disposition towards a solution and that spontaneous healing reactions (SHRs) are the gateway to the solution. Addressing the cause of chronic symptom manifestation requires an understanding of SHRs and their role as part of

* Correspondence: Johan O Steenkamp, Private Practice, PO Box 35077, Menlo Park, 0102, South Africa. E-mail: jos@intekom.co.za.

the system's autonomic self-regulation of unconscious/trauma material towards healing, integration and balance.

The writing of this article was prompted by decades of work with clients and their SHRs in SHIP®. Precursors to the birth of SHIP® in the mid-1980s were the concept of self-regulation promoted by Autogenic Training and the intuition that dis-eases are part of an internal healing plan where the internal wisdom of the client's system will point the way (3, 4). The SHIP® psychotherapeutic setting facilitates a healing space within which clients are activated through their trauma-activating events gathered from autobiographical information, and other activators discovered during the development of SHIP® (4). Clients in SHIP® are asked to refrain from voluntary action while they are lying on the psychotherapy bed. Because the clients remain passive in the face of SHIP® activation, clients' SHRs are exposed and facilitated towards completion of previously uncompleted responses.

The function of this article is to present a SHIP® perspective on SHRs that may assist practitioners of trauma psychotherapy. It could also stimulate further research on SHRs, leading to a greater understanding of TSM and its treatment.

To open a debate on SHRs, the author will focus on the following research questions:

- What are the etiological constituents of SHRs?
- What are the characteristics and natural disposition of SHRs?
- Could mapping of SHRs locate unconscious territory?

Explanations and discussions on the etiology, characteristics and mapping of SHRs will be introduced in the following paragraphs. This will incorporate other authors' views. For the sake of brevity and in deference to the journal parameters the focus where possible will be on concise explanations.

EXPLANATIONS AND DISCUSSIONS ON THE ETIOLOGY, CHARACTERISTICS AND MAPPING OF SHRS

Some basic etiological determinants are clarified below to create a platform for the discussion on SHRs. These etiological factors are classified into energy-chemical communication, autonomic self-regulation, the HPA axis protection system and trauma.

Energy-chemical communication

According to the quantum perspective the universe is a holistic information matrix constituted of extensive and dynamic intertwined, interdependent and integrated energy fields. The building blocks of the universal matrix, the quantum atom structures, each have their own unique energy signature of miniature energy radiating universes with vibrating, spinning vortices (5). This forms the medium in which chemical communication is generated. All material structures are collectively made up of assemblies of atoms called molecules (6, 7), and molecules are the smallest units of meaning in chemistry (8).

According to SHIP® theory, the individual specific field (ISF) is the person's holographic field within the universal matrix that harbours all past, present and potential future experiences, both intra- and inter-systemically (1, 3, 4). Intra-systemic experience involves all energy-chemical information during impulse transmission that links internal systems into a multidirectional communication web. This internal web forms the substrate of the manifestations that allow the ISF to experience itself in its interactions and translations with the inter-systemic external world.

Proteins, the stuff of life such as enzymes, are the essential molecular physical building blocks of the intra-systemic domain that determine the cell's structure and behaviour, and catalyse processes of chemical change (5, 8). Nerve impulses start at cellular level and the cell membrane, also referred to as the brain of the cell, functions as an interface for certain proteins. Cell death is imminent in the absence of its membrane or if the membrane does not allow the translation of environmental signals (5, 8). Integral membrane proteins (IMPs) embedded within either side of the cell membrane are the fundamental physical subunits of the cell's intelligence/awareness mechanism and chemical communication (5). IMPs are divided into two classes that function as an autonomic stimulus-response mechanism regulating information transportation or signal transduction across either side of the membrane (5, 8). This allows nutrients, waste products, and other forms of information molecules, necessary for the smooth functioning of the cytoplasm, to be transported through the membrane. Signals can be sent down the tendril that releases the chemicals through the membrane into the synaptic cleft on their journey to neighbouring neuron dendrites. The two functional classes of protein complexes that link reception of environmental stimuli to response-generating pathways are the receptor and effector protein reflexive perception switches (5):

- *Receptor proteins (awareness oriented)*: These IMPs are the cell's sense organs and function as physical sensation nanno-antennae tuned to respond to specific environmental stimuli (vibrating energy fields and physical stimuli). Some IMPs extend inwards from the membrane surface and monitor the internal world of the cell while others extend outwards, monitoring external signals. Cells possess a uniquely tuned receptor protein for every environmental signal. When a specific molecule is in the cell's vicinity a specific receptor locks onto it. This locking-on changes the receptor's electromagnetic charge and the protein shifts into its active conformation, entering the environmental data into the cell. This in turn stimulates the effector proteins, altering their molecular angles.
- *Effector proteins (action oriented)*: Effector proteins are the creators of physical sensation and engage in action-generating life-sustaining cellular behaviour responses. There are different kinds of behaviour control effector proteins for different actions. In active mode the effector proteins ensure the smooth functioning of the cell through open action, such as shuttling information from one side of the membrane to the other (transport proteins) or facilitating cell energy production to empower biological processes (channel proteins).

The two classes of protein complexes cause expansion or contraction of the cell membrane, determining the shape and size of the molecules able to pass through it (9). Constant changes in the shape of protein conformations, which can occur thousands of times per second, are exploited by cells to empower specific metabolic and behavioural functions that support life. The complex behaviour of a living cell is collectively created through the simultaneous interactions of tens of thousands of reflexive perception IMP switches in the functioning membrane, each directly reading an individual environmental signal. Cell survival depends on the ability to adjust dynamically to an ever-changing environment. If movement stops functions stop. When the number of these IMPs is maximised, awareness is increased, which translates to greater resilience and survivability (5). Consciousness depends on IMP flow – the more molecular conversations the greater consciousness (8, 10).

Complementary environmental signals are required to animate the protein's movement (5). Cells are impaired when the environment is less than optimal. Epigenetics ("control above the genes") is the science of how environmental signals select and regulate the protein-gene activity (5, 7-9, 11-17):

> Genes are physical memories, a molecular record, of an organism's learned experiences and evolution. Current external life affects this memory bank – when a gene product is needed, the quality of external signals from the environment outside of the cell will set in motion a set of energy-chemical instructions. The receptor-effector complex acts as a molecular switch: The acceptance of environmental signals by the receptors stimulates the effector proteins to activate the reading of genes by un-wrapping the protein sleeve around the DNA. Certain genes within the human DNA will be switched on and express while others will remain inactive. The expression of a gene is therefore not an emergent property of the gene itself and the brain appears to be naturally driven by both genetic information and the impact of experience. It is the perception of the environment that causes cells to change their structure and behaviour. Constant remoulding and modification of genes without changing their basic DNA code is complemented by other environmental influences and life experiences (e.g., nutrition, stress) that all contribute to the change in brain structure and the shaping of biology.

Epigenetic mechanisms may compromise the internal process of autonomic self-regulation.

Autonomic self-regulation

Autonomic self-regulation within the ISF can be defined as a self-organisational interactive feedback process that emerges from the nature of the properties of the ISF. It incorporates fine tuning devices for multiple energy-chemical correction and integrative functions that move the system towards its optimal healthy blueprint and maximal complexity (1, 8, 13).

The brain is the main controlling role player in autonomic self-regulation. Through the nervous system and its protein-activated reflexive perception switches the brain perceives, monitors and interprets environmental signals, and responds by organizing and coordinating appropriate behavioural responses in all the cells in the system (5). In view of the discussions that follow, a concise summary is presented of the Triune Brain Model of the evolutionary development of the brain (18):

- The first and oldest area, which is fully developed at birth, consists of the primitive systems responsible for survival, the ongoing autonomic self-regulatory firing patterns of important basic life-affirming processes, including the regulation of heart rhythms, respiration, states of alertness and sleepiness, and aspects of the fight/flight/freeze response. These deeper structures are referred to as the reptilian brain (the arousal system) and consist of the brainstem, medulla, pons, and a section of the cerebellum.

- The limbic system or mid-brain (the interpretive system of the brain consisting of the hippocampus, amygdale, hypothalamus and thalamus) and the basal ganglia are the second part of the brain to develop. This region, which is fully developed at birth although not fully functional, is a primary source of stimulus evaluation and is involved in attachment, memory and meaning regulation (especially processing events into factual and autobiographical forms), emotion and the fight/flight response.
- The largest section of the brain, the cortical regions, is the third part to develop. It consists of areas such as the left and right prefrontal cortex, the orbito-frontal areas and the anterior cingulate. Most of the cortical regions (needed for higher thought processes) develop after birth and are affected by the constant interplay between the internal and external environments (13, 16).

The connections between the reptilian and limbic brains that organize our lower reflexive sensorimotor processing and responses to sensory stimuli can function independently of top-down regulation, whereas top-down processing depends on the lower levels. All autonomic self-regulation is controlled and organized by signals sent from the connections and close collaboration of the more primitive brain regions via the neural pathways to every individual muscle or organ (19, 20). The body is continuously detecting signals from its quantum field and neurons of these lower levels switch on distinct gene combinations whose responses are initially concerned with movement and the responsibility for carrying out tasks in different locations (21). The hypothalamus within the limbic zone enables such direct influences on the body (13, 22).

The hypothalamus-pituitary-adrenal (HPA) axis protection system

The body has two protection systems that form part of autonomic self-regulation: the HPA axis for the perception of external threats and the immune system for internal threats such as those caused by bacteria and viruses (5). In preparation for the discussion on SHRs further on in this paper, the focus in the following paragraphs will be on the HPA axis.

Perception exists in conjunction with the potential for action. During initial threat perception information processing of the higher mode, the cortical region, is deactivated so that the deeper reflexive survival regions of the brain, the brainstem and limbic regions, can take immediate, automatic and instinctual control. Stimulation of the immediate reflexive response initiates the motor behaviours necessary for fight/flight as follows (2, 5, 10, 16, 17, 22-28):

Sensory input is sent to the *locus coeruleus*, a part of the brainstem and the anatomical core of the physiological arousal mechanism (stress responses) in the central nervous system; the *locus coeruleus* is a principle site for brain synthesis of norepinephrine. Norepinephrine is the neurotransmitter responsible for delivering messages to the rest of the brain about the need to prepare for emergencies. The *locus coeruleus* is therefore involved in intensive alertness modulation and autonomic reflexes. During stress neurons of the *locus coeruleus* evaluate the threat value of the sensory input and initiate and mediate the arousal response by secreting increasing levels of norepinephrine. The enhanced norepinephrine postsynaptic responsiveness in the neuronal pathway will stimulate arousal in parts of the brain such as the amygdale, which mediates processing of arousal-based memories.

The activated amygdale quickly assesses and evaluates the emotional content of the external activating event and initiates the following two fight/flight response sequences:

- Outside of conscious awareness and via the release of neurotransmitters the amygdale mediates the regulation of the autonomic nervous system's (ANS) preparation for bodily execution. The somatic nervous system takes over from the ANS, and the hypothalamus (the master hormone regulator within the limbic regions that functions as a way station for signals originating elsewhere in the brain) and pituitary gland (the master gland of the endocrine system) sense and coordinate the flow of behaviour-regulating signals within the cellular community. The hypothalamus receives the environmental threat and activates sympathetic acceleration of the initial involuntary activation by stimulating and engaging the HPA stress hormonal axis through a signal sent to the pituitary gland. The pituitary gland launches the body's organs into action by sending a signal to the adrenal glands (adrenal alarm). In endocrine response the adrenal stress hormones coordinate the flight/fight function of the body's organs. Adrenal stress hormones (epinephrine and norepinephrine) released in the blood, constrict the blood vessels of the digestive tract. This forces nutrient-rich blood to flow preferentially to the muscles of the arms and legs and stimulates the life-sustaining reflexive behaviour of the hindbrain, providing the person with great physiological power to retaliate and to get to safety.
- The amygdale sends the information to the hippocampus, which assigns a cognitive meaning to the information and then sends messages to the orbitofrontal cortex (OFC). The OFC activates the HPA stress hormonal axis to organize the autonomic and endocrine responses, increase the sympathetic discharge and inhibit parasympathetic tone (through the brainstem). The OFC functions as the master regulator (of the limbic system, the ANS, and the HPA axis) in processing arousal-based information and modulating autonomic regulation and homeostasis. Finally, from there the information will be sent to the cerebral cortex, which organizes complex survival behaviour.

When the fight/flight response discharges the arousal of the sympathetic nervous system successfully, everything returns to normal. In the absence of threat the HPA axis remains inactive. In the face of trauma an adaptive sequence of events unfolds.

Trauma

During a trauma-activating event the person experiences a perception of powerlessness to retain complete integrity (4). When fight/flight defence possibilities are mobilized but cannot be carried through, their natural progression is aborted through parasympathetic firing that takes over from the sympathetic system and creates a state of collapse (16, 21, 23). The information remains stuck as non-integrated energy-chemical material in the deeper brain arena and cannot be relayed to the limbic system or neocortex through the thalamus (which serves as a relay port through which much of perceptual input passes). This shutting off of the initiated stress response holds the neuroendocrine stress reaction (endogenous, stress-responsive neural hormones such as cortisol, epinephrine, and norepinephrine) in a time-frozen state of hyper-aroused fight/flight energy activation (2, 4). Although the information loop has gone into freeze or "play dead" response mode (23), it still seems to involve an intensely engaged sympathetic system, since muscles have become tense and stiff, heart rate is elevated, and sensory awareness is increased to hypervigilance (21). Trauma equals disrupted neurotransmitter impulses and neuroendocrine stress hormones that were unable to discharge through the synapses to ensure the passing of impulses from one neuron to the next.

The freeze response has a short-term life-saving function, but the disrupted flow of vital energy due to the long-term freeze of activated stress-responsive neural hormones disrupts brain efficiency (4, 13). When the membrane's receptor proteins are left intact and its effector proteins are immobilized, the result is cell coma (5). Additional trauma (developmental trauma or shock trauma) accumulated after the initial trauma-activating event can add to the length of the trauma-chain that feeds excessive disruption of autonomic self-regulation.

Compromised neural integrity affects all physical organ systems. The state of disrupted autonomic self-regulation predicts the health problems and manifestation of dis-ease (1, 2, 29). Trauma-induced long-term non-alignment with the natural healthy blueprint disposition of free-flowing energy within the ISF will put the client at risk of developing trauma-spectrum manifestation or TSM (1, 16, 23). The following chronic dis-eases (TSM) have been documented as arising from epigenetic mechanisms and trauma (4, 30-36):

> Growth inhibition, higher risks and rates of infections and some autoimmune dis-orders (e.g., systemic lupus erythematosus and cancer), cerebrovascular dis-eases (e.g., stroke), coronary artery/cardiovascular dis-eases, liver dis-eases, skin dis-eases, chronic lung dis-eases, irritable bowel syndrome, obesity, chronic pain, osteoporosis, dysautonomia (syndromes like fibromyalgia, somatisation dis-order, and chronic fatigue syndrome), preterm labour, ovarian dysfunction and early menopause, ADD and ADHD, PTSD and Complex PTSD, diabetes, mood disorders (such as problems which affect regulation and relatedness – depression, psychoses, and sociopathic dis-orders), fragmentation of memory and disintegration of sense of self, diminished conscious awareness and reduced intelligence, and other neural dysfunctions.

Variations of TSM could possibly originate in particular brain areas due to neurobiological abnormalities caused by the shut-down or abnormal switching on of certain genes.

Initially, before trauma entered the picture, the brain experienced raw, rich and direct unbiased sensation (4, 22). Trauma disrupts this picture; a perceptual sense of injustice in the face of powerlessness is an inhibitor of consciousness. Enhanced energy activated in the brain shape-shifts into unconscious procedural memory territory, the primary storage place of survival-based information (16). Consistent panelbeating through external influences leads to a further recession of expression and free-flowing energy of other potentialities and possible coping configurations. The adapted coping that defines also confines owing to a loss of the complete experience of ongoing sensation of the now (1, 6). Spontaneity is sacrificed to inhibition and subsequent rigidity, and clarity gives way to projection. The survival journey from the original raw and direct sensation to a narrowing in consciousness characterised by assembled and moulded perception equals a change in the physical structure of the brain (22). Life experiences have altered the natural free firing patterns within the brain's neural tracts and the ISF's natural self-organizational executive functioning towards complexity (1, 13, 21). Autonomic self-regulation has been compromised in favour of unconsciousness.

TSM is an ISF systemic 911 call focusing attention on the fact that the person is living a compromised life (1). It is part of the ISF's innate natural disposition to manifest its inherent potential, and SHIP® theory proposes that SHRs is the energy-chemical lifeline of trauma-healing in favour of living a conscious and uncompromised life with free access to all internal potentialities (1, 4).

Spontaneous healing reactions (SHRs)

The author of this article proposes that SHRs are the reflexive reaction link (apart from all the other neural complexities) between receptor and effector proteins and trauma. SHRs are at the heart of autonomic self-regulation and manifest continuous involuntary, interconnected energy-chemical reflexive perception reactions in favour of internal balance (1). During a trauma-activating event information is received by the receptor proteins and some of the initial reflexive reactions are not distributed by the effector proteins, but the kinetic energy is kept on-hold and frozen into unconscious timeless potential energy. The disruption in autonomic self-regulation implies that the complete processing and assimilation of sensorimotor activations to the trauma-activating event have not taken place (9, 21).

Migration to a state of connectedness depends on the enigmatic wisdom of the SHRs. When activated through external associative activators to the initial trauma, the lower regions of the brain drive the continuous selective fragmented executive release of the unfreezing stored procedural memory (1, 21). In addition, autonomic self-regulation, because of its natural detoxifying process, evokes these typical bottom-up flashback somatic experiences and responses of trauma memory into consciousness (16). The limbic system (ANS) selectively regulates and exposes the person to this fragmented release of SHRs by converting energy-chemical communication into sensations (3), operating as if the danger is still imminent – which in fact it is, since unfreezing is only taking place now. It is noteworthy that neurons of the *locus coeruleus* are viewed by some as the first or second leg in the pathophysiology of the TSM circuit (26). Research has shown that chemical stimulation of norepinephrine release from the *locus coeruleus* can induce somatosensory flashbacks in TSM sufferers (2). This implies that SHRs have norepinephrine as a constituent.

SHRs can be compared with the sensations one has when one's leg "awakes" from "sleeping" – all the pins and needles and peculiar sensations signify the opening of the blocked neural communication channels. SHRs lead to the completion of the initial on-hold neuroendocrine stress reaction. This equates to the flow of energy within the ISF – the reverse movement, or freeze discharge, of timeless potential energy to in-the-moment kinetic energy. Release and completion of involuntary SHRs reciprocally lead to integration of trauma, a disappearance of TSM and the realignment of the psychobiology to its natural free flow energy disposition. SHRs restore the integrity within the ISF. This results in a reciprocal movement to spontaneity, self-assertiveness and an access to full potential. SHIP® facilitates such life-changing results with former TSM sufferers who have gone through spontaneous healing of their trauma, and has developed a wide variety of activators to activate and expose frozen SHRs (1).

The questions remain: What can SHRs teach us? Can their neural origin provide clarity on the etiology of certain dis-eases and their possible prevention or eventual healing? This article focuses on opening this debate. Potential pointers may be discovered when mapping SHRs. SHIP® categories of SHRs will be listed in order to create a platform for the discussion on mapping.

Categories of SHRs

The author of this article has noted in excess of 2000 varieties/combinations of SHRs that serve to extinguish internal trauma. It is quite common in SHIP® for a chain reaction of SHRs to follow initial activation, signifying energy release of the trauma-chain.

The two main sensory systems that are involved during the manifestation of SHRs and that are well developed by birth are the exteroceptive and interoceptive sensory systems. The categories of SHRs within these systems are based on experiential research and literature on the flashback fragments of clients' trauma memory (10, 13, 16, 21, 24, 27, 29, 37):

The exteroceptive sensory system (perception – awareness-oriented) consists of nerves that receive and transmit information from the exterior environment of the body by way of the eyes, ears, tongue, nose, and skin – these are the primary senses that warn the person of impending threat. SHRs in this system would include the following:

- *Visual* – such as seeing various images (e.g., spots, balls, wavy patterns, colours, written words, or realistic images of previous incidents), or tunnel vision, or de-realization and micropsia (distortions in visual perception).
- *Auditory* (audition) – such as hearing an incessant ringing in the ears, or a zooming sound around the whole body, or somebody calling the client's name, or a tune going round and round in the client's head, or other sounds.
- *Taste* (gustation) – such as the taste of blood, or metal, or semen, or a bitter or acid or an acrid taste.
- *Smell* (olfaction) – something very definite such as the smell of petrol, or oil, or ether, or anaesthetic, or a hospital, or perspiration, or an attic, or an old cupboard, or perfume, or copper bangles, or the client's childhood home, or somebody's body odour from long ago.
- *Touch* – such as hot or cold sensations.

The interoceptive sensory system (somatosensory – action-oriented) consists of nerves that receive and transmit information from the interior environment of the body (from the viscera - organs of the chest and abdomen), muscles and connective tissue. SHRs in this system would include the following:

- *Proprioception* – the kinesthetic sense (of the body's spatial and internal states, which enables a person to locate all the parts of his or her body in space, and the force, timing and speed of muscle movement), and the visceral sense (which gives feedback on body states such as heart rate, respiration, digestive muscles, internal temperature, muscular tension and visceral discomfort) through nociceptors and thermoceptors: sensations such as a sharp pain in the ears, or a pressure on the ears or a strange feeling in the ears, or twitches or tics or cramping in any muscle area or tremors or turning movements of parts of the body such as the head and neck (involuntary and self-perpetuated muscle fasciculations), or the feeling that there is a tight steel band around the head or chest, or feeling someone holding the client, or someone putting pressure on any part of the body, or being strangled by someone, or someone tightening a corset around the client's middle, or a feeling of a blanket around the shoulders, or tightness in the throat, or hypoglycaemic feelings, or a spiky pain sensation anywhere in the body, or a hollow feeling in the pit of the stomach, or pressure inside or on top of the head, or jaw clenching, or heart palpitations, or suffocation, or excessive sweating, or numbness, or fever-related feelings similar to delirium, or pins-and-needles sensations, or reddening of the skin, or a flickering in the eyes, or eyes jumping, or a lot of movement behind the eyes, or squinting, or burning discomfort in the bladder, or pain in the breasts.
- *Vestibular responses* – a subset of proprioception located in the inner ear. The vestibular responses indicate which way is up and help the body sustain a balanced posture and maintain a comfortable relationship with gravity: sensations such as confusion and disorientation, or being off-balance, or experiencing vertigo or spinning in any direction and motion sickness, or lying skew or swaying, or falling through the psychotherapy bed, or somersaulting in a swimming pool and not being able to tell top from bottom, or that one's body is bumping up and down, or levitating, or being sucked backwards head first into a vortex, or flying backwards and upside down, or floating in water.
- *Depersonalization* – related to, and sometimes in conjunction with, vestibular responses, and manifesting as body distortion and out-of-body experiences: sensations such as the brain sinking deep down, or body decreasing in size and the environment increases in size, or feeling that the head is shaped like a block, or the body or hands or feet or ears or other parts feel inflated and distorted, or body parts feel separate/ disjointed from each other and do not feel like a unit, or arms have switched positions, or organs are too large for the body, or the body feels asymmetrical or cylindrical or twisted in the middle with the stomach facing down and the top half of the body facing upwards, or that the arms are short and the legs long, or the face feels pointed like a long beak, or a person feels like a triangle with a hole in the middle and falling to the left, or de-realization experiences (that time is standing still or moving very fast).

- *Emotional feelings* – closely linked to proprioception, the combination of sensations and the urge for physical activation is experienced as an emotion: each basic emotion (fear, anger, shame, sadness, disgust, frustration, or happiness) is an integral experience of the body and has an accompanying set of discrete underlying body sensations (e.g., sadness manifesting as a burning in the throat) stimulated by pattern activity in the brain. Emotional SHRs have the common originator of a loss of complete experience due to trauma. Loss is always sad, it implies an internal knowledge that something should have been different; it is released through crying, which is a basic deep neural release present since infanthood.

Clinical practice shows two distinct interoceptive SHR release avenues: various possibilities and combinations of any SHRs found within the four interoceptive categories (suggesting the inter-relatedness), or with the absence of emotional feelings. In either case, and whether implicit or in combination with explicit memory, the result is the relief of TSM.

Mapping of the different types of SHRs will be done in the next section in view of the hypothesis that SHRs are reflexive reactions that unfreeze accumulated neurotransmitter impulses and neuroendocrine stress hormones. This exercise might indicate the location of origin of SHRs, where initial trauma found its unconscious nestling place in the brain.

Mapping of SHRs

SHIP® categories of SHRs were confirmed by the work of others who noted that activity in sensory regions of the brain may mediate perception and the specific nature of this firing may signify the different aspects of perceptual information – this led to the following mapping of the SHIP® SHRs categories (16-18, 22, 25, 29, 38, 39):

The exteroceptive sensory system:

- *Visual* – vision and its messages are routed from the visual cortex to the *locus coeruleus*; high levels of activation in the amygdale and low levels in the fusiform area (that specializes in deciphering specific visual stimuli) result in a possible dysfunction in the visual cortex through periodic fragmented effector release and projection of internal trauma.
- *Auditory* – auditory messages are sent from the auditory cortex to the cochlear nucleus in the medulla from which fibres project to the medulla level, the midbrain level and the thalamus; from the thalamus auditory fibres project to the primary auditory cortex in the temporal lobe for detection of the auditory stimulus, and from there the auditory message is sent to the auditory association areas for interpretation.
- *Taste* – the gestation pathway leads from the taste bud receptors on the surface of the tongue to the solitary nucleus in the medulla, after which the information is propagated to the amygdale, hypothalamus and thalamus; from the thalamus the gustatory information travels to the primary gustatory cortex located in the frontal insula for conscious interpretation.
- *Smell* – except for olfaction all sensory information travels through the thalamus before it reaches the cortex: smell is detected by the olfactory cortex from which it

has a direct connection to the amygdale and the primitive emotional and unconscious fear responses to threat. Like vision, smell and its messages, are routed to the *locus coeruleus*.

- *Touch* – sensory receptors carry a stimulus (vibration, tactile sensation and proprioception information) along nerve fibres to where they synapse with the first order neuron in the dorsal root ganglion and from there into the spinal cord through the dorsal nerve roots; after entering the spinal cord the nerve fibres terminate by synapsing with a spinal second-order neuron that eventually runs through the brainstem (succeeding through the medulla, pons and midbrain) and terminates by synapsing with cells/neurons in the thalamus; third-order sensory neurons in the thalamus carry the sensations to the somatosensory cortex in the parietal lobes.

The interoceptive sensory system – both the limbic system and the basal ganglia are responsible for the activation of patterns of sensory responses to external cues and set the trajectory of protection:

- *Proprioception* – the kinesthetic and visceral systems involve all autonomic self-regulatory processes of the body and its organs: the abdominal viscera have unique neural connections with parts of the brainstem and the limbic system (made possible by the somatic nervous system that sets up a continuum between the brain and the musculoskeletal system). Many musculoskeletal reflexes are automatic and are governed unconsciously by neural pathways in the spinal cord and brainstem. Vasomotor control is governed by reciprocal alternating of dominance of the sympathetic and the parasympathetic parts of the ANS, the motor cortex (where commands to move the muscles are generated) and the somatosensory cortex (a map of the body). Nerve input to the somatosensory area generally comes from the thalamus deeper in the brain. Each part of the brain is assigned a particular spot in the somatosensory cortex for processing and with less cortical space due to trauma a body part becomes more alienated – fragmented SHR release through that body part could possibly restore functionality.
- *Vestibular responses* – many brainstem reflexes that influence posture are instinctual and hardwired in the brain before birth: vestibular nuclei in the pons-medulla junction receive information about balance and equilibrium from the inner ear, midbrain, pons and cerebellum.
- *Depersonalization* – the parietal cortex in the brain helps define bodily boundaries and this could form part of the neural regions associated with the experience of identity. It has been postulated that the thalamus could be shut down during certain somatically oriented therapies, allowing input from the deeper structure of the most basic self at the brainstem level to flow directly and alter how a person perceives the body's boundary – the suggestion is that the enhanced release of SHRs stimulates a part of the parietal cortex, causing the body boundary distortion until there is eventual integration and increased neural alignment towards the healthy blueprint disposition. The sense of self is influenced by memory formation and space-time relation. It is the point of reference in life, and although memory is not stored in the hippocampus the hippocampus is necessary for processing memory (it receives input

from and sends efferents to both the amygdale and the cortex) and for conceptualizing and coordinating this memory in space-time before the eventual lower activation is recorded as explicit memory in the cortex – a trauma-induced shrunken and dysfunctional hippocampus disorientates the experience of space-time and affects the sense of self and boundary specificity.

- *Emotional feelings* – the biology of emotion in the body and brain is called affect and is largely a subcortical process with a decrease in information processing in neocortical systems during intense emotional states. Immediate, automatic and unconscious emotional responses follow a direct route - the sensory information is sent to the thalamus from where it is transmitted to the amygdale. The amygdale is responsible for reflexive autonomic components of emotion, such as uncomfortable emotion and distress (e.g., changes in heart rate); the central nucleus of the amygdale projects to a variety of brain structures, including the brainstem; large bundles of neurons run between certain regions of the amygdale and the prefrontal cortex and eventual emotional control and similar high-order cognitive function is then done by the prefrontal region, which plays a key role in regulating emotions; the anterior cingulate cortex (part of the limbic system and a central station for processing top-down and bottom-up stimuli) has extensive connections with different brain structures within the limbic system and brainstem that orchestrate and play a key role in processing the autonomic, neuroendocrine, visceral behavioural response coordination and expression of emotion (activation and modulation), enabling more response flexibility for both bodily input and affective responses. The hypothalamus works in collaboration with the limbic system in the expression of emotion and sends signals to the body to generate many of the visceral and hormonal changes that frequently accompany emotion. Disruption in the functioning in the anterior cingulate may provide a neural basis for problems with emotional regulation, as well as a generalized problem with physiological arousal and emotional numbing. A key area of the brain for self-awareness is the insula in the cerebral cortex, which sends signals to the visceral organs during emotion and monitors the body through reception of signals related to pain, temperature, visceral sensations, and the state of the blood vessels.

The author of this article has often observed when dealing with clients in SHIP® that exteroceptive sensory experiences are the key to opening the perception of interoceptive energy – awareness leads to action. This could indicate that the interoceptive SHRs are the deeper embedded truncated trauma energy-chemical release. With some clients the interoceptive SHRs are immediate, while with others they are introduced through activation of exteroceptive SHRs such as visual memory of people, events, or archetypal images. The above mapping suggests that interoceptive SHRs can largely be traced to the lower brain regions – the cortical processes in the higher brain regions could not receive and process the trauma material successfully because of disrupted autonomic self-regulation. Taken together with the proposal that SHRs are the reflexive reaction link between receptor and effector proteins and trauma, this has an interesting implication: TSM could possibly originate from curtailed reflexive behaviour in the spinal cord, brainstem and limbic regions. This should be seen in conjunction with genetic susceptibility and supplemented by additional complementary environmental constituents such as climate, diet, exercise, and other constituents of everyday life.

Conclusion

The author of this article has presented different constituents and characteristics of SHRs. It is proposed that SHRs show qualities of disrupted neurotransmitter and neuroendocrine stress hormone responses, and that trauma is born through this disruption. Mapping of the different categories of SHRs indicates that SHRs probably originate in the deeper reflex-oriented brain structures. This implies that trauma-spectrum manifestation (TSM – which includes most chronic dis-eases) could originate due to curtailed reflexive behaviour. SHRs may be defined as subcortical somatic flashbacks attempting to rectify the disruption in autonomic self-regulation caused by an energy-chemical induced unconscious. The suggestion is that TSM may be reversible through a process such as SHIP® that resurrects and facilitates interaction with the dark night of the deep brain regions. This allows the enigmatic SHRs to unleash the trauma shackles of unconsciousness and to complete the unfreezing journey towards integration and optimal autonomic and conscious functioning. Further neural-biochemical research on SHRs is needed to verify the proposal on SHRs and the implication that the neural wound can heal itself within the appropriate psychotherapeutic healing space.

References

[1] Steenkamp JO. Introducing an Integrated SHIP® trauma-spectrum model on the etiology, characteristics and natural disposition of trauma-spectrum manifestations (TSM). J Pain Manage 2014;(7)1:47-59.
[2] Van der Kolk BA, Saporta J. The biological response to psychic trauma: Mechanisms and treatment of intrusion and numbing. Anxiety Res (UK) 1991;4:199-212.
[3] Steenkamp JO, Van der Walt MJ, Schoeman-Steenkamp EM, Strydom I. Introducing SHIP® as a psychotherapeutic model to access the body memory of traumatised clients: Depathologising expressions of trauma. S Afr J Psychol 2012;42(2):202-13.
[4] Steenkamp JO. A SHIP® perspective on creating a healing space for the integration of trauma. J Altern Med Res 2013;5(3):179-93.
[5] Lipton BH. The biology of belief: Unleashing the power of consciousness, mind and matter. Carlsbad: Hay House, 2009.
[6] Oschman JL. Trauma energetics. J Bodywork Movement Ther 2006;10(1):21-34.
[7] Kehoe J. Quantum warrior: The future of the mind. Vancouver: Zoetic, 2011.
[8] Ball P. Molecules: A very short introduction. New York: Oxford University Press, 2001.
[9] Church D. The genie in your genes. USA: Energy Psychology Press, 2007.
[10] Steenkamp JO. SHIP®, Spontaneous Healing Intrasystemic Process: The age-old art of facilitating healing, 17th Impression. Pretoria: JOS, 2002.
[11] Nijhout HF. Metaphors and the role of genes in development. Bioessays 1990;12(9):441-6.
[12] Ridley M. Nature via nurture. New York: Harper Collins, 2003.
[13] Solomon MF, Siegel DJ. Healing trauma: Attachment, mind, body, and brain. New York: Norton, 2003.
[14] Pray LA. Epigenetics: Genome, meet your environment. Scientist 2004:14-20.
[15] Silverman PH. Rethinking genetic determinism: With only 30,000 genes, what is it that makes humans humans? Scientist 2004:32-3.

[16] Scaer R. The trauma spectrum: Hidden wounds and human resiliency. New York: Norton, 2005.

[17] Davidson RJ. The emotional life of your brain: How its unique patterns affect the way you think, feel, and live – and how you can change them. UK: Hodder Stoughton, 2012.

[18] MacLean PD. The triune brain in evolution: Role in paleocerebral functions. New York: Penguin, 1990.

[19] Grawe K. Neuropsychotherapy: How neurosciences inform effective psychotherapy. New York: Taylor Francis, 2007.

[20] Maupin C. CFS and autonomic dysfunction. 2014. Accessed 2014 Feb 22 Jul 11. URL: http://www.cfidsreport.com/Articles?CFS/Autonomic_Nervous_System_Dysfunction.htm.

[21] Ogden P, Minton K, Pain C. Trauma and the body: A sensorimotor approach to psychotherapy. New York: Norton, 2006.

[22] Siegel DJ. The mindful brain: Reflection and attunement in the cultivation of well-being. New York: Norton, 2007.

[23] Porges SW. Love: An emergent property of the mammalian autonomic nervous system. J Psychoneuroendocrinology 1998;23:837-61.

[24] Rothschild B. The body remembers: The psychophysiology of trauma and trauma treatment. New York: Norton, 2000.

[25] Rothschild B. The body remembers casebook: Unifying methods and models in the treatment of trauma and PTSD. New York: Norton, 2003.

[26] Bracha HS, Garcia-Rill E, Mrak RE, Skinner R. Postmortem locus coeruleus neuron count in three American veterans with probable or possible war-related PTSD. J Neuropsychiatr Clin Neurosci 2005;17(4):503-9.

[27] Levine PA. Healing trauma: A pioneering program for restoring the wisdom of your body. Boulder: Sounds True, 2005.

[28] Rothschild B. 8 Keys to safe trauma recovery: Take-charge strategies to empower your healing. New York: Norton, 2010.

[29] Bremner JD. Does stress damage the brain? Understanding trauma-related disorders from a mind-body perspective. New York: Norton, 2005.

[30] Nathanielsz P. Life in the womb. New York: Promethean, 1999.

[31] Christensen D. Weight matters, even in the womb: Status at birth can foreshadow illnesses decades later. J Sci News 2000;158:382-3.

[32] McEwen B, Lasley EN. The end of stress as we know it. Washington, DC: National Academic Press, 2002.

[33] Holden C. Future brightening for depression treatments. Science 2003;302:810-3.

[34] Gluckman PD, Hanson MA. Living with the past: Evolution, development, and patterns of disease. J Science 2004;305:1733-6.

[35] Kopp MS, Réthelyi J. Where psychology meets physiology: Chronic stress and premature mortality – the Central-Eastern European health paradox. Brain Res Bull 2004;62:351-67.

[36] Segerstrom SC, Miller GE. Psychological stress and the human immune system: A meta-analytic study of 30 years of inquiry. Psychol Bull 2004;130(4):601-30.

[37] Van der Kolk BA, MacFarlane I, Weisaeth L. Traumatic stress: The effects of overwhelming experience on the mind, body, and society. New York: Guilford, 1996.

[38] Gutman S. Neuroscience: Quick reference for rehabilitation professionals, 2nd Edition. USA: Slack, 2008.

[39] Zillmer EA, Spiers MV, Culbertson WC. Principles of neuropsychology, 2nd Edition. USA: Wadsworth, 2008.

Submitted: November 20, 2014. *Revised:* December 31, 2014 *Accepted:* January 08, 2015.

In: Pain Management Yearbook 2015
Editor: Joav Merrick

ISBN: 978-1-63484-515-1

Chapter 3

LONG-TERM OUTCOMES OF CAUDAL EPIDURAL STEROID INJECTIONS IN MANAGING CHRONIC LOW BACK PAIN AND RADICULOPATHY IN PATIENTS WITH PREVIOUS LUMBAR SURGERY

Gregory G Billy[1,*], MD, Ji Lin[2], BA, Mengzhao Gao[3], MAS, and Mosuk Chow[3], PhD

[1]Department of Orthopaedics and Rehabilitation,
Penn State Orthopaedics, State College, PA, US
[2]Penn State College of Medicine,
Milton S Hershey Medical Center, Hershey, PA, US
[3]Department of Statistics, Eberly College of Science,
Pennsylvania State University, University Park, PA, US

Persistent pain following lumbar spinal surgery can be a significant problem for both patients and their treating physicians. The caudal epidural approach is commonly utilized with patients who are on anticoagulation or who have had prior lumbar surgery to treat radicular pain originating from the lumbar 5 (L5) or sacral 1 (S1) levels. Objective: To evaluate and determine the efficacy of caudal epidural steroid injections (ESI) in managing pain in patients with previous lumbar surgery (PLS) and radiculopathy. Study group: Retrospective clinical outcome analysis. Methods: Retrospective review of patients undergoing caudal ESIs for radiculopathy from January 1, 2006 to August 30, 2013, a total of 288 injections were analyzed. Results: The percentage improvement and relief duration for the PLS patients was compared to a cohort group of non-surgical patients undergoing caudal ESIs. The percentage improvement for the two groups was compared using the two-sample t-test for injections number 1 to 3. There was no significant difference between the two groups. For analysis of relief duration, the distribution is skewed and the medians for the two groups were compared using the Mann-Whitney test. There was no significant difference of the medians between the two groups. Conclusions: Efficacy following a caudal ESI for treating radicular pain in

[*] Correspondence: Gregory G Billy, MD, Department of Orthopaedics and Rehabilitation, Penn State Orthopaedics, 1850 East Park Avenue, Suite 112, State College, PA 16803, United States. E-mail: gbilly@hmc.psu.edu.

patients with a previous history of back surgery is not significantly different from patients without a previous history of back surgery. Fluroscopically guided caudal epidural steroid injection is an effective short to intermediate treatment for radicular pain in post lumbar surgical patients with chronic radiculopathy.

Keywords: caudal, epidural steroid injections, effective, radiculopathy, post-surgical patients

INTRODUCTION

Persistent pain following lumbar spinal surgery can be a significant problem for both patients and their treating physicians to manage. It is estimated that greater than 500,000 lumbar spinal fusions and laminectomies take place each year in the United States (1). Despite advances in surgical technology complications following surgeries have not declined and can include persistent pain with a frequency estimated to be between 8-40% (2-5). The etiologies of this persistent pain can vary and are felt to include: myofascial pain, foraminal stenosis, pseudoarthrosis, neuropathic pain, recurrent disc herniation, facet joint pain and sacroiliac join pain (6-7).

Over the years a number of potential treatments with varying evidence of efficacy for post-surgical pain have been advocated including anterior lumbar interbody fusion, spinal cord stimulation, oral and intrathecal medications, percutaneous adhesiolysis and caudal epidural steroid injections (8-13). The efficacy of the caudal ESI has been debated, but most studies have shown the injection to be helpful for treatment of chronic spinal pain and radiculopathy and also helpful in the management of persistent pain in post -surgical patients (14-18). The studies vary in regards to their efficacies, but most studies conclude additional investigation including long term follow up is needed. Our group wishes to further explore the efficacy of caudal ESI injections in post-surgical patients over a seven year period.

METHODS

The medical charts of patients who underwent a caudal epidural steroid injection for management of chronic low back pain and radiculopathy from January 1, 2006 to August 30, 2013 were reviewed. The patients who underwent the caudal approach were almost exclusively patients with prior history of lumbar surgery(ies) or patients on anticoagulation.

The caudal epidural approach is commonly utilized with patients who are on anticoagulation or who have had prior lumbar surgery to treat radicular pain originating from the lumbar 5 (L5) or sacral 1 (S1) levels. There may be concern with holding the anticoagulation in patients placing them at an increase of a thromboembolic event. The caudal ESI approach can be done without the need to hold the anticoagulation medication. Additionally, in patients with prior lumbar surgeries in which the dura has been entered the caudal approach is the route of choice to avoid potential injection into the thecal space.

All patients were evaluated in an academic clinic for their complaints of low back pain with radiculopathy. The patients had failed conservative treatments. Patients prior to their injection had a lumbar MRI performed within 6 months of the injection; the MRI study was reviewed by a neuroradiologist and a pain specialist. The MRI was reviewed in regards to its pathology and evidence of a radiculopathy involving the L5 or S1 levels. Patient history included evaluation of their pain history including their diagnosis, the duration of their symptoms and assessment of their pain levels, lowest pain and highest pain level by means of the visual analog scale (VAS). A total of 136 patients underwent a caudal epidural injection during this time period.

Procedures

All injections were performed at a surgi-center and were done by a single practitioner. They were done with fluroscopic guidance using a c-arm (GE OEC 9800 Plus/9900 Elite, GE Healthcare, Wauwatosa, Wisconsin, USA). The injections were performed by placing a 25 gauge 3 ½ inch spinal needle (BD Medical, Franklin Lakes, New Jersey, USA) in through the sacral hiatus and advancing into the sacral canal under lateral fluroscopic guidance. The superior endpoint of the needle tip was the S2 level. The patient was then injected with 5 ml of preservative free 0.9% sodium chloride (Hospira Inc., Lake Forest, Illinois, USA) and 40mg/ml of methylprednisolone acetate injectable suspension, USP (Pharmacia and Upjohn Co, Division of Pfizer Inc., New York, New York, USA).

Outcome measures

Following the injection patients were scheduled for follow-up visits, typically 4 weeks post injection. At their follow up visit their percentage improvement in pain and current lowest and highest VAS pain scales since their injection were assessed. The return of pain was documented in their charts. Complete data for follow up visit was able to be completed on 278 patient injections.

RESULTS

The data was analyzed for both percentage of improvement following a caudal ESI and if the injection did provide relief then the relief duration (in weeks) was then analyzed. The SAS version 9.3 statistical package (SAS Institute INC., Cary, North Carolina, USA) was used for the statistical analysis.

The percentage improvement was categorized into four groups: 0-29%, 30-49%, 50-70% and 80-100%. The distributions of percentage improvement for all the subjects are shown in Figure 1.

This graph is comprehensive and it shows that there is a considerable decrease in the number of patients who take more than three injections. It is important to note that the highest percentage of responses is in the 80-100% category for first three injections, showing the effectiveness of the injection. The graph also suggests that there is not much difference between the two groups for injections with enough sample size to merit a statistical comparison. Table 2 compares the mean percentage of improvement for the two groups by two sample t-test. The result shows the two means are not significantly different for injections 1 to 3. Table 3 lists the count and percentage of subjects that get significant pain relief (50% or more) for two groups.

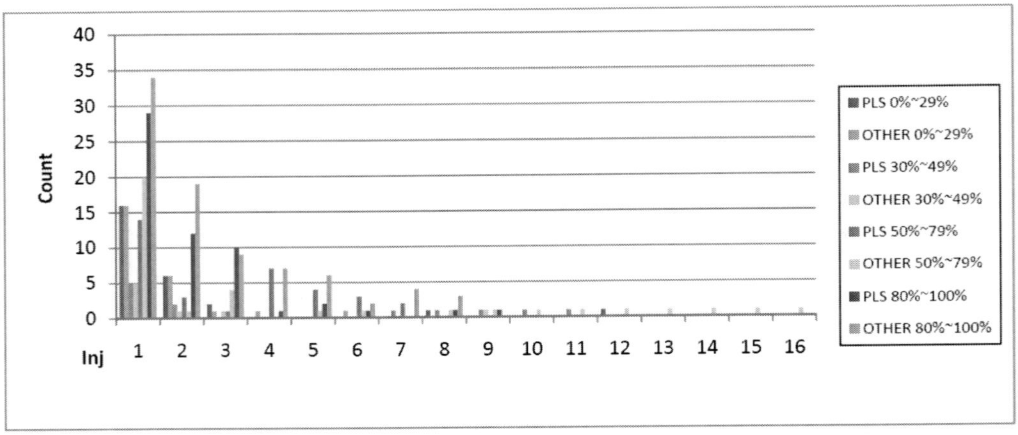

Figure 1. Injection Response Rates.

Table 1. Demographic information on subjects

	PLS group N = 64	Other group N = 72	Total N = 136
Age (years)			
Mean ± SD	60.39 ± 16.26	70.58 ± 14.61	65.79 ± 16.19
Range	23 to 91	28 to 95	23 to 95
Gender			
Male (%)	30 (48.39)	32 (51.61)	62 (45.59)
Female (%)	34 (45.95)	40 (54.05)	74 (54.41)
Duration of symptoms (weeks) before the first visit			
Mean ± SD	75.17 ± 112.25	53.69 ± 62.54	63.80 ± 89.74
Range	1 to 520	1 to 200	1 to 520

Table 2. Comparison of the percentage of improvement for the two groups

Injection #	PLS	Other	Difference	p-value
1	0.5609 ± 0.3676 (n=64)	0.5861 ± 0.3408 (n=72)	-0.0252	0.6793
2	0.5935 ± 0.3788 (n=23)	0.6942 ± 0.3567 (n=26)	-0.1008	0.3427
3	0.7077 ± 0.3220 (n=13)	0.6833 ± 0.2152 (n=15)	0.0244	0.8135

Note: Data expressed as mean ± standard deviation, sample size is in bracket.

Table 3. Count and % of Significant pain relief in each group, % in bracket

Injection #	PLS		Other		Total	
	sig. improvement	sample size	sig. improvement	sample size	sig. improvement	sample size
1	43 (67.18)	64	52 (72.22)	72	95 (69.85)	136
2	15 (65.21)	23	20 (76.92)	26	35 (71.42)	49
3	11 (84.61)	13	13 (86.67)	15	24 (85.71)	28
4	8 (100)	8	7 (87.50)	8	15 (93.75)	16
5	6 (100)	6	7 (100)	7	13 (100)	13
6	4 (100)	4	3 (75)	4	7 (87.5)	8
7	2 (66.67)	3	4 (100)	4	6 (85.71)	7
8	1 (33.33)	3	4 (100)	4	5 (71.43)	7
9	1 (50)	2	1 (50)	2	2 (50)	4
10	0 (0)	1	1 (100)	1	1 (50)	2
11	0 (0)	1	1 (100)	1	1 (50)	2
12	0 (0)	1	1 (100)	1	1 (50)	2
13		0	1 (100)	1	1 (100)	1
14		0	1 (100)	1	1 (100)	1
15		0	1 (100)	1	1 (100)	1
16		0	1 (100)	1	1 (100)	1

Table 4. Correlation between percentage of improvement and VAS PAIN score difference between post- and pre- injections

Injection #	PLS		Other	
	Post high - pre high	Post low - pre low	Post high - pre high	Post low - pre low
1	-0.66966 (<0.0001)	-0.48114 (<0.0001)	-0.56462 (<0.0001)	-0.18972 (0.1104)
2	-0.66377 (0.0006)	-0.09925 (0.6523)	-0.55885 (0.0030)	-0.27050 (0.1814)
3	-0.80367 (0.0009)	-0.13287 (0.6652)	-0.58071 (0.0232)	-0.41598 (0.1230)

Note: p-value in bracket.

Here we see that the percentages are good for most injections when the sample size is not too small.

The VAS pain values were also analyzed. They were examined in regards to the correlation between the percentage improvement and pre-injection highest level of pain, post-injection highest level of pain, pre-injection lowest level of pain, and post-injection lowest level of pain. We found the correlation between percentage of improvement and the difference between post-injection low and pre-injection low, for injections #1-3 where the sample size of both groups are large enough for statistical inference to be meaningful. Also, the correlation between the percentage of improvement and the difference between post-injection high and pre-injection high are reported. The Pearson correlation coefficients are summarized in Table 4. The difference between post-injection high and pre-injection high is more correlated with the percentage improvement for both groups.

The other important variable to consider is length of relief duration. The boxplot for both the post lumbar surgery group and other group is summarized in Figure 2. For the relief duration (in weeks), since the distribution is skewed, we compare the medians using the Mann-Whitney test for the two groups for injections 1 to 3 where the sample sizes are large enough to merit statistical inference. There is no significant difference between the two groups as indicated by the Table 5. In Table 6, we list the medians for both groups for all injections to provide an overall summary of the data.

It is also of interest to note that the average number ± standard deviation of procedures per year for subjects in the PLS group is 1.37±0.67 and 1.33±0.61 for the other group. The p-value for the 2 sample t –test is 0.718 and there is no significant difference between the two groups.

Table 5. Relief duration (in weeks)

Injection #	PLS	Other	Difference	p-value
1	18 (n=64)	32.5 (n=72)	-8	0.1490
2	20 (n=23)	13 (n=26)	4	0.4895
3	17 (n=13)	23 (n= 15)	-9	0.1405

Note: the p-value is obtained by Mann-Whitney test, sample size is in bracket.

Table 6. Median of relief duration (in weeks) for both groups on all injections

Injection #	PLS	Other
1	18 (64)	32.5 (72)
2	20 (23)	13 (26)
3	17 (13)	23 (15)
4	12.5 (8)	17 (8)
5	14 (6)	16 (7)
6	14.5 (4)	12 (4)
7	36 (3)	13 (4)
8	14 (3)	14 (4)
9	14.5 (2)	14.5 (2)
10	14 (1)	10 (1)
11	23 (1)	13 (1)
12	0 (1)	16 (1)
13		14 (1)
14		10 (1)
15		18 (1)
16		18 (1)

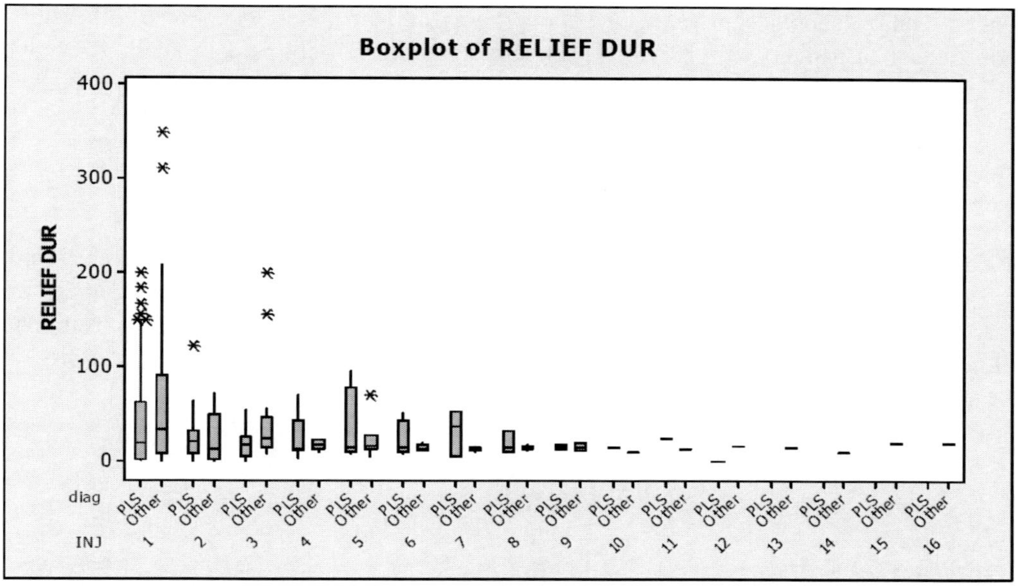

Figure 2. Relief Duration Responses (in weeks) Comparisons.

Discussion

We were able to analyze a total of 288 injections over a seven year period whereas other studies have analyzed much smaller sample sizes over a shorter period of time. In addition, a single practitioner did all of the injections under fluroscopy following the same protocol and consistency with the injection medications. Other studies have shown variation into the technique utilized, and some were done without the use of fluroscopy. The sample size used showed no difference in the prior lumbar group with its matched controls in terms of both symptom length and intensity. Historically, the post-surgical patients are felt to be a difficult group to treat and studies have suggested significant underlying psychiatric factors and psychological illness (19, 20). Our analysis showed this group responds in a very similar fashion to caudal ESIs as does the nonsurgical group.

A limitation of this study is it is a retrospective review of clinical data. When compared to previously published studies our response rates were greater than previously reported rates for spinal stenosis patients with 35-54% of patients obtaining greater than 50% of pain relief for 12 months or longer (21, 22). The difference was felt more to be reflective of limiting the injections to patients who would be more likely to respond with radicular pain>axial pain.

Our results support the role of ESI in the treatment algorithm of managing chronic low back pain and radiculopathy in patients with previous back surgery (23). There is a significant emphasis in this age of cost containment to demonstrate both efficacious and cost effective treatments. Recent analysis was able to show positive results in the cost utility analysis in post lumbar surgery syndrome patients with epidural steroid injections and our results are in agreement with such findings (24).

Caudal ESI under fluroscopic guidance is a safe and effective option to manage persistent chronic low back pain and radiculopathy in patients with previous back surgery. The majority of patients enjoyed both short and long term relief following their injections. This study demonstrates that patients with previous back surgery and persistent pain are likely to obtain benefit from a caudal ESI.

ACKNOWLEDGMENTS

The study was approved by the Pennsylvania State University Institutional Research Board (protocol 43025EP). The project described was supported by the National Center for Research Resources and the National Center for Advancing Translational Sciences, National Institutes of Health, through Grant UL1TR000127. The content is solely the responsibility of the authors and does not necessarily represent the official views of the NIH.

REFERENCES

[1] Rajaee SS, Bae HW, Kanim LE, Delamarter RB. Spinal fusion in the United States. Spine. 2012;37(1):67-76.

[2] Chan CW, Peng P. Failed back surgery syndrome. Pain Med 2011;12(4):577-606.

[3] Weir BK, Jacobs GA. Reoperation rate following lumbar discectomy. An analysis of 662 lumbar discectomies. Spine 1980;5(4):366-70.

[4] Martin BI, Mirza SK, Comstock BA, Gray DT, Kreuter W, Deyo RA. Reoperation rates following lumbar spine surgery and the influence of spinal fusion procedures. Spine 2007;32(3):382-7.

[5] Martin BI, Mirza SK, Comstock BA, Gray DT, Kreuter W, Deyo RA. Are lumbar spine reoperational rates falling with greater use of fusion surgery and new surgical technology. Spine 2007;32(19):2119-26.

[6] Schofferman J, Reynolds J, Herzog R, Covington E, Dreyfuss P, O'Neill C. Failed back surgery: etiology and diagnostic evaluation. Spine J 2003;3(5):400-3.

[7] Thomson S. Failed back surgery syndrome – definition, epidemiology and demographics. BJP 2013;7(1):56-9.

[8] Raphael JH, Southall JL, Gnanadurai TV, Treharne GJ, Kitas GD. Long-term experience with implanted intrathecal drug administration systems for failed back syndrome and chronic mechanical low back pain. BMC Musculoskelet Disord 2002;3:17.

[9] Boswell MV, Trescot AM, Datta S, Schultz DM, Hansen HC, Abdi S, et al. Interventional techniques: evidence-based practice guidelines in the management of chronic spinal pain. Pain Physician 2007;10(1):7-11.

[10] Kumar K, Taylor RS, Jacques L, Eldabe S, Meqlio M, Molet J, et al. Spinal cord stimulation versus conventional medical management for neuropathic pain: a multicenter randomized controlled trial in patients with failed back surgery syndrome. Pain 2007;132(1-2):179-88.

[11] Simon A, Seizeur R, Person H, Forlodou P, Dam Hieu P, Besson G. Anterior lumbar interbody fusion for treatment of failed back surgery syndrome: a retrospective study of 46 cases. Neurochirurgie 2009;55(3):309-13.

[12] Manchikanti L, Singh V, Cash KA, Pampati V. Assessment of effectiveness of percutaneous adhesiolysis and caudal epidural injections in managing post lumbar surgery syndrome: 2-year follow-up of a randomized, controlled trial. J Pain Res 2012;5:597-608.

[13] Schu S, Slotty PJ, Bara G, von Knop M, Edgar D, Vesper J. A prospective, randomized, double-blind, placebo-controlled study to examine the effectiveness of burst spinal cord stimulation patterns for the treatment of failed back surgery syndrome. Neuromodulation 2014 Jun 19. Doi: 10.1111/ner.12197.

[14] Manchikanti L, Singh V, Cash KA, Pampati V, Datta S. Preliminary results of a randomized, equivalence trial of fluroscopic caudal epidural injections in managing chronic low back pain: part 3-post surgery syndrome. Pain Physician 2008;11:817-31.

[15] Manchikanti L, Cash KA, McManus CD, Pampati V, Abdi S. Preliminary results of a randomized, equivalence trial of fluroscopic caudal epidural injections in managing chronic low back pain: part 4-spinal stenosis. Pain Physician 2008;11:833-48.

[16] Manchikanti L, Singh V, Cash KA, Pampati V, Datta S. Management of pain of post lumbar surgery syndrome: one-year results of a randomized, double-blind, active controlled trial of fluroscopic caudal epidural injections. Pain Physician 2010;13(6):509-521.

[17] Iversen T, Solberg TK, Romner B, Wilsgaard T, Twisk J, Anke A, et al. Effect of caudal epidural steroid or saline injection in chronic lumbar radiculopathy: multicenter, blinded, randomized controlled trial. BMJ 2011;343:d5278.

[18] Parr AT, Manchikanti L, Hameed H, Conn A, Manchikanti KN, Benyamin RM, et al. Caudal epidural injection in the management of chronic low back pain: a systematic appraisal of the literature. Pain Physician 2012;15(3):E159-98.

[19] Lond DM, Filtzer DL, BenDebba M, Hendler NH. Clinical features of the failed-back syndrome. J Neurosurg 1988;69(1):61-71.

[20] Thomson S, Jacques L. Demographic characteristics of patients with severe neuropathic pain secondary to failed back surgery syndrome. Pain Pract 2009;9(3):206-15.

[21] Botwin K, Brown LA, Fishman M, Rao S. Fluroscopically guided caudal epidural steroid injections in degenerative lumbar spine stenosis. Pain Physician 2007;10(4):547-8.

[22] Barre L, Lutz GE, Southern D, Cooper G. Fluroscopically guided caudal epidural steroid injections for lumbar spinal stenosis: a retrospective evaluation of long term efficacy. Pain Physician 2004;7(2):187-93.

[23] Anderson SR. A Rationale for the treatment algorithm of failed back surgery syndrome. Curr Rev Pain 2000;4(5):395-406.

[24] Manchikanti L, Falco FJ, Pampati V, Cash KA, Benyamin RM, Hirsh JA. Cost utility analysis of caudal epidural injections in the treatment of lumbar disc herniation, axial or discogenic low back pain, central spinal stenosis, and post lumbar surgery syndrome. Pain Physician 2013;16(3):E129-43.

Submitted: October 29, 2014. *Revised:* December 20, 2014. *Accepted:* January 08, 2015.

In: Pain Management Yearbook 2015
Editor: Joav Merrick
ISBN: 978-1-63484-515-1

Chapter 4

COPING WITH PAIN IN CHILDREN AND ADOLESCENTS WITH MILD TO MODERATE INTELLECTUAL DISABILITIES: OBSERVATIONS IN CLINICAL SETTING

Marc Zabalia*, Corinne Grasménil and Anaïs Saëlen

Laboratoire Psychologie des Actions Langagières et Motrices (EA 4649), Université de Caen Basse-Normandie, Caen, France

Little is known about pain coping strategies in children with mild and moderate intellectual disabilities. Objectives: The aim of this study is to identify coping skills in clinical settings and the health-providers' role in children's coping behaviors. Method: Eighteen medical procedures were video recorded involving fourteen children aged from 8 to 23 years and with 8 years-old mean developmental age. Data were collected with the Pediatric Pain Coping Inventory-French version and the Child-Adult Medical Procedure Interaction Scale-Revised. Pain was rated with the Faces Pain Scale-R. Results: No coping strategies were found in children and adolescents with mild and moderate intellectual disabilities. Health-providers did not encourage any kind of coping behaviors. Nevertheless, they provided information about pain and the running of the event and gave the children an active role in the interview. Conclusions: Further studies are needed to see how this population could be supported by the use of coping to increase their abilities to deal with pain.

Keywords: pain, coping strategies, intellectual disabilities, children, adolescents

---

* Correspondence: Professor Marc Zabalia, Université de Caen Basse-Normandie. CS 14032, F-14032 CAEN cedex 5, France. E-mail : marc.zabalia@unicaen.fr.

INTRODUCTION

There are few investigations about coping skills in people with intellectual disabilities when experiencing pain. This population is excluded from many studies, because somatic disorders, sensory deficits or behavioral problems make them difficult-to-assess patients. Yet people with intellectual disabilities suffer more often from complications and may experience more painful situations than the general population (1). Various types of pain can be experienced, including pain related to medical procedures: injections, surgery, orthosis (2) or related to chronic conditions of intellectual disability: muscle spasms in case of spasticity (3) temporomandibular disorders associated with Down's syndrome that produce headaches, neck and back pain (4). The pain appears to be a common experience in people with intellectual disabilities, but they are also likely to experience different kinds of pain. Limited intellectual potential suggests they will cope differently than expected.

The coping skills are the adjustment, confrontation or adaptation processes to deal with stress or pain. Research about pain coping strategies in children with typical development has highlighted specific strategies. Studies have suggested that there are passive and active ways to cope with pain and that these help people more effectively to deal with pain. Active strategies such as seeking for distraction are considered optimal and most effective to decrease the pain. Passive strategies such as avoidance, catastrophizing or seeking social support are considered less relevant because the person in pain cannot manage directly to cope with the painful phenomenon (5-7). Only one study focused on coping strategies in children and adolescents with intellectual disability. With the French version of the Pediatric Pain and Coping Inventory, PPCI (8) translated by Spicher (9), Zabalia and Duchaux (10) showed that children with intellectual disabilities more frequently use seeking social support strategy to cope with pain. This strategy is not considered as optimal in normal conditions. But in the context of intellectual disability, it is the most likely efficient behavior because these children are not able to manage unassisted. However, the use of this strategy can be unfavorable to the patients because it can be understood as low reactivity to pain rather than as a relevant strategy (11).

To increase our pain management protocols in the population with intellectual disabilities, we need to understand which factors are involved in coping skills. Many studies have assessed the role of age and gender on the coping strategies (12-16). Varni and colleagues (17) have shown that grown-up children seek less social support but they use more cognitive self-instructions. Differences in gender were found in the literature (13-15, 18). During the cold pressor test, women focused on their emotional state while men focused on their sensations. Fearon, McGrath and Achat (19) found evidences in gender differences in pre-school children. In a painful situation, girls cry and are angry while boys try to stay stoic and underreport pain.

Coping strategies are not innate behaviors. They are defined by individual and environmental elements. For example, there are relationships between parental influences and the child coping styles (20). Research has examined how the behavior of sick children could be affected by parental education (21). The results suggest that children are more likely to adopt the role of a sick child if they receive comfort during illness. In another study, parent-child interactions influence children's adjustment to pain during an experimental procedure. Reid, McGrath and Lang (22) and Frank, Blount, Smith and colleagues (23) showed that the presence and the comfort of a parent could hamper the ability of children to cope during a painful medical procedure. Coping may vary as a function of the child's painful experiences. This may be due to the fact that repeated pain generates awareness. But there are also environmental influences on the choice of coping strategies. Experiencing repeated pain can provide opportunities to learn how to develop and test various strategies.

The aim of the study is to better understand the pain coping strategies used by children and adolescents with intellectual disabilities during a painful procedure. First, we expected that children and adolescents with intellectual disabilities would use coping strategies to deal with pain. Secondly, we expected that health-providers would be involved in promoting or inhibiting the coping strategies as a function of the relevancy of their support.

METHODS

Initially, heads of the institutes were contacted by phone. The objective of this initial contact was to briefly introduce the project and the research team. This contact enabled to provide appointment interviews with principals involved in the study in order to deepen the study sets and get their agreement or not to participate in this project. In a second step, a contact was made with professionals able to work with the lab team order to present the study and evaluate with them the feasibility of the project. Thirdly work focuses on more organizational exchanges on the study allowed to work on making contact with families, set the days of presence of the psychologist in charge of study, and how to submit the study to the children and physically organize the room to record pain assessment interviews.

Pain assessments were conducted by health-providers during a painful procedure and were video recorded. Recording was carried out by a psychologist with expertise in the population with intellectual disability during the 2012 year.

An information form recorded the child's characteristics and the reason for consultation, familiarity with the health-provider, painful or anxious state at the time of consultation. The pain coping strategies actualized by the child during the consultation were rated by two independent coders on randomized videos to calculate an index of reliability (Intraclass Correlation Coefficient). The involvement of health-providers and parents in the coping process was assessed with the Child-Adult Medical Procedure Interaction Scale-Revised, CAMPIS-R (24). Health-providers assessed the child's pain using the Faces Pain Scale-R (25).

Inclusion criteria

- Children with intellectual disabilities with a proven diagnosis.
- Children understand and speak French
- Children are able to take part in an interview

Exclusion criteria

- Children do not give their consent to participate in the interview
- During the interview, the children seem uneasy or uncomfortable
- During the interview, the children seem to have difficulty understanding

We hypothesized that children and adolescents with mild and moderate intellectual disability would use strategies to cope with pain in clinical situations. Secondly, we hypothesized that health-providers would influence the choice of pain coping strategies by promoting or by inhibiting it.

Participants

The children population consisted of 14 children and adolescents (9 boys and 5 girls) aged 8-23 years (mean chronological age 16,9 years) with mild to moderate intellectual disabilities (age range between developmental age 1 year and 14 years, mean developmental age : 8 years). All children were able to understand the language, even if they could not express themselves verbally. Some children experienced several pain assessments (for different painful events). We recorded a total of 18 pain assessments.

Assessments were made by 9 health-providers (nurse, medical doctor, physiotherapist, special-need educator). In three cases, the child was accompanied by his mother. All health-providers were well-known to the children.

During the pain assessment interviews, the intensity of the child's pain was assessed by the Faces Pain Scale-Revised. Twelve assessments were done and six assessments could not be carried out due to a visual impairment or misunderstanding of the instructions. The mean pain intensity obtained was 3, 42/10 (n = 12, SD = 3, 96). It was a moderate pain score.

Results

Thirteen PPCI-F questionnaires were completed by the parents of the child. A questionnaire was not accepted in the study due to the lack of response to several questions. The graph below shows the mean factor scores of the types of strategies used by the 13 children with intellectual disability. Factor scores were obtained through standard score tables. Our results show that our sample mainly used the problem solving strategy and seeking social support strategy. On the other side, cognitive self- instructions and research for distraction strategies were used less frequently or not at all (see Figure 1).

Quantitative data analysis

The CAMPIS studies to whom adults are speaking (see Figure 2).

The comparison between the number of Adult to child's verbal expressions and the number of Adult to adult's verbal expressions shows significant difference (chi^2 [1] = 91, 00, $p < 0.001$). The health-provider interacted more with the child than the other adults present at the time of the procedure. The difference is also significant when the category Adult to either adult or child is linked with the category Adult to child (chi^2 [1] = 265.52, $p < 0.001$). The difference is not significant between Adult to Adult and Adult to either adult or child (chi^2 [1] = 0.19, $p > 0.05$).

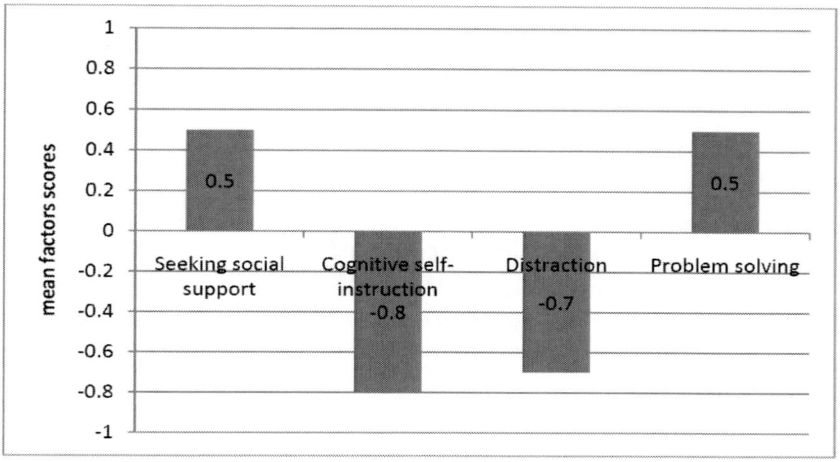

Figure 1. Mean PPCI-F factors scores in children with mild and moderate intellectual disabilities.

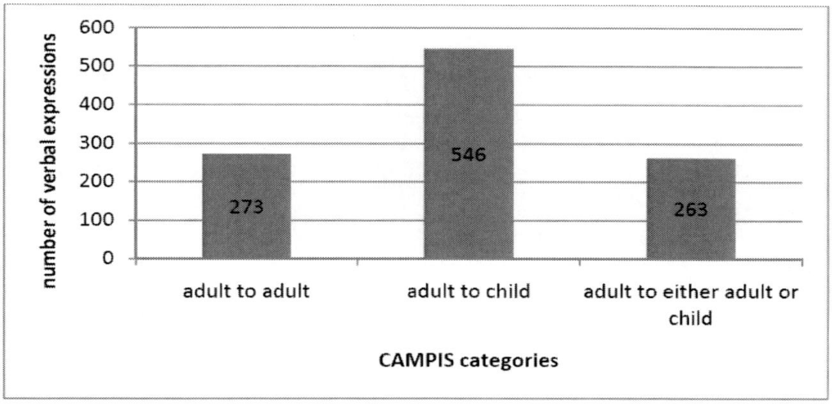

Figure 2. Number of healthcare-providers' verbal expressions.

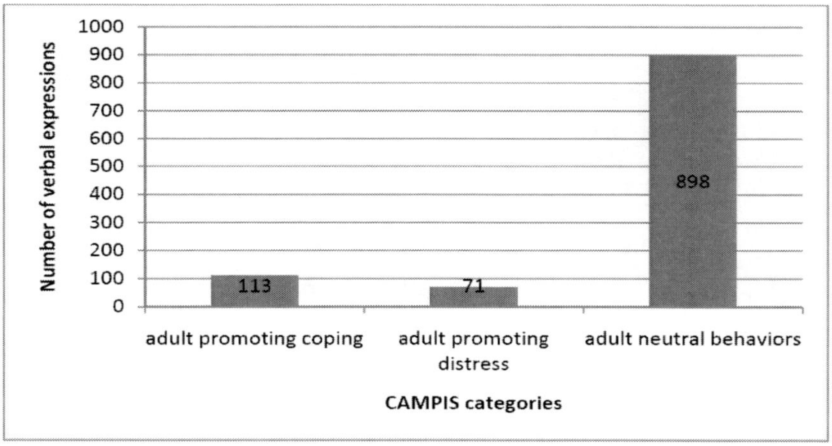

Figure 3. Categories of healthcare-providers' behaviors.

Regarding the types of verbal expressions used by adults (adult promoting coping; adult promoting distress; adult neutral behaviors) neutral verbal expressions were mainly used (Figure 3). There was a significant difference (chi^2 [1] = 609.52, $p < 0.001$) between adult promoting coping and adult neutral behaviors, between adult promoting distress and adult neutral behaviors as well (chi^2 [1] = 705.81, $p < 0.001$). There was a significant difference between verbal expressions of adults encouraging the use of coping strategies and verbal expressions resulting in the distress in children (chi^2 [1] = 9, 59, $p < 0.01$). Overall, what the healthcare-provider says to the child (in the category adult neutral behaviors) covers topics on the child's health and medical procedure. The three items with the majority of verbal expressions are "Child's general conditions related talk" (203 items), "Procedure-related talk to adults" (202 items) and "Checking child's status" (169 items). Verbal expressions promoting pain coping strategies (adult promoting coping) expressed mainly distraction and humor.

The CAMPIS scale examines the verbal expressions used by children and puts them in three categories: child neutral behaviors, child distress behaviors and child coping behaviors (Figure 4). The data indicate that children primarily use neutral behaviors compared to the other two categories. The difference is significant between child neutral behaviors and child coping behaviors (chi^2 [1] = 44.480, $p < 0.001$). The difference is also significant between child neutral behaviors and child distress behavior (chi^2 [1] = 65,504, $p < 0.001$). Coping behaviors and distress behaviors were used similarly, there was no significant difference (chi^2 [1] = 2.456, $p > 0.05$). As for the healthcare-provider's words, we observed more expressions of the child on his medical condition "Child's general conditions related talk" (109 items) and "Child Informs about status" (78 items).

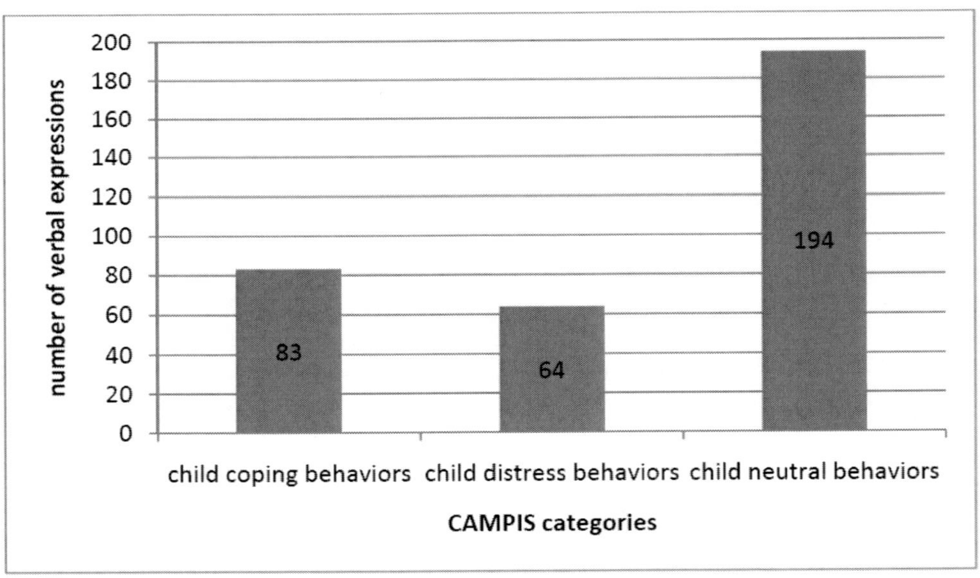

Figure 4. Categories of child's behaviors.

Qualitative data analysis

The analysis of the health-providers' verbal expressions shows that one of the two most recorded item is "Child's general conditions related talk" (18, 76%). This item includes comments and questions about the child's health. For example, the health-provider asks the child if he has recently seen his physician, if medication was prescribed or if the parents give him his medication, he also asks about the diet of the child and or the quality of sleep. Health-providers seek information on health and pain ("will they redo infiltration?").

The second frequent item is "Procedure-related talk to adults" (18, 67%), which includes comments relating to the child's health or medical procedures addressed to other adults present during the procedure ("yeah because he is on morphine anyway!"). The item "checking child's status" (15,62%) is also often picked up ("it hurts or not?"). Verbal expressions "Notice of procedure to come" announcing the upcoming medical procedure (8,5%) are also present ("I'll make you a little dressing, do you agree ?"). The other items observed are "Demands to engage in procedural activity" (6, 93%) which includes verbal expressions directed at the child asking him/her to engage in an activity related to the medical procedure. Items "humor directed to child" (3, 6%) and "non-procedure related talk to child" (6, 56%) are those which include verbal expressions promoting distraction.

The health-provider talks significantly more about the child's pain management (27%). He explains what he will doing "we can put a band with an alcohol pad"; "Don't move, I'll stick to you, okay?"). Consolation (21%) consists mainly of distraction ("so, what did you do yesterday?"). For assessing the pain itself (18%), the health-provider asks the child ("do you hurt anywhere?)"). During the assessment, he checks several times if the child is ill. The adults also assess the pain intensity with the Faces Pain Scale. Pain location is located (18%) as "ah in the throat, yesterday was already the throat that hurts you." The cause of pain (11%) is less understood. Statements and expressions accompanying pain (4%) are poorly addressed ("Were you surprised?" "Were you scared?")

In the children's speech, the verbal expressions more frequently used belonged to the item "Child's general conditions related talk" (31, 96%). The child spoke of his current or previous health state "Because sometimes it hurts when I sit." The item "Child informs about status" (22, 87%) combines verbal expressions informing the state during the evaluation of the child such as "this is always the way my thigh still hurts "or "I feel nothing." The item "nonprocedural -related talk by the child" (19, 06%) includes verbal expressions referring to various topics unrelated to pain assessment and medical procedures. Children sometimes use humor (4, 99%). Behavioral distraction techniques are unfrequently used. Children verbalize their pain (3, 23%) "It burns me" and sometimes seek information about the medical procedure (3, 52%) ("Do we put a dressing?"). Only one child cried during the whole pain interview.

DISCUSSION

Results show that parents of children with intellectual disabilities know the strategies their child uses to cope with pain. Children seem to be able to use these strategies when in painful situations. Scores of PPCI-F show that children use mainly seeking social support and problem solving. Our results are in agreement with our previous works (10, 26, 27). According to parents, children use coping strategies when they are painful. Indeed, we observed few strategies that could be identified. We can assume that adults overestimate the capacities of children with developmental disabilities.

Whatever their cognitive level, children showed few strategies during the interviews although the intensity of the pain was moderate. The regulation capacities of children did not seem modified by stress. Children having access to verbal communication showed capacities s to verbalize their pain. These children were also able to comment about their health state and not only the pain. For example, they could speak about their medication. In addition, children who could communicate seemed could use the Faces Pain Scale-Revised. Other studies have shown that children with developmental disabilities can express and locate their pain (28) and assess it with a simple tool (29, 30).

We expected that adults would show behaviors promoting pain coping strategies in children. But our data show that adults do not explicitly promote pain coping strategies in children, helping them to cope with pain and stress except for some non-procedural related speech. It is difficult to assess the precise impact of health-providers on the child's behavior. Many studies highlight the impact of adults' behaviors on the level of pain perception in the child with typical development. Reid, McGrath and Lang (22) show the importance of parents' support to help their child to cope with chronic pain. As Blount and colleagues (31) had shown in a context of acute pain, Reid and colleagues (7) showed that behaviors such as discouragement and excuses produce a loss of capacity on pain coping in children. With encouragements and distraction the child will mobilize the skills he has to cope with pain. Our data show that the health-providers do not encourage the use of pain coping strategies in children. Yet, adults spontaneously use distraction and incentives to enhance pain coping strategies in young normal children in a kindergarten (32).

Nevertheless, the adults provide information to the child and consider him as a partner. Health-providers give information about the pain and the procedure. Spafford, von Baeyer and Hicks (33) studied the effect of the information provided by the parents on the level of the child's pain. Providing information about the event that will occur resulted in a decrease in the pain intensity assessed by the child. In our study, adults do not show explicit behavior to promote pain coping strategies, but they provide information. In addition, health-providers involved the child during the consultation. They communicated with the children with intellectual disability according to their language skills. The adult speaks primarily to the child and not with the other adults who are present during the consultation. The child seems to be considered able to express his pain and to talk about his health state. He is considered as a full partner. It is only very recently that children are involved during the medical consultation (34), this does not seem to be the case for adults with intellectual disabilities who are not considered capable of speaking by themselves. According to a study, general practitioners usually ask their educator about their health and their symptoms, and do not tell the patient of the upcoming medical procedure (35). In our study, health-providers identify the pain, ask about the intensity and location and explain the upcoming medical care. Garth, Murphy and Reddihough (36) also showed that children with cerebral palsy could be involved in consultation.

In seeking information and providing explanations, the adults can better understand the child's pain. While the literature shows the beneficial effect of distraction on pain intensity and coping skills (31, 37), we observed very little of these behaviors in our study.

CONCLUSION

Some time back, professionals doubted about the existence of pain perception in people with intellectual disabilities compared to the general population. Today, it is recognized that they feel pain but we still do not know how they can deal with the pain and how we can support them and help them to cope. Our results show that the child does not always mobilize the coping strategies when he immediately experiences pain. Contrary to the observations in the general population, the adult does not systematically support the use of coping strategies. However, the integration and involvement of the child in the consultation appears to promote better pain management by providing elements of understanding and by helping the child to anticipate the painful event.

ACKNOWLEDGMENTS

Authors would like to acknowledge the Dr Chantal Wood for her help to improve the quality of English language. This work was supported by the Fondation de France under Grant ENG 15188. Authors have no conflict of interest.

REFERENCES

[1] McGrath PJ, Rosmus C, Camfield C, Campbell MA, Hennigar A. Behaviours caregivers use to determine pain in non-verbal, cognitively impaired individuals. Dev Med Child Neurol 1998;40:340-3.

[2] Breau LM, McGrath PJ, Camfield C, Rosmus C, Finley GA. Preliminary validation of an observational pain checklist for persons with cognitive impairments and inability to communicate verbally. Dev Med Child Neurol 2000;42:609-16.

[3] Hunt A, Burne R. Medical and nursing problems of children with neurodegenerative disease. Palliat Med 1995;9:19-26.

[4] Hennequin M, Faulks D, Roux D. Accuracy of estimation of dental treatment need in special care patients. J Dent 2000;28:131-6.

[5] Bennett-Branson SM, Craig KD. Postoperative pain in children: Developmental and family influences on spontaneous coping strategies. Can J Behav Sci 1993;25:355-83.

[6] Piira T, Hayes B, Goodenough B, von Baeyer CL. Effects of attentional direction, age, and coping style on cold-pressor pain in children. Behav Res Ther 2006;44:835-848.

[7] Reid GJ, Lang BA, McGrath PJ. Primary juvenile fibromyalgia: Psychological adjustment, family functioning, coping and functional disability. Arthritis Rheum 1996;40:752-60.

[8] Varni JW, Seid M, Kurtin PS. PedsQL 4.0: reliability and validity of the Pediatric Quality of Life Inventory version 4.0 generic core scales in healthy and patient populations. Med Care 2001;39:800-12.

[9] Spicher P. Traduction francophone et validation du Pediatric Pain Coping Inventory (PPCIF). Douleur Analg 2003;16(1):3-14.

[10] Zabalia M, Duchaux C. Stratégies de faire-face à la douleur chez des enfants porteurs de d?ficience intellectuelle. Revue Francophone De La Defic Intellect 2006;17:53-64. [French]
[11] Hunt A, Mastroyannopoulou K, Goldman A, Seers K. Not knowing-the problem of pain in children with severe neurological impairment. Int J Nurs Stud 2003;40:171-83.
[12] Unruh AM, Ritchie J, Merskey H. Does gender affect appraisal of pain and pain coping strategies? Clin J Pain 1999;15:31-40.
[13] Sallfors C, Hallber LR, Fasth A. Gender and age differences in pain, coping and health status among children with chronic arthritis. Clin Exp Rheumatol 2003;21:785-93.
[14] Keogh E, Herdenfeldt M. Gender, coping and the perception of pain. Pain 2002;9:195-201.
[15] Hodgins MJ, Lander J. Children's coping with venipuncture. J Pain Sympt Manage 1997;3:274-85.
[16] Bursztein C, Steinberg T, Sadeh A. Sleep, sleepiness, and behavior problems in children with headache. J Child Neurol 2006;21:1012-9.
[17] Varni JW, Rapoff MA, Waldron SA, Gragg RA, Bernstein BH, Lindsley CB. Effects of perceived stress on pediatric chronic pain. J Behav Med 1996;19:515-28.
[18] Keefe FJ, Lefebvre JC, Egert JR, Affleck G, Sullivan MJ, Caldwell DS. The relationship of gender to pain, pain behavior, and disability in osteoarthritis patients: the role of catastrophizing. Pain 2000;87:325-34.
[19] Fearon I, McGrath PJ, Achat H. 'Booboos': the study of everyday pain among young children. Pain 1996;68:55-62.
[20] Sweet SD, McGrat, PJ, Symons D. The roles of child reactivity and parenting context in infant pain response. Pain 1999;80:655-61.
[21] Walker LS, Zeman, JL. Parental response to child illness behavior. J Pediatr Psychol 1992;17:49-71.
[22] Reid GJ, McGrath PJ, Lang BA. Parent-child interactions among children with juvenile fibromyalgia, arthritis, and healthy controls. Pain 2005;113:201-10.
[23] Frank NC, Blount RL, Smith AJ, Manimala MR, Martin JK. Parent and staff behavior, previous child medical experience, and maternal anxiety as they relate to child procedural distress and coping. J Pediatr Psychol 1995;20:277-89.
[24] Blount RL, Cohen LL, Franck NC, Bachanas PJ, Smith AJ, Manimala MR, et al. The child-adult medical procedure interaction scale-revised : An assessment of validity. J Pediatr Psychol 1997;22(1):73-88.
[25] Hicks CL, von Baeyer CL, Spafford PA, Van KI, Goodenough B. The Faces Pain Scale - Revised: toward a common metric in pediatric pain measurement. Pain 2001;93:173-83.
[26] Zabalia M, Breau LM, Burkitt CC, Boinet E, Gauché C. Stratégies de faire face à la douleur chez des adolescents atteints de déficience intellectuelle. Douleurs 2010;11:165-70. [French]
[27] Burkitt C, Breau LM, Zabalia M. Parental assessment of pain coping in individuals with intellectual and developmental disabilities. Res Dev Disabil 2011;32(5):1564-71.
[28] Fanurik D, Koh JL, Harrison RD, Conrad TM, Tomerlin C. Pain assessment in children with cognitive impairment. An exploration of self-report skills. Clin Nurs Res 1998;7:103–19.
[29] Benini F, Trapanotto M, Gobber D, Agosto C, Carli G, Drigo P, et al. Evaluating pain induced by venipuncture in pediatric patients with developmental delay. Clin J Pain 2004;20:156-63.
[30] Zabalia M, Corfec S. Reconnaissance des émotions et évaluation de la douleur chez des enfants et adolescents porteurs de Trisomie 21. Enfance 2008;60(4):357-69. [French]
[31] Blount RL, Corbin SM, Sturges JW, Wolfe VV, Prater JM. James LD. The relationship between adults' behaviour and child coping and distress during BMA/LP procedures: a sequential analysis. Behav Ther 1989;20:585-601.
[32] Zabalia M, Martel K, Dykstra F. Exprimer la douleur: analyses qualitatives d'interaction adulte/enfant au sein d'une créche. Douleur Analg 2010;23:233-8. [French]
[33] Spafford P, von Baeyer CL, Hicks CL. Expected and reported pain in children undergoing ear piercing: A randomized trial of preparation by parents. Behav Res Ther 2002;40:253-66.
[34] Tates K, Elbers E, Meeuwese L, Bensing J. Doctor-parent-child relationships: a "pas de trios." Patient Educ Couns 2002;48:5-14.

[35] Wullink M, Veldhuijzen W, Van Schrojenstein Lantman - de Valk, HMJ, Metsemakers JFM, Dinant GJ. Doctor-patient communication with people with intellectual disability - a qualitative study. BMC Fam Pract 2009;10(82):1-10.

[36] Garth B, Murphy GC, Reddihough DS. Perceptions of participation: child patients with a disability in the doctor-parent-child partnership. Patient Educ Couns 2009;74:45-52.

[37] McMurtry CM, Chambers CT, McGrath PJ, Asp E. When "don't worry" communicates fear: Children's perceptions of parental reassurance and distraction during a painful pediatric medical procedure. Pain 2010;150:52-8.

Submitted: November 26, 2014. *Revised:* December 27, 2014. *Accepted:* January 08, 2015.

In: Pain Management Yearbook 2015
Editor: Joav Merrick

ISBN: 978-1-63484-515-1

Chapter 5

PERCEPTUAL MINDFULNESS AND IMAGERY FOR CHRONIC PAIN AND SKIN DISORDERS IN A BUSY COLLEGE POPULATION

Felice L Bedford**, PhD
Department of Psychology,
University of Arizona, Tucson, Arizona, US

Perceptually-oriented training, consisting of an abbreviated "body scanning" exercise of mindfulness along with visual imagery, was assessed for its benefit to chronic conditions in a busy population. While mindfulness interventions are a promising non-invasive psychological approach for managing pain and other conditions, they require a big time commitment from patients. This can decrease compliance and therefore effectiveness. The experiment also sought to assess whether individual differences in imagery ability influence effectiveness and to contribute to the development of paradigms in mindfulness research from t unique perspective of the field of Perception. A brief course of 12-minute training was developed and given to college students with mostly chronic pain or skin conditions of 3 weeks to 18 years duration (mean=6.8 years). Matched subjects without the intervention served as a wait-list control group. Dependent measures consisted of change in participant ratings on symptom severity (semi-objective measure), assessments of the value of the intervention (subjective measure) and independent ratings of photos (objective measure). Results included high ratings for training satisfaction, ease, and compliance, a positive relation between imagery ability and improvement, and a difference between experimental and control groups in severity of symptoms for high visualizers only. Interestingly, high imagers in the control group may have shown worsening of symptoms.

In conclusion, brief training is effective in high imagers, and the audio training file can be easily distributed to patients. A novel innovative theory for "mind-body" healing based on perceptual adaptation to vision-immune system conflicts is offered.

* Correspondence: Felice Bedford, PhD, Department of Psychology, University of Arizona, PO Box 210068, Tucson, AZ 85721, United States. E-mail: bedford@u.arizona.edu.

Keywords: psychoneuroimmunology mindfulness, meditation, visual imagery, guided imagery, prism adaptation, perception, perceptual adaptation, cross-modal conflict, pain, skin disorder

INTRODUCTION

Perception psychologists are infrequent contributors to the field of psychoneuroimmunology. However, common alternative treatments in medicine for pain and other chronic conditions are inherently perceptual in nature (1). The purpose of the present study was to investigate a combination of two especially perceptual interventions, the "body scanning" exercise of mindful meditation along with imagery, also frequently used in mindfulness practice for healing and well-being (2–4).

In body scanning, the practicer closes her eyes and focuses attention on successive parts of the body feeling for the precise sensations (5). The application of attention is relentless in that any mind-wandering is repeatedly guided back to the body. This exercise suggests a role for perception generally and "body schema" specifically. Attention is indispensible to the act of perception. Attention controls the sensory input – what gets in and what does not (6). Without sensory input, perception of the world cannot occur. The consequences of such arguably unnaturally enhanced and sustained attention of mindfulness meditation, however, has not been investigated in the field perception. Body schema has also long been a concept in the field of perception (7). Proprioceptors in the joints and muscles relay positional information enabling the construction of the body envelope without the use of vision; thermoreceptors, nocioreceptors and mechanoreceptors in the skin add additional sensations.

Guided imagery as medical treatment has its roots in clinical therapies, yet visual imagery has a rich history in the field of perception and its use in medical interventions can benefit from such accumulated knowledge. For instance, images conjured in the mind have been shown to stimulate the same brain hardware as real vision (8); this suggests imagined vision can substitute for real vision, if needed. In addition, ability to from visual images has been found to vary markedly across individuals (9, 10) and may therefore contribute to individual differences in the effectiveness of mindfulness treatment.

The purpose of the present experiment was to test a short course of mindfulness training for its effectiveness on managing chronic illness that would be of sufficient ease and brevity to appeal both to patients and to scientists. By extracting and concentrating the perceptual components of mindfulness, we seek to streamline what would otherwise be a major undertaking for a patient on the order of months or even years for thorough meditation study. College students were selected as a population that has little tolerance for extra chores in an already busy schedule. Pain was targeted as an object of treatment because our piloting revealed it to be a frequent complaint among students, especially women, in an otherwise healthy population. A second purpose was to contribute to the development of paradigms in mindfulness-related research (11) especially from the perspective of the field of perception. Therefore, chronic skin problems were also selected as an object of treatment to be amenable to photographs for the development of non-invasive objective measures of training effectiveness. Finally, imagery ability was assessed to determine its effect on outcomes.

Methods

A total of 47 undergraduate college students (mean age 19.8 years) were enrolled with chronic ailments. The two largest subgroups were comprised of pain (migraine headaches, tension type headaches, injury related, arm, knee, herniated lumbar disk, other back, abdominal, endometriosis, arthritis; neck pain, unknown) and skin disorders (dermatitis, warts, acne, psoriasis, unspecified rash, involving hands, arms, and/or face).

Table 1 shows details of the population from which participants were recruited. Notable is the high number of students with frequent headaches, twice as high for woman, and likewise, the high incidence of Type A personality which is a known risk factor for subsequent disease. Duration of condition ranged from 3 weeks to 18 years with a mean of 6.8 years.

Intervention

A 12-minute audio file was created consisting of half body-scanning and half imagery. The body scan exercise was adapted from Jon Kabat-Zinn's (5) mindfulness meditation program, except that it lasted 6 minutes rather than 45 minutes and was performed seated rather than supine. A participant's attention was first directed to the left foot with instructions to feel the sensations, followed by such mindfulness on successive parts of the body ascending to the head. Following a few seconds of imagined breathing of fresh air in and stale air out, instructions were given to the participant to feel the body heavily against the chair, which provided the transition to imagery for the second half of the training. The imagery was compiled from a variety of exercises in use (12–15) including our own and included mentally going to a favorite place, experiencing the surroundings, looking at the affected part through a magnifying glass, seeing the ailment under attack, and visualizing full healing.

The initial training took place in the lab in a one-on-one session with each participant. Participants were then instructed to practice subsequent sessions at home either with or without the provided audio file guidance and to be documented in a log over a 3-week period at least 8 more times for at least 10 minutes each time, for a total of approximately 90 cumulative minutes.

Table 1. Percent of students responding "True" on the Screening Questionnaire

		Skin hands/arms	Skin face	Headache frequent	Pain chronic	AI	Sinus frequent	Chronic any	Interest in training?	Type B personality	Type A personality
Female	604	9.4	22.2	39.1	8.8	1.8	19.7	17.7	40.2	65.6	46.2
Male	385	5.5	26.8	15.6	7.0	0.8	17.7	16.1	38.7	70.4	39.5

Procedure

Participants were assigned alternately within condition (pain, skin, other) and gender to either an experimental group with the mindfulness intervention or a "wait-list" control with just the passage of time (and the hope of future intervention). Participants in both groups were asked 14 questions about the condition and stress including severity of symptoms right now on a scale from 1 ("completely normal") to 25 ("as bad as I've ever had it"). A photo was taken for those with skin conditions. We expected that individual difference in imagery ability (9) might affect the effectiveness of an imagery-heavy intervention (See also 16). Consequently, experimental group participants were asked at the end of the first training session for a rating of the vividness of their immediately preceding images ranging from 1, "couldn't see anything," to 10, "like it was really there." Participants of both groups returned in 3 weeks to retake the questionnaire, answer a question concerning general imagery ability, and have another photo taken, if applicable. Experimental group participants were also asked questions about their experience: Did they think others would be able to engage in this practice and to rate (on a 10-point scale) how easy it was to follow the instructions, to get themselves to actually practice, if it had benefit for improving their specific chronic- illness symptoms they were working on, had benefit for other symptoms, had benefit for reducing stress, and two additional questions on visual imagery during the home sessions.

Photographs

Following the experiment proper, 51 independent observers rated pairs of photos for severity. They were blind to whether each photograph was from pretest (appearing on the left half the time) or posttest, whether from experimental or control group, or the purpose of the photo judging. Mean of all observer ratings was used for each photo and the difference between mean pretest and posttest severity ratings for each photo served as a measure of "photo improvement" or "photo decline."

RESULTS

Nearly all experimental-group participants (95.8%) thought that others would be able to engage in the training and gave relatively high ratings on a 10-point scale for ability to follow the instructions (8.0) and get themselves to practice (7.2). Remarkably, they also almost all (92%) reported at least a tiny subjective benefit on their specific symptoms they were working on (rating of 2 or higher) although interestingly, rated the benefit for other things, usually stress, higher than for their specific symptoms (mean=8.0 on stress vs. 4.8 on specific symptoms, $t(23)=7.54$, $p<.001$). Also notable was a finding of higher ratings for strength of "vivid imagery generally during the technique" (7.9) compared to specifically being able to "visualize the ailment completely healed" (5.8), a significant difference ($t(23)=4.51, p<.001$). Conclusions were not altered by separate consideration of pain and skin subgroups; these were equal on rating for visualizing the condition completely healed and higher for pain than skin subgroup on rating for benefit to specific symptoms at 6.0 (pain) vs. 4.0 (skin condition).

Compliance

Three participants from the experimental group and 2 participants from the control group did not return for the follow-up appointment; all 5 were those with scheduled returns for the last week of the semester.

Experimental group, imagery ability and pre-post-test change on symptom severity
There was a substantial correlation between the imagery vividness rating taken during the very first training session and the change in the pretest to posttest severity rating of symptoms after the 3 weeks of training (r (22)= -.43, p<.05, Pearson's product-moment correlation, 2-tailed test). See Figure 1. Change in self-report of symptoms (the rating of how bad symptoms are right now on a scale from 1 to 25) is a semi-objective dependent measure despite being self-reported because of the delay between tests and the presence of other questions. That is, posttest response is largely independent of pretest response because it is unlikely subjects remembered the exact score they gave previously. Thus, participants with the most vivid visual imagery showed the greatest improvement in severity of symptoms. Note improvement is reflected by a lowering of severity rating score. The correlation appeared both in women (-.42, n=16) and men (-.52, n=8) and for both skin conditions (-.62, n=10) and pain (-.46, n=9). There is no evidence the result is an artifact of outliers, of averaging men and women, or of participants rating everything highly.

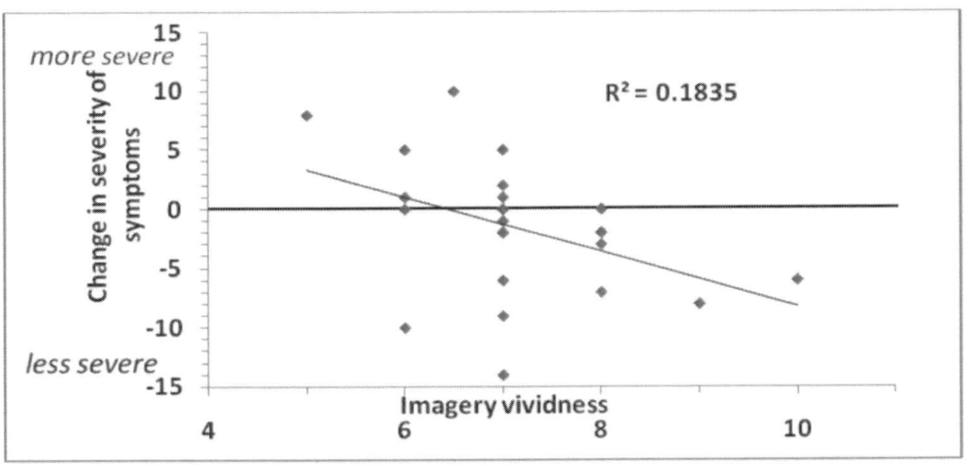

Figure 1. Participants' imagery ability from the very first training session predicts who will improve from the brief mindfulness intervention.

Experimental group vs. control group
A split sample of the top half visualizers from the experimental group and from the control group revealed a difference in the change between pretest and posttest-rated severity of symptoms between the two groups (Figure 2) of 18.2% with improvement in the former and worsening in the latter. The difference did not quite reach significance (t(19) = 2.0, p=.06, two-tailed) with the small sample size. For the entire sample including the bottom visualizers,

a difference between experimental and control groups was not found (Δ=1.2%) with both groups showing a small improvement (5.2%, 4.0% respectively) from pretest to posttest.

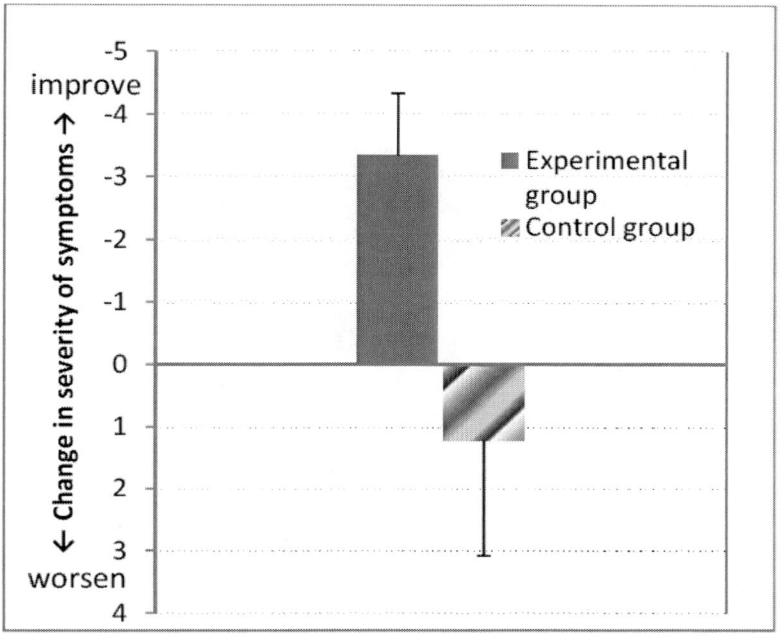

Figure 2. Symptom change in the mindfulness intervention (experimental group) and the waiting non-intervention (control group) in the top half of visualizers.

Control group, imagery ability and pre-post-test change on symptom severity
In the control group, the relation between imagery ability (as measured by the posttest rating on ability to form visual images) and changes in severity was in the opposite direction ($r(16) = +.462$, $p<.05$). This result tentatively suggests that natural spontaneous images without training in high imagers may help sustain chronic conditions.

Gender

Women showed a trend for greater improvement in both the experimental group (mean change for women, -2.0; men -1.0) and the control group (women, -1.3; men +0.3). Note that lower severity scores reflect greater improvement.

Photographs

A total of only 12 pairs of photos in the experimental group and 5 pairs in the control group limited analyses. In the experimental group, there was a trend towards a positive relation between photo improvement and imagery ability ($r(10)=.43$) and between photo improvement and reduction in stress ($r(10)=.49$, $p\approx.10$). That is: 1) the higher the vividness of imagery in participants, the greater the improvement in skin condition as rated by outside observers and 2) the more stress was reduced in participants by posttest, the greater the improvement in visible skin condition. Considered across both experimental and control groups, the correlation between photo improvement and stress is statistically significant ($r(15)=.52, p<.02$), and may reflect that stress, well known to affect skin conditions, is a predictor of improvement that is independent of the effect of an imagery/body scan intervention. See Figure 3 for photos of pre-post change in two of the experimental group participants; anecdotally one of these participants remarked that she tried everything for warts and this was the first thing that helped. Photographic evidence of change is a promising objective outcome measure for the intervention when conditions have visible components (see also (4)).

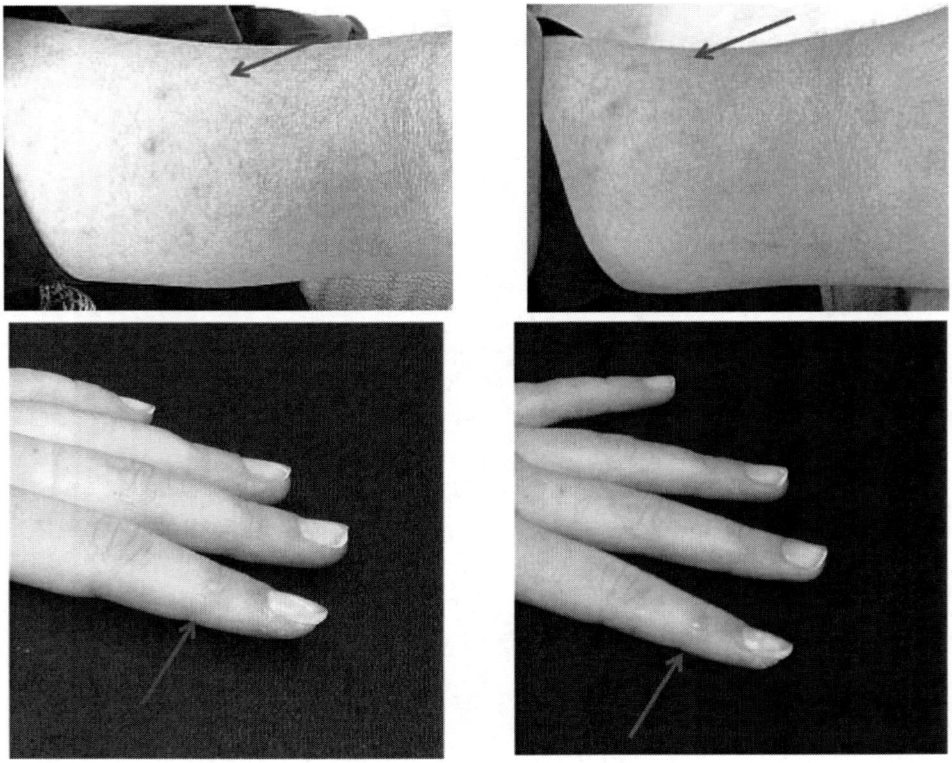

Figure 3. Photos before (pretest) and after (posttest) the mindfulness intervention in two participants. Visible changes after only three weeks are subtle. Participant's self-assessment of improvement may precede changes visible to outside observers. Top: Pretest is on the left. Bottom: Pretest is on the right.

Discussion

The experiment was successful in implementing a streamlined mindfulness paradigm for mind-body healing that ordinary busy people can engage in and find satisfying. The vast majority of participants subjectively felt this training was of some benefit, especially for stress. This is a notable result because of high patient dissatisfaction with conventional treatments for chronic pain and other conditions.

The experiment also found that people able to form vivid visual images during training had a reduction in severity of symptoms (less pain and/or reduced skin abnormality) as measured by a more objective test, despite not much more than an hour and a half of cumulative practice. Participants without strong imagery, however, did not show this improvement. The relation between vividness of imagery and improvement is consistent with the literature, in which a relation between the two was reported for warts (16) and for immune system activation in breast cancer patients (12). The present study extends those findings to other skin conditions and to pain. Additionally, the study finds the imagery-healing relation with just a single-item imagery vividness assessment administered at the outset of training and with minimal mindfulness training for healing. This suggests that a brief prescreening imagery test is both feasible and of value to identify individuals who would most benefit from an abbreviated 90-minute cumulative course of training of the sort used in this experiment. Individuals scoring low in imagery ability might instead require longer periods of training to achieve measurable symptom reduction or require greater assistance with forming images.

Few psychological theories exist for how and why mindfulness training works to promote physical healing. Recently, I put forth an innovative new theory from the perspective of the field of perception in the theoretical journal Psychological Bulletin (1, 17). According to the theory, mind-body healing is merely an example of the very common perceptual adaptation that occurs following conflict between sensory modalities. Such cross-modal perceptual adaptation has been extensively researched in the perception literature; for example, in the phenomenon known as prism adaptation (or spatial adaptation), the sensory modalities of vision and proprioception are made to conflict with one another and the result is a change in one modality or the other (18–20). As applied to mindfulness and healing, the theory builds on the claim that the immune system is another sensory modality, like vision or proprioception (17, 21, 22). A visual image then of one's self fully healed and healthy, along with an immune system that has erroneously detected an antigen, would reflect a conflict between perceptual modalities. As with prism adaptation, mindfulness creates a conflict between sensory systems, except in this context, according to Bedford's theory, there is a conflict between vision and the immune system organ rather than between vision and proprioception. As with prism adaptation, a conflict suggests an error and one of the modalities must change.

In the present experiment, the cross-modal conflict purported to occur is brought about by the training in which the visual images generated by the participant indicate that a bodily region of interest is fully healed and healthy while the immune system modality continues to detect that something is wrong. Acquired immunity is involved in many skin diseases and in both inflammatory and neuropathic pain (23). (In pain, for instance, opoid brain receptors are also found in the immune system whilepain modulating endorphins, i.e., neuropeptides produced in the brain, are also produced by the immune system.) As in prism adaptation, a conflict between modalities leads to change because it is indicative of an error in perceptual systems. One or the other modality must change to remove the error, which also brings the modalities back in agreement (24). When that required change occurs to the immune system, the mindfulness intervention will be judged successful. While such a change may still seem to some to reflect an attainment of an extraordinary "mind-body connection," it is instead ordinary adaptation between sensory systems. The chemical messengers of the immune organ (cytokines) and of the nervous system (neurotransmitters) were once thought separate but have been shown to be shared (21, 25). The shared ligands can provide the physical mechanism for instantiating the conflict-induced change proposed by the theory.

Note that this process will only be successful to the extent the participant is able to generate the images of health to conflict with the immune system. Consistent with this is the finding that only high imagers in the group that received training appeared successful, as well as the finding that participants who received training scored lower on ratings of ease of visualizing the medical condition fully healed compared to forming other kinds of visual images (such as of their favorite place). It may not be easy to visualize the counterfactual, which is precisely what is required for effective change. Additionally, among high imagers that did not receive the training, there was an apparent worsening of symptoms. Without the guidance to form images of healing, natural spontaneous imagery may be doing exactly the opposite. If images that conflict with the immune system can make symptoms better than we would expect that images consistent with a chronic illness should make things worse. High visual imagers may be contributing to the chronicity of their symptoms by reinforcing through imagery a problem that may not even still exist.

Attention as well as imagery is critical for success. The unnaturally sustained and focus attention of mindfulness is important in order to strengthen and modulate which modality will change in the conflict. In prism adaptation, it has been shown that attention to one modality - e.g., through manipulating when the hand is visible (19) - leads to changes in the other modality. In addition, increasing the signal to a modality - e.g., through arm vibration (26) - increases the amount of adaptation. Thus, immune system change will be more likely with a strong and attentive signal of vision (and perhaps felt body position), the other modalityin the immune-vision conflict. Mindfulness can provide this attentional boost.

The procedure of the intervention in the present experiment is to some extent guilty of throwing everything at the wall to see what sticks. It lumped together body scanning and imagery and used several types of imagery. Its purpose was to extract the notably perceptual components of mindfulness in attempt to streamline mindfulness training for pain and other chronic conditions in a busy population with little patience for months of difficult practice. Refinements of the types of images trained, as well as assessing separate contributions of body scanning and imagery, should now be possible. One intriguing avenue of pursuit concerns the nature of images that are useful for pain. While it is sensible to visualize a red rash faded to the color and texture of normal skin, what does one, and what should one, visualize for the absence of pain? An advantage of visual imagery over actual vision is its ability to conjure things that do not exist.

The present experiment can hopefully serve as a launch of a new approach to mindfulness-based interventions for illness and well-being: We are calling this *perceptual repair*. At present, the 12-minute audio training can be easily distributed by practitioners to patients electronically or in the office.

ACKNOWLEDGMENTS

Thanks to Whitney McNeil, Sabrina Peterson, and Benjamin Travis for assisting with data collection. This work was supported by a mini grant from SBSRI (Social and Behavioral

Research Institute) at the University of Arizona. Audio file of the intervention is available from the author.

REFERENCES

[1] Bedford FL. A perception theory in mind-body medicine: guided imagery and mindful meditation as cross-modal adaptation. Psychol Bull Rev 2012;19(1):24–45.
[2] Miller GE, Cohen S. Psychological interventions and the immune system: a meta-analytic review and critique. Health Psychol 2001;20(1):47–63.
[3] Elomaa MM, de C. Williams AC, Kalso EA. Attention management as a treatment for chronic pain. Eur J Pain 2009;13(10):1062–7.
[4] Kabat-Zinn J, Wheeler E, Light T, Skillings A, Scharf MJ, Cropley TG, et al. Influence of a mindfulness meditation-based stress reduction intervention on rates of skin clearing in patients with moderate to severe psoriasis undergoing phototherapy (UVB) and photochemotherapy (PUVA). Psychosom Med 1998;60(5):625–32.
[5] Kabat-Zinn J. Full catastrophe living: Using the wisdom of your body and mind to face stress, pain, and illness, Fifteenth anniversary Edition. New York: Random House, 2005.
[6] Posner MI. Orienting of attention. Q J Exp Psychol 1980;32(1):3–25.
[7] Head H, Holmes HG. Sensory disturbances from cerebral lesions. Brain 1911-1912;34:102–254.
[8] Farah MJ. Is visual imagery really visual? Overlooked evidence from neuropsychology. Psychol Rev 1988;95(3):307–17.
[9] Marks DF. Visual imagery differences in the recall of pictures. Br J Psychol 1973;64(1):17–24.
[10] Marks DF. New directions for mental imagery research. J Ment Imag 1995;19(3-4):153–67.
[11] Baer RA. Mindfulness training as a clinical intervention: A conceptual and empirical review. Clin Psychol Sci Pract 2003;10(2):125–43.
[12] Eremin O, Walker MB, Simpson E, Heys SD, Ah-See AK, Hutcheon AW, et al. Immuno-modulatory effects of relaxation training and guided imagery in women with locally advanced breast cancer undergoing multimodality therapy: a randomised controlled trial. Breast Edinb Scotl 2009;18(1):17–25.
[13] Carrico DJ, Peters KM, Diokno AC. Guided imagery for women with interstitial cystitis: results of a prospective, randomized controlled pilot study. J Altern Complement Med 2008;14(1):53–60.
[14] La Roche MJ, Batista C, D'Angelo E. A content analyses of guided imagery scripts: a strategy for the development of cultural adaptations. J Clin Psychol 2011;67(1):45–57.
[15] Menzies V, Taylor AG, Bourguignon C. Effects of guided imagery on outcomes of pain, functional status, and self-efficacy in persons diagnosed with fibromyalgia. J Altern Complement Med 2006;12(1):23–30.
[16] Spanos NP, Stenstrom RJ, Johnston JC. Hypnosis, placebo, and suggestion in the treatment of warts. Psychosom Med 1988;50(3):245–60.
[17] Bedford FL. The missing sense modality: the immune system. Perception 2011;40(10):1265–7.
[18] Harris CS. Perceptual adaptation to inverted, reversed, and displaced vision. Psychol Rev 1965;72(6):419–44.
[19] Redding GM, Wallace B. Adaptive spatial alignment. London: Taylor Francis, 2013.
[20] Welch RB. Perceptual modification adapting to altered sensory environments. New York: Academic Press, 1978.
[21] Blalock JE. The immune system as the sixth sense. J Intern Med 2005;257(2):126–38.
[22] Blalock JE. The immune system as a sensory organ. J Immunol 1984;132(3):1067–70.
[23] Ren K, Dubner R. Interactions between the immune and nervous systems in pain. Nat Med 2010 Oct 14. URL: http://dx.doi.org.ezproxy2.library.arizona.edu/10.1038/nm.2234.

[24] Bedford FL. Keeping perception accurate. Trends Cogn Sci 1999;3(1):4–11.
[25] Irwin M, Vedhara K. Human psychoneuroimmunology. Oxford: Oxford University Press, 2005.
[26] Kravitz JH, Wallach H. Adaptation to displaced vision contingent upon vibrating stimulation. Psychon Sci 1966;6(10):465–6.

Submitted: July 27, 2014 *Revised:* January 02, 2015. *Accepted:* January 11, 2015.

In: Pain Management Yearbook 2015
Editor: Joav Merrick

ISBN: 978-1-63484-515-1

Chapter 6

RADIO-FREQUENCY ABLATION ASSISTED CEMENTOPLASTY OF A LYTIC ACETABULAR LESION

Leigha Rowbottom[1], BSc(C), Elizabeth David[2], MD, Rachel McDonald[1], BSc(C) and Edward Chow[2,*], MBBS

[1]Rapid Response Radiotherapy Program, Department of Radiation Oncology, Odette Cancer Centre, Sunnybrook Health Sciences Centre, University of Toronto, Toronto, Ontario, Canada

[2]Department of Interventional Radiology, Sunnybrook Health Sciences Centre, University of Toronto, Toronto, Ontario, Canada

Bone metastases may cause severe debilitating pain that significantly impacts mobility and decreases quality of life. In particular, osteolytic lesions may create a significant potential fracture risk in weight bearing regions and if left unattended may necessitate complex orthopedic surgical intervention. Radiofrequency ablation (RFA) assisted cementoplasty is an efficacious method in palliating and stabilizing such lesions and can produce durable pain control in cancer patients. RFA alone imparts significant improvements in pain reduction; however, if used in adjunct with cementoplasty, it improves stabilization and may enhance pain relief. The combination of RFA assisted osteoplasty or vertebroplasty with radiation may have a synergistic effect that combines pain control with the added benefit of stabilization. We present the case of a prostate cancer patient with a focal lytic deposit in the acetabular region causing severe and pain on weight bearing, resulting in loss of mobility.

Keywords: bone metastases, radiofrequency ablation, cementoplasty

* Correspondence: Professor Edward Chow MBBS, MSc, PhD, FRCPC, Department of Radiation Oncology, Odette Cancer Centre, Sunnybrook Health Sciences Centre, 2075 Bayview Avenue, Toronto, ON, Canada. E-mail:Edward.Chow@sunnybrook.ca.

INTRODUCTION

Bone metastases are a frequent occurrence in cancer patients and often cause debilitating pain that may impair quality of life and reduce mobility (1). Many palliative cancer patients are prescribed analgesics in order to cope with the complications of bone metastases, however they also tend to have side effects and the medications may not adequately manage pain (2). Radiotherapy is an efficacious method of relieving pain induced by bone metastases in upwards of 80% of patients. In certain cases, radiofrequency ablation (RFA) can be used to palliate symptoms experienced by cancer patients with osteolytic bone metastasis. In general, patients experience immediate pain relief that typically lasts upwards of 7 months (3). An RFA procedure involves the insertion of an electrode that subsequently delivers heat to destroy the affected tissue (4). Cement is then injected into the cavity for enhanced stability. In certain cases, RFA assisted cementoplasty may be technically successful, but may not improve clinical symptoms regarding pain. However, stability and prevention future deformity has been achieved. Radiotherapy can be administered before or after RFA assisted vertebroplasty.

In the following report, the case of an elderly prostate cancer patient with extensive bony involvement treated with RFA assisted percutanous cementoplasty is presented. The procedure resulted in reduced fracture risk due to cement filling; the patient did not have worsened pain and proceeded with adjuvant irradiation therapy.

CASE REPORT

A 69 year old male with aggressive prostate cancer with bone metastases was admitted to hospital for increasing pain and inability to cope at home. Three weeks prior the patient was able to fulfill all activities of daily living and was highly active, playing badminton weekly. The attending medical oncologist referred him to the Rapid Response Radiotherapy Program at the Odette Cancer Centre in Toronto in November 2014. The patient presented to the clinic with severe bilateral pelvic pain, which he scored to be a 10 on a scale of 0-10 at its worst, and inability to weight bear on right side. The patient was taking 240 mg of codeine per day to palliate his symptoms.

Upon admission a CT scan of the chest, abdomen and pelvis was ordered, which revealed a large lytic lesion in the posterior aspect of the right acetabulum measuring 19mm. The radiologist deemed this lesion at risk of fracture (Figure 1). Due to fracture risk, both Orthopedic and Interventional Radiology teams were consulted on the case. The possible treatment options were to proceed with a total right hip arthroplasty or radiofrequency ablation (RFA) assisted percutaneous cementoplasty. As this was an isolated lesion, the patient was not keen on pursuing a complex surgical option and arthroplasty was excluded. Of notable concern was a possible cortical breach medially; however, when undergoing a cementoplasty in the pelvis cortical breaches are only of concern if there is communication with the joint. We also postulate that the use of RFA prior to cement injection may aid in the creation of a cavity and a decrease in the creation of cement leaks. It was determined that the best course of action was to proceed with RFA assisted percutaneous cementoplasty. The procedure was carried out the following day with no complications and no soft tissue cement leaks. A 2 cm RFA probe was used (Baylis) followed by injection of 2 cc of cement (Kyphon). There was good filling of the lesion on the post procedural CT (Figure 2).

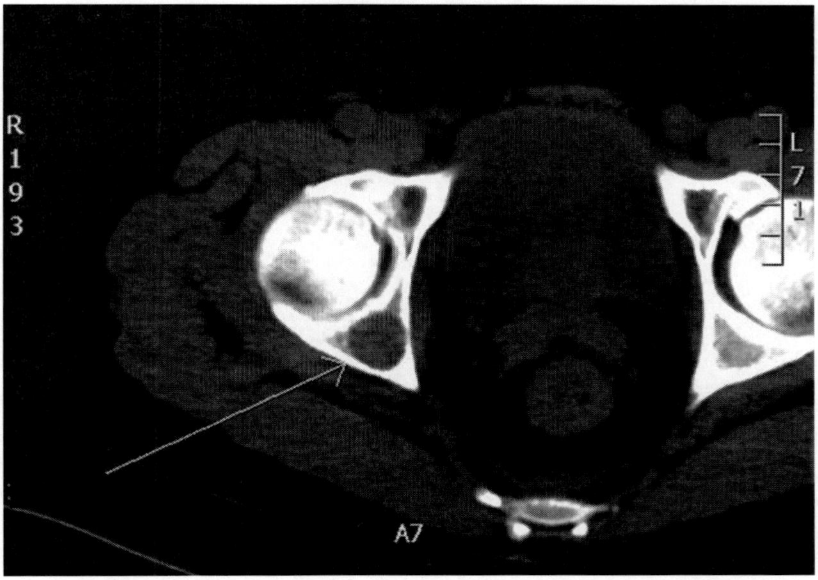

Figure 1. CT image of lytic acetabular lesion before undergoing radiofrequency ablation (RFA) assisted percutanous cementoplasty.

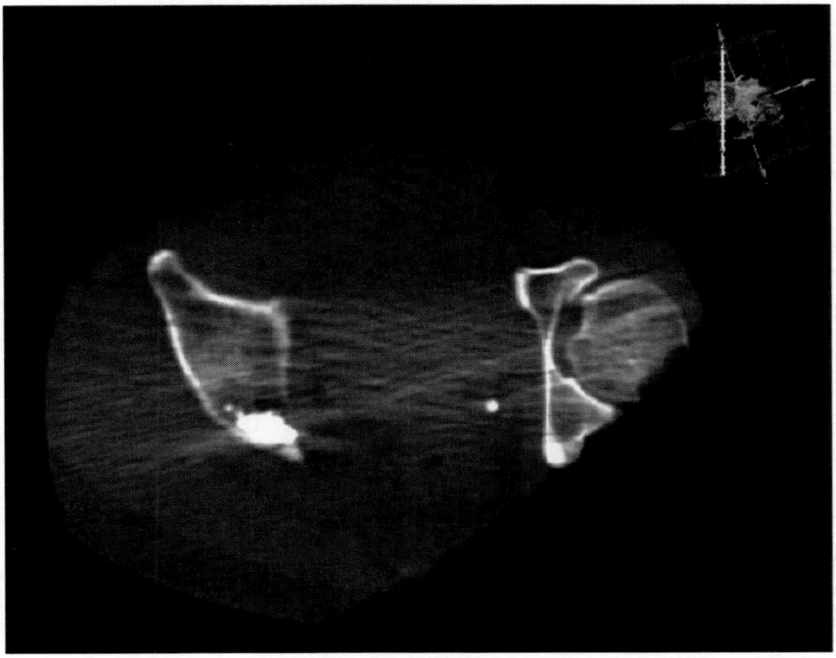

Figure 2. Post-procedural imaging displays good cement filling of the lytic acetabular lesion.

No periprocedural complications occurred and the patient was able to weight bear immediately following the procedure and tolerated mild stretches of walking. The patient returned to referring hospital with the intent to return to the Odette Cancer Centre for post procedure radiation. One week post-surgery the patient had no worsened pain and rated the worst pain as a 7 on 0-10 scale, 5 days post-cementoplasty. The patient underwent a course of irradiation 1 week post-cementoplasty of 20 Gy in 5 fractions to further palliate his residual symptoms.

Discussion

Bone metastases are a common complication of metastatic cancer, which may have debilitating consequences on completion of daily activities and quality of life. In particular, osteoytic lesions may result in significant pain burden, neuropathic symptoms, pathological fractures, and decreased mobility (3). Patients with lytic bone metastases have various treatment options in order to improve pain and promote healing of destroyed bone, such as radiation or interventional techniques. RFA assisted percutanous cementoplasty often relieves pain rapidly in patients experiencing severe bone metastases related pain (3). This technique was determined to be the optimal treatment to reduce pain and improve mobility for this patient.

RFA is a focal ablative therapy that may be used to treat patients with bone metastases. Individuals with sclerotic lesions may not be effectively treated with RFA therapy, as RFA energy is not optimally delivered to sclerotic bone with conventional unipolar devices (1). However, with bipolar devices this does not seem to be an issue. RFA assisted percutaneous cementoplasty was one of the potential therapeutic options for this patient. As the patient had an acetabular lytic lesion at risk for fracture, RFA assisted cementoplasty provided bone stabilization and reduced fracture risk. Patients who receive RFA treatment typically have improved pain rapidly after procedure completion.

Belfiore et al. examined 12 patients with 13 painful osteolytic lesions who underwent RFA therapy without complications resulting in immediate pain relief in 9 out of 12 patients; however, 2 patients had pain recurrence within the first week (5). Lane et al. observed 54 RFA assisted cementoplasties, 14 of which were for an acetabular lesion. Procedures in 36 patients resulted in total technical success and mean reduction of pain from 7.2 to 3.4, on the Visual Analog Scale (VAS) (6). Both studies concluded that RFA and RFA assisted cementoplasty are safe and effective means of relieving pain in palliative cancer patients (5, 6).

In this report, the presented patient presented with typical debilitating pain induced by lytic bone metastases. Various multidisciplinary treatment options were discussed in order to determine the appropriate treatment to optimize the patient's pain management. To fully palliate his symptoms, the patient underwent RFA assisted cementoplasty to the acetabular lesion by an interventional radiologist followed by irradiation. It is essential that physicians use multidisciplinary approaches to fully manage patient symptoms.

CONCLUSION

Radiofrequency ablation assisted (RFA) percutanous cementoplasty is typically an efficacious method at relieving pain in palliative cancer patients. In patients with good performance status, it may be used as a first line therapy to palliate pain associated with lytic bone metastases. In cases where activities of daily living and normal mobility are significantly hindered, it may represent a means of improving quality of life. Post-cementoplasty irradiation may be adjuvantly used to promote further healing and palliation of pain.

ACKNOWLEDGMENTS

We thank the generous support of Bratty Family Fund, Michael and Karyn Goldstein Cancer Research Fund, Pulenzas Cancer Research Fund, Joseph and Silvana Melara Cancer Research Fund, and Ofelia Cancer Research Fund.

REFERENCES

[1] Belfiore G, Tedeschi E, Ronza FM, Belfiore MV, Zeppetella G, Rotondo A. Radiofrequency ablation of bone metastases induces long-lasting palliation in patients with untreatable cancer. Singapore Med J 2008;49(7):565–70.

[2] Harris K, Pugash R, David E, Yee A, Sinclair E, Myers J, et al. Percutaneous cementoplasty of lytic metastasis in left acetabulum. Curr Oncol 2007;14:4–8.

[3] Iannessi A, Amoretti N, Marcy P, Sedat J. Percutaneous cementoplasty for the treatment of extraspinal painful bone lesion, a prospective study. Diagnostic and Interventional Imaging 2012;93(11):859–70.

[4] Lane MD, Le HBQ, Lee S, Young C, Heran MKS, Badii M, et al. Combination radiofrequency ablation and cementoplasty for palliative treatment of painful neoplastic bone metastasis: Experience with 53 treated lesions in 36 patients. Skeletal Radiol 2011;40:25–32.

[5] Peyser A, Applbaum Y. Radiofrequency ablation of bone tumors. Curr Orthop Pract 2009;20:616–21.

[6] Smith, H. S. Painful bony metastases. Ann Palliat Med 2012;1(1):14-31.

Submitted: November 12, 2014. *Revised*: December 12, 2014. *Accepted:* January 08, 2015.

In: Pain Management Yearbook 2015
Editor: Joav Merrick

ISBN: 978-1-63484-515-1

Chapter 7

Spinal cord compression in a patient with malignant spindle cell carcinoma: A case report and review of the literature

Stephanie Cheon, BHSc(C), Paul Cheon, MD(C), Leigha Rowbottom, BSc(C), Erin Wong, BSc(C), Rachel McDonald, BSc(C), Natalie Pulenzas, BSc(C), Nicholas Lao, BMSc(C) and Edward Chow*, MBBS
Sunnybrook Health Sciences Centre, University of Toronto,
Toronto, Ontario, Canada

A 59-year-old female patient presented to the hospital with a pathological fracture of the right femur after a fall on her right hip. MRI of the lumbar spine showed a burst fracture of the T11 and T12 vertebra with retropulsion and impingement of the spinal cord. CT of the thoracic spine discovered compression of the superior T11 endplate. Pathology of the T12 tumor concluded malignant spindle cell carcinoma. Herein, we present the case and review the literature of spinal cord compression (SCC) caused by spindle cell tumors.

Keywords: spinal cord compression, malignant spindle cell carcinoma, spindle cell tumor

Introduction

Spinal cord compression (SCC) presents itself through back pain in approximately 96% of afflicted patients and through weakness in 80% of patients (1). Neurological signs and symptoms of SCC, such as motor impairment, scoliosis, impaired bladder function, constipation, and impaired cutaneous sensibility can present after several weeks of pain (2, 3).

* Correspondence: Professor Edward Chow MBBS, MSc, PhD, FRCPC Department of Radiation Oncology, Odette Cancer Centre, Sunnybrook Health Sciences Centre, 2075 Bayview Avenue, Toronto, ON, Canada. E-mail: Edward.Chow@sunnybrook.ca.

Approximately 10% to 20% of patients with metastatic spinal disease develop epidural SCC, of which 70% occur in the thoracic spine (4). Suspicion of epidural SCC is investigated with imaging studies, such as plain radiography, magnetic resonance imaging (MRI) and computed tomography (CT) (4). MRI is the preferred technique of choice for its sensitivity and specificity in diagnosing epidural SCC (5). Radiotherapy, chemotherapy, and surgery are treatment options (6) that prevent the progression of malignant SCC, which has the potential to lead to neurological damage (7) and permanent paralysis (8).

Spindle cell tumors causing SCC are very rare, and only 14 cases have been reported to date in the literature (9-22). However, spindle cell carcinomas with SCC specifically have not been identified in the literature, suggesting they are even rarer. Due to the lack of literature on spindle cell carcinomas with SCC, we review the broader scope of literature regarding spindle cell tumors resulting in SCC.

Spindle cell carcinoma is a rare and highly malignant variant of squamous cell carcinoma (23) that is rarely found in the breast and head and neck region, but when found are most common in the upper aerodigestive tract, larynx, and hypopharynx and less so in the oral cavity (24, 25). Its presentation is often a large tumor with cyst formation, and histologically appears as sheets of spindle-shaped cells (24). The literature suggests both favorable and poor prognoses of spindle cell carcinomas. Early detection and subsequent polypectomy of the tumor likely lead to a favorable prognosis (26), whereas a highly malignant tumor can result in a poor prognosis due to its high local recurrence or distant metastasis rate (27). Herein, we report the instance of a patient with malignant spindle cell carcinoma presenting with SCC.

CASE REPORT

A 59-year-old female patient presented to the emergency department in June 2014 with increasing weakness and inability to ambulate after suffering a fall onto her right hip. The patient had a history of falls and subsequent ongoing back pain, increasing weakness, and decreased mobility.

The patient was initially admitted for a pathological fracture of the right femur, where a CT scan showed permeative bone destruction in the pelvis and right femur with extensive soft tissue replacement of the medullary canal of the right femur. These findings suggested an underlying malignancy, most likely representing myeloma or metastatic disease. Surgical fixation of the proximal femur was performed, and the pathology was consistent with malignant spindle cell neoplasm.

Furthermore, a CT scan of the abdomen and pelvis showed numerous solid liver lesions and multiple nodules in the adrenal glands. An additional CT of the chest showed extensive lytic metastases, and pulmonary nodules were found scattered throughout both lungs. MRI of the lumbar spine showed a burst fracture of the T11 and T12 vertebra with bony retropulsion and impingement of the spinal cord.

Due to the resulting back pain and the inability of the patient to ambulate, a spine surgeon was consulted. The patient was operated on for posterior stabilization, spinal decompression, and biopsy in June 2014. Laminectomy of T11-T12 was performed. Pathology from the surgical decompression concluded malignant spindle cell carcinoma as the likely diagnosis. Following surgery, postoperative radiation treatment to the surgical site at T11-T12 and lesion at T4 was recommended. However, the patient's condition deteriorated and eventually succumbed to the disease in July 2014.

DISCUSSION

The aforementioned case describes the instance of malignant spindle cell carcinoma resulting in SCC, causing significant barriers to ambulation in an elderly patient. A literature search was conducted in PubMed, OVID, MEDLINE, and Web of Science, and 14 articles discussing cases of spindle cell tumors causing SCC were found. A summary of our results including the details and outcomes can be found in Table 1. Lack of literature suggests the rarity of spindle cell tumors resulting in SCC, while the complete absence of literature suggests the rarity of spindle cell carcinomas resulting in SCC. Spindle cell carcinomas themselves are rare: for instance, they only comprise 2 to 3% of all laryngeal cancers (28), and 0.3 to 1.3% of all lung malignancies (29). Comparably, SCC is not as rare, as 15,367 metastatic SCC-related cases were identified within a 9-year period in the United States (30). This suggests the even greater rarity of spindle cell carcinomas with SCC presentation, rather than the rarity of each individual condition.

Of the 14 cases reported in the literature, 7 cases (16-22) presented patients with a malignant peripheral nerve sheath tumor, which is a form of spindle cell sarcoma (31). Furthermore, the location of the spinal metastasis causing SCC varied.

Table 1. Spinal Cord Compression in Individuals with Spindle Cell Tumors

First Author (Year)	Patient Characteristics	Symptoms	Outcome
Ochiai H (9) (2009)	75 yr female, malignant fibrous histiocytoma in thoracic spine.	Compression fracture causing progressive gait disturbance with bilateral leg weakness. Destruction of vertebral bodies at T7 and T8.	Decompressive surgery, laminectomy from T7-T9, and vertebroplasty performed, resulting in resolved weakness of lower extremities, ability to walk without a cane, and discharge.
Talan-Hranilović J (10) (2007)	31 yr male, intraspinal extradural mass lesion, histological lesion was a spindle cell haemangioma.	Bilateral leg weakness.	Laminectomy and complete removal of tumorous lesion performed, resulting in uneventful postoperative recovery, with regression of sensory disturbance and improved leg weakness.

Table 1. (Continued).

First Author (Year)	Patient Characteristics	Symptoms	Outcome
Abdullah JM (11) (2002)	28 yr male, thoracic spinal cord tumor T7.	Progressive paraparesis over 6 months.	Limited field radiotherapy followed by systemic interferon therapy performed, resulting in neurological improvement and 48-month survival with growth restraint at primary site. Residual neurological deficit persists.
Malek AM (12) (1997)	33 yr male with intradural extramedullary mass at T7-T8.	Back pain, progressive myelopathy, lower extremity dysthesias.	Surgical intervention performed.
Arnesen MA (13) (1992)	56 yr female, spindle cell sarcoma.	Cord compression from lesion of thoracic spine.	N/A.
Kurtkaya O (14) (2001)	70 yr female, solitary fibrous tumor at T3.	Progressive right leg weakness over 30 days.	Laminectomy performed, resulting in uneventful postsurgical period, no strength deficits, and discharge. No neurological deficits presented 12 months after surgery.
Zeng X (15) (2012)	63 yr male, extradural mass at L4.	Six-month history of progressive weakness and numbness on left lower extremity and eventually weakness.	Laminectomy performed at L3-L5. At 30-month follow up patient suffered from persistent, mild dysesthesias of the left foot, no other neurological deficits. No residual or recurrent tumor detected by MRI.
Baek WS (16) (2005)	39 yr female with malignant peripheral nerve sheath tumor (MPNST) of the gluteal mass, leading to metastases to cervicothoracic cord.	Two-week history of painless right lower extremity numbness and weakness, on admission developed urinary and bowel retention.	Treated with Decadron and discharged to hospice centre, died 2 months later.

First Author (Year)	Patient Characteristics	Symptoms	Outcome
Gnanalingham K (17) (2004)	59 yr female, intraosseous MPNST of the thoracic spine.	Midthoracic back pain, paraparesis, T4 sensory level, and destructive lesion at T3 with cord compression.	Decompressive laminectomies, tumor debulking, and instrumentation performed. Surgical excision incomplete and spine stabilized. Patient developed metastatic deposits in spine and femur despite adjuvant radiotherapy.
Suzuki K (18) (2014)	45 yr female, MPNST of the lumbar spine.	One-month history of severe lower back pain, pain radiating to left leg. Compression of spinal canal resulting from osteolytic lesion at L4.	Decompressive laminectomies and extradural tumor resection were performed, but progressive hypoesthesia and motor weakness of the legs presented two weeks later. Spondylectomy of L4 was then performed, but tumor recurred 1 month after surgery. Despite adjuvant chemotherapy, the patient died due to intramedullary dissemination and carcinomatous meningitis 8 months after initial consultation.
Yeap E (19) (2010)	11yr female, retroperitoneal MPNST involving L1.	Six-week history of low back pain and spinal cord compression from collapse of and soft tissue mass at L1.	Posterior decompression, instrumentation, and fusion were performed. Unresectable parts of tumor remained after concurrent discectomy. Despite radiotherapy and chemotherapy, patient died due to multiple metastases 3 months following the last surgery.

Table 1. (Continued).

First Author (Year)	Patient Characteristics	Symptoms	Outcome
Patnaik A (20) (2012)	75 yr male, primary intraosseous MPNST of thoracic spine.	Three-month history of rapidly progressive weakness of lower limbs, definite sensory level at L2 level for all modalities of sensation. Erosion of L3 and spinal cord compression due to an intraspinal component.	L3 laminenctomy was performed, intraspinal part excised, and extraspinal part of tumor removed.
Miyakoshi N (21) (2007)	75 yr woman, MPNST arising from intraosseous region of thoracic spine.	Two-week history of severe back pain, progressive hypethesia, and motor weakness in both legs. Spinal cord compression due to epidural mass arising from intraosseous lesion of T7.	Decompression surgery and posterior stabilization was performed. Despite radiotherapy following recurrence of symptoms, patient died six months following initial clinical presentation from respiratory failure due to invasion of mass into thorax and multiple lung metastases.
Senapati SB (22) (2013)	a) 75 yr male, MPNST in spine. b) 35 yr female, MPNST in spine.	a) History of rapidly progressing swelling over back with burning sensation and paraparesis. Grade 0.5 power around all joints in lower limb and diminished sensation of all modalities below L3 level. L3 destruction by soft tissue mass and epidural cord compression. b) Three-month history of severe lower back pain radiating to both thighs, paraparesis, and bowel bladder involvement. Destruction of L5 by soft tissue mass and epidural cord compression.	a) Near total excision of paraspinal and intraspinal components, and local radiotherapy. Patient did not demonstrate signs of local or distant metastasis at six-month follow up. b) Near total excision of paraspinal and intraspinal components, and local radiotherapy. Patient died at six-month follow-up due to lung metastasis and related complications.

Characteristic of our own case, 8 out of 14 cases (9-14, 17, 21) presented SCC at the level of the thoracic vertebrae as the most common location of SCC, followed by 5 out of 14 cases (15, 18-20, 22) that showed SCC at the level of the lumbar vertebrae. The one remaining case (16) had SCC at the cervical and thoracic vertebral levels.

For cases where symptoms of SCC were noted (9-12, 14-22), common findings were lower limb weakness and back pain, which are consistent with the symptoms of the patient we present. Following clinical presentation of SCC symptoms, spindle cell tumors were discovered simultaneously with SCC, as with our patient and all cases in Table 1, with the exception of one case (9-15, 17-22). This case (16) presented a patient whose spindle cell tumor was discovered prior to SCC. The reason for this deviation may lie in the difference in origin of the spindle cell tumor. The majority of cases examined patients with spindle cell tumors originating from the spine, directly leading to SCC, providing reason for both being discovered simultaneously (9-15, 17-22). In contrast, the anomalous case presented a patient with a spindle cell tumor originating from the gluteal mass, which metastasized to the cervicothroracic cord, then resulted in SCC, thus accounting for the discovery of the spindle cell tumor (gluteal mass) before SCC.

Details regarding the intervention methods for spindle cell tumors and SCC were unavailable for 2 of 14 cases (12, 13). Eleven of the 12 remaining cases (9-11, 14-21) and the patient we present showed commonalities in the intervention methods used; decompression surgery was the most common intervention, of which 7 cases specifically performed laminectomies (9, 10, 14, 15, 17, 18, 20). Radiotherapy was also a shared intervention between our patient and 5 of the 12 cases (11, 17, 19, 21, 22). Although not performed on our patient, other intervention methods among the cases included chemotherapy (17, 19) and surgical removal of the tumorous lesion (10, 17, 18, 20, 22).

The outcome of intervention was unavailable for 3 of 14 cases (12, 13, 20). Four of 11 remaining cases (9, 10, 14, 15) showed symptom relief following intervention. However, 6 of 11 cases (11, 16-19, 21) showed eventual recurrence of symptoms. One publication (22) reported one patient had experienced improvement in symptoms, while the second patient had recurrence of symptoms. Death resulted within 2 to 48 months following intervention (11, 16, 18, 19, 21, 22), in which 3 of these 6 cases were the result of metastases (19, 21, 22), similar to our patient. Interestingly, with the exception of one case that presented symptom relief as a result of intervention (22), radiotherapy and chemotherapy were not used where patients experienced an improvement in their symptoms. Instead, radiotherapy (11, 17, 19, 21, 22) and chemotherapy (18, 19) were often the choices of intervention for cases that resulted in recurrence of symptoms, potentially suggesting their palliative intentions, such as that of our own patient.

CONCLUSION

The incidence of spindle cell tumors and in particular, spindle cell carcinomas resulting in SCC are very rare and represent a niche patient group. Appropriate monitoring must be undertaken in order to adequately treat the debilitating neurological complications resulting from SCC. Commonalities between cases reported and the case presented here may indicate trends for SCC caused by spindle cell tumors. It may be pertinent to document such presentations in order to determine the true incidence and successful treatments for afflicted individuals.

ACKNOWLEDGMENTS

We thank the generous support of Bratty Family Fund, Michael and Karyn Goldstein Cancer Research Fund, Pulenzas Cancer Research Fund, Joseph and Silvana Melara Cancer Research Fund, and Ofelia Cancer Research Fund.

REFERENCES

[1] Gilbert RW, Kim JH, Posner JB. Epidural spinal cord compression from metastatic tumor: diagnosis and treatment. Ann Neurol 1978;3(1):40-51.
[2] National Collaborating Centre for Cancer (UK). Metastatic spinal cord compression: diagnosis and management of patients at risk of or with metastatic spinal cord compression. Cardiff (UK): National Collaborating Centre for Cancer (UK); 2008.
[3] Simon T, Niemann CA, Hero B, Henze G, Suttorp M, Schilling FH, Berthold F. Short- and long-term outcome of patients with symptoms of spinal cord compression by neuroblastoma. Dev Med Child Neurol 2012;54(4):347-52.
[4] Kilmo P Jr, Schmidt MH. Surgical management of spinal metastases. Oncologist 2004;9(2):188-96.
[5] Mavrogenis AF, Pneumaticos S, Sapkas GS, Papagelopoulos PJ. Metastatic epidural spinal cord compression. Orthopedics 2009;32(6):431-9.
[6] Daw HA, Markman M. Epidural spinal cord compression in cancer patients: diagnosis and management. Cleve Clin J Med 2000;67(7):497,501-4.
[7] Byrne TN. Spinal cord compression from epidural metastases. N Engl J Med 1992;327:614-9.
[8] Cole JS, Patchell RA. Metastatic epidural spinal cord compression. Lancet Neurol 2008;7(5):459-66.
[9] Ochiai H, Kawano H, Shimao Y, Hayashi T, Yamada H. Malignant fibrous histiocytoma of the thoracic spine manifesting as rapidly progressive compressive myelopathy. Neurol Med Chir (Tokyo) 2009;49(9):438-41.
[10] Talan-Hranilović J, Vucić M, Sajko T, Bedek D, Tomić K, Lupret V. Spinal spindle cell haemangioma: an atypical location. Acta Neurochir (Wien) 2007;149(3):325-8.
[11] Abdullah JM, Mutum SS, Nasuha NA, Biswal BM, Ariff AR. Intramedullary spindle cell hemangioendothelioma of the thoracic spinal cord--case report. Neurol Med Chir (Tokyo) 2002;42(6):259-63.
[12] Malek AM, Weller SJ, Price DL Jr, Madsen JR. Solitary fibrous tumor presenting as a symptomatic intraspinal mass: case report. Neurosurgery 1997;40(4):844-7.
[13] Arnesen MA, Jones JW. Spindle cell neoplasm of the thoracic spine. Ultrastruct Pathol 1992;16(1-2):29-34.
[14] Kurtkaya O, Elmaci I, Sav A, Pamir MN. Spinal solitary fibrous tumor: seventh reported case and review of the literature. Spinal Cord 2001;39(1):57-60.
[15] Zeng X, Li B, Wang X. Solitary fibrous tumor of the lumbar spine: case report and review of the literature. J Neurol Sci 2012;29(3):623.
[16] Baek WS, Pytel P, Undevia SD, Rubeiz H. Spinal cord metastasis of a non- neurofibromatosis type-1 malignant peripheral nerve sheath tumor: an unusual manifestation of a rare tumor. J Neurooncol 2005;74(2):183-5.
[17] Gnanalingham K, Bhattacharjee S, O'Neill K. Intraosseous malignant peripheral nerve sheath tumor (MPNST) of the thoracic spine: a rare cause of spinal cord compression. Spine (Phila Pa 1976) 2004;29(18):402-5.

[18] Suzuki K, Yasuda T, Hori T, Watanabe K, Kanamori M, Kimura T. An intraosseous malignant peripheral nerve sheath tumor of the lumbar spine without neurofibromatosis: case report and review of the literature. Oncol Lett 2014;7(6):1965-9.

[19] Yeap E, Singh D, Hussain A, Ramanujam T, Sithasanan N. Retroperitoneal malignant peripheral nerve sheath tumor associated with vertebral involvement and spinal cord compression. The Internet Journal of Orthopedic Surgery 2010;16(1):1.

[20] Patnaik A, Mishra SS, Senapati SB, Patra SK, Tripathy K, Burma S. Primary intraosseous malignant peripheral nerve sheath tumor of spine with a giant paraspinal and retrospinal subcutaneous extension. Surg Neurol Int 2012;3:157.

[21] Miyakoshi N, Nishikawa Y, Shimada Y, Okada K, Yoshida M, Enomoto K, Itoi E. Intraosseous malignant peripheral nerve sheath tumor with focal epithelioid differentiation of the thoracic spine. Neurol India 2007;55(1):64-6.

[22] Senapati SB, Mishra SS, Dhir MK, Das S. Malignant peripheral nerve sheath tumor in spine: two case reports. South Asian J Cancer 2013;2(3):141.

[23] Katase N, Tamamura R, Gunduz M, Murakami J, Asaumi J, Tsukamoto G, Sasaki A, Nagatsuka H. A spindle cell carcinoma presenting with osseous metaplasia in the gingiva: a case report with immunohistochemical analysis. Head Face Med 2008;4:28.

[24] Maemura M, Yuichilino, Oyama T, Hikino T, Yokoe T, Takei H, Horiguchi J, Ohwada S, Nakajima T, Morishita Y. Spindle cell carcinoma of the breast. Jpn J Clin Oncol 1997;27(1):46-50.

[25] Biradar MV, Dantkale SS, Abhange RS, Kamra HT, Khushboo B. Spindle cell carcinoma of the tongue: a rare variant of squamous cell carcinoma. Ecancermedicalscience 2014;8:447.

[26] Boamah H, Ballard B. A case report of spindle cell (sarcomatoid) carcinoma of the larynx. Case Rep Med 2012;2012:1.

[27] Su HH, Chu ST, Hou YY, Chang KP, Chen CJ. Spindle cell carcinoma of the oral cavity and oropharynx: factors affecting outcome. J Chin Med Assoc 2006;69(10):478-83.

[28] Völker HU, Scheich M, Höller S, Ströbel P, Hagen R, Müller-Hermelink HK, Eck M. Differential diagnosis of laryngeal spindle cell carcinoma and inflammatory myofibroblastic tumor – report of two cases with similar morphology. Diagn Pathol 2007;2:1.

[29] Terada T. Spindle cell carcinoma of the lung: frequency, clinical features, and immunohistochemical studies of three cases. Respir Med CME 2010;3(4):241-5.

[30] Mak KS, Lee LK, Mak RH, Wang S, Pile-Spellman J, Abrahm JL, Prigerson HG, Balboni TA. Incidence and treatment patterns in hospitalizations for malignant spinal cord compression in the United States, 1998-2006. Int J Radiat Oncol Biol Phys 2011;80(3):824-31.

[31] Baek WS, Pytel P, Undevia SD, Rubeiz H. Spinal cord metastasis of a non-neurofibromatosis type-1 malignant peripheral nerve sheath tumor: an unusual manifestation of a rare tumor. Neurooncol 2005;74(2):183-5.

Submitted: November 25, 2014. *Revised:* December 31, 2014. *Accepted:* January 08, 2015.

In: Pain Management Yearbook 2015
Editor: Joav Merrick

ISBN: 978-1-63484-515-1

Chapter 8

BONE METASTASES IN A PATIENT WITH SEVERAL PRIMARY CANCER ORIGINS: A CASE REPORT

Xixi Wu[1], BSc, Nick Lao[1], BMSc(C), Xiaojing Zhang[2], Erin Wong[1], BSc(C), Marko Popovic[1], BHSc(C), Natalie Pulenzas[1], BSc(C), Sherlyn Vuong[1], BSc(C), and Edward Chow[1,*], MBBS, PhD

[1]Rapid Response Radiotherapy Program,
Department of Radiation Oncology, Odette Cancer Centre,
Sunnybrook Health Sciences Centre, University of Toronto,
Toronto, Ontario, Canada
[2]Department of Bone and Soft Tissue Tumor,
Liaoning Cancer Hospital and Institute, Dalian Medical University,
Shenyang, Liaoning, China

Bone is one of the common metastases from thyroid and lung cancers. The objective of this report is to explore which primary cancer caused bone metastases in a patient first diagnosed with thyroid cancer, then uterine cancer. A 60-year-old female presented with a pathologic fracture in the right distal femur. Bone metastases from thyroid cancer or new lung cancer from the most recent biopsy were the most likely differential diagnosis. A bone scan and medical imaging reports showed diffuse metastatic disease. An MRI showed pathologic fracture through the right distal femoral metaphysis without soft tissue extension. CT scan of the chest showed right lower lobe mass and nodular densities in the right upper lobe with right pleural effusion and right lower lobe atelectasis. Bronchoscopy demonstrated that there was no obvious endobronchial lesions and active bleeding except atelectasis. A collapse of the right middle and lower lobe area was noted. CTs of chest, abdomen and pelvis showed extensive metastatic disease and unclear primary malignancy that may be breast or lung. Ultrasound of breast demonstrated no convincing evidence for malignancy. The pathological result of cecal biopsy was

[*] Correspondence: Professor Edward Chow MBBS, MSc, PhD, FRCPC Department of Radiation Oncology, Odette Cancer Centre, Sunnybrook Health Sciences Centre, 2075 Bayview Avenue, Toronto, ON Canada. E-mail: Edward.Chow@sunnybrook.ca.

metastatic adenocarcinoma that its appearance was consistent with a metastatic carcinoma of the lung or thyroid origin. Uterine cancer and lung cancer may be the second and third primary malignancies in this thyroid cancer patient. It was unclear which primary malignancy metastasized to bone. This leads to difficult choices for treatment of the patient's disease.

Keywords: thyroid cancer, uterine cancer, lung cancer, bone metastases, fracture

INTRODUCTION

Bone is one of the most common locations for metastases. While any type of cancer is capable of forming metastatic tumors within bone, the microenvironment of the marrow tends to favor particular types of cancer, including prostate, breast, lung and thyroid cancers. Bone metastases are classified as osteolytic, osteosclerotic or mixed lesions and can dramatically increase the risk of pathological fractures. Bone pain is often the first symptom of a bone metastasis. Cancer growing in the spine can put pressure on the spinal cord. This can affect the nerves, causing loss of mobility, muscle weakness, numbness, and trouble urinating.

Bone metastases can be found by a number of tests including bone scan, bone biopsy, X-ray, CT, MRI, PET-CT, alkaline phosphatase (ALP). Treatments include chemotherapy, endocrine therapy, radiation, surgery and bisphosphonates. Bisphosphonates can only improve the quality of life with no life-prolonging benefits. It is important for oncologists to design patient's treatment plan (surgery or radiotherapy) based on fracture risk of bone metastases.

In this report, we present the case of an 60-year-old woman diagnosed with the first thyroid cancer, and then uterine cancer and had a hysterectomy done five years ago, the patient had a pathological fracture of her distal femur three weeks ago and was confirmed with bone metastases from unclear primary malignancies: lung or breast cancer by medical imaging and lung or thyroid cancer by surgical biopsy.

CASE REPORT

A 60-year-old female presented with a 3-week history of right distal thigh pain and to the emergency room. At this time, she was found to have a pathologic fracture in the right distal femur by a plain film. Then she was admitted for workup and fixation of her distal femur. She was first diagnosed with thyroid cancer, second diagnosed with uterine cancer and had a hysterectomy 5 years ago.

The patient has symptoms of cough and CT scan of the chest showed right lower lobe mass and nodular densities in the right upper lobe with right pleural effusion and right lower lobe atelectasis. Bronchoscopy demonstrated that there was no obvious endobronchial lesions and active bleeding except atelectasis and collapse of the right middle and lower lobe area. Ultrasound guided right thoracentesis diagnosed suspicious for malignancy of right pleural fluid. Endoscopy proved a nonspecific abnormality in the cecum although there was on CT of the circumferential thickening in the ascending colon. The pathological result of cecum biopsy was metastatic adenocarcinoma that its appearance was consistent with a metastatic carcinoma of the lung or thyroid origin.

Bone scan and medical imaging reported show diffuse metastatic disease. Especially, there were mixed lytic and sclerotic lesions bilaterally throughout the length of the humerus. There was mild endosteal permeation in the mid shaft of the right humerus over approximately 3 cm that would be a mild increased fracture risk. MRI showed pathologic fracture through the right distal femoral metaphysis without soft tissue extension. There was no enhancing lesion in brain and ventricles on CT brain. CTs of chest, abdomen and pelvis showed extensive metastatic disease and unclear primary malignancy that may be breast or lung. Ultrasound of breast demonstrated no convincing evidence for malignancy. Overall, the combined clinical indications, medical imaging reports and pathological results were extensive bone metastases with pathologic fracture in right distal femur. The patient suffered from thyroid cancer first, then uterine cancer, followed by bone metastases from lung cancer or thyroid cancer.

DISCUSSION

In summary, we report the findings of a 60-year-old female, initially diagnosed with thyroid cancer, followed by a secondary diagnosis of uterine cancer 5 years ago, recently diagnosed bone metastases with a pathological fracture of her distal femur from lung cancer or thyroid cancer. This case represents a rare instance of thyroid cancer, then uterine cancer, followed by bone metastases from lung cancer or thyroid cancer. That is the big question as an oncologist how to treat the patient.

Thyroid carcinoma represents 1.6% of all male cancers and 5% of female ones (1). Most thyroid cancers have well histopathological differentiation. Generally the prognosis is favorable and the survival rate is over 90% at 10 years after diagnosis. Lung and bone are the most common sites of metastasis from thyroid cancer (2). But the bone metastases from thyroid cancers have a relatively favorable prognosis. Comprehensive therapeutic strategies including surgery, radioiodine, external beam radiation therapy and embolization should be considered for most thyroid cancers patients (3).

The discovery of asynchronous or synchronous double or multiple malignancies in patients is not uncommon. The co-occurrence of second primary malignancy could be randomly occurring or association with risk factors such as environmental, genetic predisposition and therapy-related. Co-occurrence ratio of thyroid cancer and second primary malignancy was high and occurred in all organ systems (4). The bone is one of the frequent metastatic sites for lung cancer. Approximately 30–40% of patients with advanced lung cancer will have bone metastases during the course of their disease, leading to death. Bone metastasis from primary lung cancer will lead to skeletal complications, including pathological fractures, spinal cord compression, hypercalcaemia and severe skeletal pain (5).

Current therapeutic approaches for bone metastases due to lung cancer include palliative radiotherapy and bisphosphonate as well as systemic therapy with chemotherapy and targeted agents (6). For bone metastasis, zoledronic acid is one of the most commonly used bisphosphonates to prevent, reduce the incidence and delay the onset of skeletal-related events. Denosumab can increase time to skeletal-related events compared with zoledronic acid (6). How should one manage the patient? It is difficulty to make the choice of treatment. Because we cannot make sure that bone metastases are from lung cancer or thyroid cancer. However, it is important to fix her right distal femur by surgery due to a pathologic fracture. Post-operation therapies include palliative radiotherapy, bisphosphonate and /or denosumab. Recommended treatment of bone metastases is usually a combination of local treatment followed by systemic treatment, such as chemotherapy, endocrinotherapy, or targeted therapy.

ACKNOWLEDGMENTS

We thank the generous support of Bratty Family Fund, Michael and Karyn Goldstein Cancer Research Fund, Pulenzas Cancer Research Fund, Joseph and Silvana Melara Cancer Research Fund, and Ofelia Cancer Research Fund.

REFERENCES

[1] Siegel R, Naishadham D, Jemal A. Cancer statistics, 2012. CA Cancer J Clin 2012;62(1):10-29.

[2] Cochetti G, Puxeddu E, Zingaro MD, D'Amico F, Cottini E, Barillaro F, et al. Laparoscopic partial nephrectomy of thyroid cancer metastasis: case report and review of the literature. Onco Targets Ther 2013;6: 355-60.

[3] Jiang L, Ouyang H, Liu X, Wei F, Wu F, Dang L, et al. Surgical treatment of 21 patients with spinal metastases of differentiated thyroid cancer. Chin Med J (Engl) 2014;127(23):4092-6.

[4] Hsu CH, Huang CL, Hsu YH, Iqbal U, Nguyen PA, Jian WS. Co-occurrence of second primary malignancy in patients with thyroid cancer. QJM 2014;107(8):643-8.

[5] Niu Y, Wen Y, Shen W, Deng L, Liu L, Zhang H. Risk factors for bone metastasis in patients with primary lung cancer: study protocol for a systematic review. BMJ Open 2014;4(7):e005202.

[6] D'Antonio C, Passaro A, Gori B, Del Signore E, Migliorino MR, Ricciardi S, et al. Bone and brain metastasis in lung cancer: recent advances in therapeutic strategies. Ther Adv Med Oncol 2014;6(3):101-4.

[7] Beck SE, Nielsen GP, Raskin KA, Schwab JH. Intraosseous synovial sarcoma of the proximal tibia. Int J Surg Oncol 2011;2011:184891. doi: 10.1155/2011/184891. Epub 2011 May 14.

[8] Zulkarnaen M, Path M, Pan KL, Shanmugam PS, Ibrahim ZA, Chan WC, Orth MS. Intraosseous synovial sarcoma of the proximal femur: case report. Malaysian Orthopaedic J 2012;6(1). http://dx.doi.org/10.5704/MOJ.1203.003.

[9] Kim KW, Park SY, Won KY, Jin W, Kim SM, Park JS, Ryu KN. Synovial sarcoma of primary bone origin arising from the cervical spine. Skeletal Radiol 2013;42(2):303-8. doi: 10.1007/s00256-012-1524-0. Epub 2012 Oct 2.

[10] Vliet M, Kliffen M, Krestin GP, Dijke CF. Soft tissue sarcomas at a glance: clinical, histological, and MR imaging features of malignant extremity soft tissue tumors. Eur Radiol 2009;19(6):1499-1511.

[11] Jung SC, Choi JA, Chung JH, Oh JH, Lee JW, Kang HS. Synovial sarcoma of primary bone origin: a rare case in a rare site with atypical features. Skeletal Radiol 2007;36(1):67-71.

Submitted: December 12, 2014. *Revised:* January 05, 2015. *Accepted:* January 12, 2015.

In: Pain Management Yearbook 2015
Editor: Joav Merrick

ISBN: 978-1-63484-515-1

Chapter 9

SPINAL CORD COMPRESSION AS INITIAL PRESENTATION OF CANCER

Anthony F Adili, MBBCh(C), Julia DiGiovanni, MBBCh(C), Nemica Thavarajah, BSc, Natalie Pulenzas, BSc(C), Nicholas Lao, BMSc(C), Sherlyn Vuong, BSc(C), and Edward Chow*, MBBS PhD

Rapid Response Radiotherapy Program,
Department of Radiation Oncology,
Odette Cancer Centre, Sunnybrook Health Sciences Centre,
University of Toronto,
Toronto, Ontario, Canada

Lung cancer is the leading cause of cancer death in Canada, with the most common sites of metastasis being the liver, adrenal gland, bone, and brain. Spinal cord compression is a debilitating complication of cancer. We report the case of an 83 year-old man with a recent diagnosis of pulmonary adenocarcinoma. The patient presented to the emergency department presenting with increasing back pain, bilateral leg pain, urinary retention, and right toe weakness. Investigations revealed stage IV primary pulmonary adenocarcinoma with extensive marrow-replacing lesions throughout the cervical, thoracic, lumbar spine resulting in spinal cord compression. The patient was not a candidate for chemotherapy, and received palliative radiotherapy and support services.

Keywords: spinal cord compression, pulmonary adenocarcinoma

---

* Correspondence: Professor Edward Chow MBBS, MSc, PhD, FRCPC Department of Radiation Oncology, Odette Cancer Centre, Sunnybrook Health Sciences Centre, 2075 Bayview Avenue, Toronto, Ontario, Canada. E-mail: Edward.Chow@sunnybrook.ca.

INTRODUCTION

Lung cancer is the leading cause of cancer death (1). Lung cancer accounted for 14% of all new cancer cases in Canada in 2014 (1). Lung cancer mortality within the last 25 years has significantly dropped, especially in men, contributing to the decline in the overall cancer death rate (1). Although lung cancer continues to have high mortality rates, early diagnosis has remained infrequent (2). There is a widely held view that lung cancer is silent until it is too far advanced (2). This may be in part due to a lack of recognition of symptoms by general practitioners, since symptoms presented before diagnosis often differ from the ones listed in evidence based-practice guidelines for the suspected cancer in question (3). The most common symptoms presented in patients include cough, pain and breathlessness. However, there tends to be up to weeks of delay before patients see a general practitioner (GP) and an even greater delay before they are referred to a specialist (3).

A study by Bowen and Rayner (2003) found that 75% of patients were not aware of the seriousness of their symptoms and had never been exposed to any information about these symptoms (3). As a result, these prolonged delays could allow the lung cancer to metastasize, with the most common sites of metastasis being the liver, adrenal gland, bone, and brain (4).

With an occurrence between 5-14%, metastatic spinal cord compression (MSCC) is a common complication of cancer (5). Surgical management is offered to selected patients with MSCC for immediate relief of spinal compression and mechanical stabilization of the vertebral column (5). Radiotherapy may be used adjuvant with surgery, or as the primary therapy when surgery is contraindicated or when palliation is the aim (5). The role of corticosteroids in the treatment of MSCC has been well indicated (5). Corticosteroids are given to patients with MSCC because they are considered to reduce tumour bulk and spinal cord swelling. As well as to relieve spinal cord pressure and therefore improve treatment outcomes (5).

Epidermal growth factor receptor (EGFR), a growth-factor-receptor tyrosine kinase, is a common component found in multiple cancer types that promote solid tumor growth (6). A study that examined the relationship between EGFR expression and cancer prognosis found patient survival rates in 52% of non-small cell lung cancer (NSCLC) studies with elevated levels of EGFR (6). The EGFR is a key biomarker that is screened for in the histological diagnosis of cancer (6, 8). Different primary treatment options may be dependent on the patient's carrier status of the mutation, varying from targeted therapy to general chemotherapy (6, 8).

We present the case of an 83-year-old male who presented to the emergency department (ED) with spinal cord compression. The patient was later diagnosed with EGFR mutation-negative stage IV pulmonary adenocarcinoma.

CASE REPORT

An 83 year-old man presented to the emergency department (ED) with one episode of a sudden onset of shortness of breath, right arm pain, and supraventricular tachycardia (SVT) which resolved spontaneously. Although the patient had never had similar symptoms, bilateral arm pain with use of the upper extremities had been noted for the past week. While in the ED, the patient was found to have a narrow complex tachycardia around 130 beats per minute (bpm), which terminated on its own. The patient was noted to be mildly volume overloaded; indicating a mild increase in fluid was discharged on Lasix and Tylenol for his back pain. He was noted to have a compression fracture of T11 on his abdominal x-ray and as such was given a prescription for calcium and vitamin D. A raised alkaline phosphatase (ALP) was noted. Past medical history included chronic lower back pain, benign prostate hyperplasia, and heavy smoking (60 pack-years and quitted in 1990). There was no family history of venous thromboembolism (VTE), and the patient had no VTE risk factors. Weight loss over the last 6 months was reported by the family, and a past history of working in construction was noted. The patient was discharged home to follow up in general internal medicine clinic, where a normal exercise stress test was arranged.

Two weeks later the patient returned to the ED due to increasing back pain with bilateral leg pain, urinary retention, and right toe weakness. On presentation to the ED he had an x-ray of his pelvis, lumbar spine, and knee. A lytic lesion in the right lesser trochanter with pathological fracture was found. A CT of his lumbar spine showed multiple lytic lesions in the thoracolumbar spine with central stenosis in T12, right neruforaminal narrowing of T11, T12, and T12 to L1, and soft tissue in the left S1 to S3 neuroforaminal area. MRI of the spine was subsequently taken which showed extensive marrow-replacing lesions throughout the cervical, thoracic, lumbar spine and a pathological lesser trochanteric fracture on the right. There were areas of extraosseous soft tissue at T8, T11, T12, S1, S2, and T2 with the latter resulting in compression of the cord and canal narrowing. An urgent CT -guided biopsy was performed, which confirmed metastatic carcinoma. A CT of the chest and abdomen demonstrated a 44mm x 25mm lesion in the medial basal right lower lobe of the lung. Peripheral sub-segmental atelectasis and consolidation was noted. Biopsy of the right iliac lesion showed metastatic adenocarcinoma forming solid and papillary structures. Immunohistochemistry staining was positive for TTF-1 and Napsin-A and negative for EGFR and ALK. Upon review with the radiologist, pathologist, and immunohistochemistry, stage IV primary pulmonary adenocarcinoma was diagnosed. Radiotherapy for the spinal cord compression, 20 Gy in five fractions to T2, T8, and T12 was given, and dexamethasone and hydromorphone was started for pain control. The patient had a poor performance status (ECOG 4) and therefore was confined to bed. He was unable to ambulate, secondary to pain with partial weight-bearing of his right leg as per orthopedics. As a result, this patient was not a candidate for chemotherapy.

Upon follow-up X-ray, a 4cm eccentric lytic lesion was found in the surgical neck of the humerus without a definite fracture. The patient received palliative radiation treatment in the right femur, 30Gy/10. The patient was discharged to home setting with palliative support services.

DISCUSSION

Globally, lung cancer is the leading cause of cancer death in men (7). The median age at diagnosis is 71 years, with 85% of all cases of lung cancer related to cigarette smoking (7). Studies have shown that cigarettes contain many carcinogens including but not limited to carbon monoxide, nitrogen oxides, hydrogen cyanides and that can results in mutations and genetic changes that contribute to the onset of lung cancer. There is an average 10-fold higher risk of lung cancer in smokers than in non-smokers, dependent on duration and amount smoked (7). Following smoking, the risk of lung cancer is increased upon exposure to asbestos, environmental smoke, radiation, radon gas, and host factors.

As in our case, spinal cord compression was one of the initial presentations of lung cancer. Spinal cord compression is an uncommon, but important complication of metastasis that needs to be treated immediately because if untreated will lead to permanent damage and paralysis, with small cell lung cancer accounting for 20-30% of primary tumors (8). Small cell lung cancer is a disease in which malignant cancer cells form in the tissues of the lung (1). There is an estimated 3.5 to 13% incidence of spinal cord compression in patients with small cell lung cancer (SCLC) (8). Successful treatment of spinal cord compression is often not achieved, with many patients remaining seriously disabled throughout the illness (8). Therefore, putting an emphasis on the recognition of patients at high risk of cord compression could allow early treatment with surgery, corticosteroids, and radiotherapy (5, 8). Early recognition and treatment of metastatic spinal cord compression have led to improved outcomes (5).

Epidermal growth factor receptor tyrosine kinase (EGFR-TK) mutation in general practice is routinely tested in patients presenting with lung cancer (9). There are many tests available to detect these mutations. These tests differ in the specific mutations that they attempt to detect, the amount of tumor cells needed for the test to work, the time that it takes to give a result, and the cost of the test (9). This test helps identify whether or not the patient will benefit from EGFR-TK inhibitor drugs such as erlotinib or gefitinib (9). EGFR-TK mutation-positive tumors gain more benefit from treatment with EGFR-TK inhibitors than from standard chemotherapy treatment. In our case the patient was EGFR- TK mutation-negative, and would benefit more from standard chemotherapy than from EGFR-TK inhibitors (9).

Acknowledgments

We thank the generous support of the Bratty Family Fund, Michael and Karyn Goldstein Cancer Research Fund, Pulenzas Cancer Research Fund, Joseph and Silvana Melara Cancer Research Fund, and Ofelia Cancer Research Fund.

References

[1] Canadian Cancer Society's Advisory Committee on Cancer Statistics. Cancer Statistics 2014. Toronto, ON: Canadian Cancer Society, 2014.

[2] Corner J, Hopkinson. J, Fitzsimmons D, Barclay S, Muers M. Is late diagnosis of lung cancer inevitable? Interview study of patients' recollections of symptoms before diagnosis. Thorax 2005;60(4):314-9.

[3] Bowen F, Rayner CFJ. Patient and GP led delays in the recognition of symptoms suggestive of lung cancer. Lung Cancer 2003;37(2):227-8.

[4] Pezzulo A, Mariotta S, Fioretti F, Uccini S. Metastasis to the colon from lung cancer presenting with severe hyponatremia and dyspnea in a young male; A case report and review of the literature. Oncol Letter 2013;5(5):1477-80.

[5] Prasad D, Schiff D. Malignant spinal-cord compression. Lancet Oncology 2005;6(1):15-24.

[6] Harper ME, Gee JM, Nicholson RI. EGFR and cancer prognosis. Eur J Cancer 2001;37 (Suppl 4):9-15.

[7] Ahn DH, Gerber DE. Lung cancer epidemiology, etiology and risk factors. In: Ganti AK, Gerber DE, eds. Lung cancer. New York: Oxford University Press, 2013:1-10.

[8] Ash CM, Goldman JM, Harper PG, Geddes DM, Souhami RL, Spiro SG et al. Spinal cord compression in small cell lung cancer: a retrospective study of 610 patients. Br J Cancer 1989;59(4):591-3.

[9] EGFT-TK mutation testing in adults with locally advanced or metastatic non-small-cell lung cancer. London: National Institute Health Care Excellence (NICE), Technology appraisal guidance 2013.

Submitted: December 27, 2014. *Revised:* January 05, 2015. *Accepted:* January 16, 2015.

SECTION TWO: PALLIATIVE CARE, QUALITY OF LIFE AND CANCER

In: Pain Management Yearbook 2015
Editor: Joav Merrick

ISBN: 978-1-63484-515-1

Chapter 10

ADVANCES OF PALLIATIVE CANCER TREATMENTS IN THE LAST EIGHT YEARS: A SELECTED LITERATURE REVIEW

Dominic Chu[1], MBBCh(C), Nicholas Chiu[1], BSc(C), Erin Wong[1], BSc(C), Nicholas Lao[1], BMSc(C), Carlo DeAngelis[2], DPharm, Rachel McDonald[1], BSc(C), Natalie Pulenzas[1], BSc(C), Julia Hamer[1], BSc(C), Marko Popovic[1], BSc,(C), Sherlyn Vuong[1], BSc(C), and Edward Chow[1,*], MBBS

[1]Rapid Response Radiotherapy Program, Department of Radiation Oncology, Odette Cancer Centre, Sunnybrook Health Sciences Centre, University of Toronto, Toronto, Canada
[2]Department of Pharmacy, Odette Cancer Centre, Sunnybrook Health Sciences Centre, University of Toronto, Toronto, Ontario, Canada

Palliative care is a comprehensive method of care management intended for patients with non-curable cancers. It aims to manage physical symptoms while also taking into account a patient's psychological, social, and emotional quality of life (QOL). We aimed to review selected recent advances in palliative care of cancer patients within the last 8 years, specifically advances in prolonging overall survival. Progression free survival, symptom palliation, and QOL were additionally studied as important secondary outcomes. We identified phase 3 randomized controlled trials attempting to improve overall survival, which were published in The Lancet, Lancet Oncology, Journal of Clinical Oncology, and The New England Journal of Medicine from January 1, 2006 to June 31, 2014. We also included studies identifying advances in progression free survival and QOL. Twenty-one studies met the inclusion criteria. These studies evaluated

[*] Correspondence: Professor Edward Chow MBBS, MSc, PhD, FRCPC Department of Radiation Oncology, Odette Cancer Centre, Sunnybrook Health Sciences Centre, 2075 Bayview Avenue, Toronto, ON Canada. Email: Edward.Chow@sunnybrook.ca.

advances in treatments regarding colorectal, prostate, breast, gastric and gastro-oesophageal, head and neck, hepatocellular, lung cancer, as well as glioblastoma. The efficacy of novel combination therapies, new single-agent therapies, as well as examining the sequencing and use of intermittent therapy were primarily noted. Fifteen of these studies showed an improvement in at least one of the aforementioned outcomes, while there were no significant improvements in any criterion in six studies. Recent therapies have either prolonged the survival or improved the quality of life in cancer patients with metastases.

Keywords: cancer, palliative care, survival, and randomised controlled trial

INTRODUCTION

Palliative care for the advanced cancer population involves the management of pain and suffering, as well as the patient's overall quality of life (QOL) (1, 2). This type of care is an increasingly important form of hospice and non-hospice care, given the rising incidence of cancer resulting from the global aging population (3).

Palliative care incorporates a multidisciplinary team of health care professionals (1-3). It involves primarily treating and managing symptoms, such as pain, cardio-respiratory symptoms, oral conditions, and constitutional symptoms; this also includes providing appropriate treatments and keeping both the patient and family highly informed (1). Such a comprehensive care system is essential for patients with both curable and non-curable cancer. Palliative care allows patients and families to better cope with the disease (1) and manage physical symptoms (3). In addition, this care may also involve aid from the psychological, social, spiritual, and functional aspects of cancer (3). This type of care is delivered primarily by family physicians and generalists, and other non-oncology specialists for core management of the patient. Oncologists offer a secondary level of care in more complex situations, often supported by an interdisciplinary team of nurses, social workers, psychologists, and spiritual counselors.

Often, oncologists utilize surgery, chemotherapy, hormonal therapy, radiotherapy, or a combination of these accompanied by strong analgesics or adjuvant analgesics as a means of pain management. All have been shown to provide beneficial symptom palliation in a variety of cancers, including improvements in QOL as well as increases in life expectancy (1, 4-6). In particular, a study done by Temel et al. (6) showed that for patients with metastatic non–small-cell lung cancer, early delivery of palliative care resulted in significant improvements in quality of life as well as mood. However, adequate utilization of these treatment modalities requires considering potential long-term complications of treatment versus expected survival estimates, which are often overly optimistic from the patients` perspective (5, 7). An accurate estimate of survival may allow for appropriate end-of-life care and help to avoid unnecessary treatment toxicities.

With substantial developments in palliative care over the last several years, advanced cancers are increasingly viewed as chronic illnesses (8). Patients are commonly placed on a continuous, lengthy regimen of chemotherapy, or radiation therapy, while maintaining a reasonable QOL.

This has shown positive effects on progression free survival, and extension of overall survival.

This study examined overall survival as a primary outcome, but also progression-free survival and QOL as secondary outcomes. We conducted a selected literature review to identify randomised controlled trials documenting recent advances in palliative treatments.

METHODS

A selected literature search was performed through the examination of literature in The Lancet, Lancet Oncology, The New England Journal of Medicine, and Journal of Clinical Oncology. Articles retrieved were published between January 1, 2006 and June 31, 2014.

Literature search results were manually assessed, and phase III randomised controlled trials, pertaining to the advancement in the palliative cancer cohort were included in this study. The type of treatment, mode of administration, and prolonged survival differences were extracted from these studies. Any non-English studies, case reports, review articles, or observational studies were not included in the results. Keywords for the search included: "cancer," "palliative care," "survival," and "randomised controlled trial."

RESULTS

A total of 21 studies were found in the aforementioned journals meeting the inclusion criteria, and were subsequently selected for this study. The majority of the randomised controlled trials describing an increased overall survival or increased progression free survival were chemotherapy based treatments.

Treatments found were targeted towards colorectal cancer, prostate cancer, breast cancer, non-small cell lung cancer, hepatocellular carcinoma, glioblastoma, gastric and gastro-oesophageal, and head and neck carcinoma.

Colorectal cancer

Phase 3 trials attempted the use of combination chemotherapy in the treatment of advanced colorectal cancer (8-9). Some colorectal cancer patients tend to undergo surgery for metastases with curative intent; however most were treated with palliative intent (8). Both studies attempted to investigate the efficacy of limiting the amount of chemotherapy to reduce toxicities, while providing at least similar survival or palliation benefit. Adams et al. examined the effects of intermittent chemotherapy, which has proven to be effective in managing breast cancer, while not reducing median overall survival. Intermittent therapy consisting of fluorouracil or capecitabine and oxaliplatin, could reduce the toxic effects of treatment, and was compared with continuous therapy of the same drugs. The study displayed that intermittent therapy could provide improved QOL and showed similar survival benefits to continuous treatment (8).

Seymour et al. investigated a similar dilemma, attempting to optimize treatment with fewer adverse effects by sequencing the use of 5-fluorouracil, oxaliplatin, and irinotecan (9). Only the study arm giving 5-fluorouracil and irinotecan from the onset of treatment showed a significantly enhanced response in median overall survival, compared to the control group giving fluorouracil until failure, then irinotecan. However, the use of single first-line 5-fluorouracil treatment with second-line combination therapy did not significantly compromise survival or overall QOL (9).

In a later study published in 2011, Seymour et al. also investigated a variety of chemotherapy options in elderly metastatic colorectal cancer patients. Treatment arms consisted of intravenous fluorouracil with levofolinate, oxaliplatin and fluorouracil, capecitabine, and lastly oxaliplatin and capecitabine. The addition of oxaliplatin to either treatment noted improved median overall survival; however, it was not significant. The use of capecitabine did not improve QOL compared to fluorouracil either. Toxicities were slightly increased with oxaliplatin, but were greater in the capecitabine treatment arm compared to fluorouracil (10).

Prostate cancer

Nine studies noted advances in prostate cancer therapy. Seven studies noted improvements in overall survival in each respective treatment modality, while two studies did not. Mitoxantrone was compared against cabazitaxel in patients with metastatic castration-resistant prostate cancer progressing following docetaxel chemotherapy (11). Mitoxantrone is a commonly chosen therapy due to its beneficial QOL outcomes, but has not provided survival improvements in chemotherapy-naïve prostate cancer patients. Trial patients underwent treatment with prednisone with either mitoxantrone or cabazitaxel. Median survival was significantly increased with cabazitaxel (15.1 months versus 12.7 months), while progression free survival also increased with cabazitaxel, despite causing neutropenia in 82% of patients (11). The management of metastatic prostate cancer after chemotherapy was also investigated through inhibition of androgen biosynthesis, with abiraterone acetate plus prednisone (12). Compared with prednisone alone, overall survival was significantly prolonged in the abiraterone acetate-prednisone arm; also secondary endpoints examining progression-free survival, PSA responses, and time to initiation of chemotherapy were considerably improved. While the use of abiraterone was associated with side effects related to elevated mineralcorticoid levels such as fluid retention, hypokalemia, hypertension, and cardiac events, patients in the abiraterone acetate-prednisone arm had less disease-related symptoms (12). A separate publication by Logothetis et al. summarized the impact of abiraterone and prednisone on palliation of pain and on improvement of occurrences of skeletal metastatic events. (15) Abiraterone treatment provided significant improvements in pain relief, delayed pain progression, and prevention of skeletal-related events, the latter of which may play a role in increasing risk of death (15). There was also a large double-blind, randomized study using enzalutamide in castration-resistant prostate cancer after chemotherapy, primarily examining overall survival.(16) This treatment was compared against placebo, and was shown to increase overall survival from 13.6 months to 18.4 months, while also improving other secondary endpoints including PSA response, QOL response, PSA progression, and time to first skeletal-related events. However, the rate of fatigue was raised in the enzalutamide group (16). Another study using Radium -223 dichloride, a bone seeking, α-particle emitting radioisotope that targets prostate cancer bone metastases, was compared against a placebo in a double-blind controlled study. (17) The study involved 921 patients receiving the best standard of care. Patients in the placebo arm had a median overall survival of 11.3 months, while patients receiving radium-223 aside from best supportive care had a median overall survival of 14.9 months (17). Another study by Widmark et al. investigated endocrine treatment with and without radiotherapy for early prostate cancer, as the survival benefits of combination therapy were still unknown (13). Faced with a cumulative incidence of 10 years for prostate cancer-specific deaths, those treated with endocrine treatment (leuprolide, and flutamide) and standard 3D conformal radiotherapy (at least a total of 70 Gy) had a 11.9% mortality rate, compared to 23.9% in endocrine therapy alone (13). PSA recurrence was considerably lower in the combination therapy group; however, there were notably more patients with urinary symptoms and erectile dysfunction. Fransson et al. performed a similar study by examining QOL in locally advanced prostate cancer patients, examining the same treatment of endocrine therapy with or without radiotherapy (14). This study noted a considerable survival benefit in the combined therapy arm along with an increase in mild toxicities. These adverse effects had a minimal effect on QOL after a four year follow-up. Mitoxantrone was the first approved agent for the treatment of castration-resistant prostate cancer due to its efficacy in mitigating pain. Docetaxel later replaced it, as using this with prednisone not only improved palliation but also improved survival. Since the approval of docetaxel for the treatment of castration-resistant prostate cancer in 2004, nine randomized phase III trials testing combinations of docetaxel with other agents failed. As an example, Tannock et al. investigated docetaxel combined with the antiangiogenic agent aflibercept versus docetaxel alone (18). Overall survival in both groups were similar, however, a higher incidence of adverse events were noted in the aflibercept group. In another trial, Quinn et al. examined docetaxel and atrasentan compared to docetaxel and a placebo (19). Median progression free survival was 9.2 months in the treatment arm, compared to 9.1 months in the placebo and median overall survival was 17.8 months in the treatment arm compared to 17.6 months. Also, patients in both groups experienced a similar amount of toxicities.

BRCA and gastric/gastro-oesophageal junction cancer

One study examining the treatment of HER2-positive breast cancer with trastuzumab. Trastuzumab has been shown in previous studies to reflect improvements in progression free survival, but not overall survival (20). This study indicated that at a 23.5 month follow-up, trastuzumab showed a 2.7% increase in overall survival compared to the observational group and displayed a 6.3% improvement in progression free survival. This major improvement in overall survival is unusual, having only been previously seen in tamoxifen trials. However, more episodes of adverse events with trastuzumab were noted relative to the observational group which included hypertension, depression, and diarrhea.

Trastuzumab efficacy has been seen in targeting the HER2 receptor protein in breast cancer, but not necessarily in other tumor types. A study by Smith et al. investigated the treatment of HER2-positive gastric or gastro-oesophageal junction cancer (21). A combination chemotherapy treatment of a fluoropyrimidine and a platinum agent are considered as a standard; a treatment of trastuzumab or without it was given with a chemotherapy regimen of cisplatin plus capecitabine, or cisplatin plus fluorouracil (21). Survival was clinically significant at 13.8 months in the trastuzumab and chemotherapy arm compared to 11.1 months without trastuzumab. Tumor response rate, duration of response, and time to progression was significantly better with trastuzumab, particularly in those with a high HER2 expression (median overall survival of 16 months). Adverse events and serious events were similar across all groups, where nausea, neutropenia, vomiting, and anorexia were most prevalent. High grade adverse effects were previously reported in the chemotherapy regimen, rather than treatment with trastuzumab and chemotherapy.

In 2014, Dutton et al. also investigated Gefitinib for the management of oesophageal cancer (22) although not targeting the HER2 receptor, but rather EGFR. This was compared against a placebo, and did not alter overall survival for the treatment group, and did not significantly improve QOL, dysphagia, or eating. Although median progression free survival was slightly improved compared to placebo, mild and severe toxicities were similar in prevalence in both groups (22).

NSCLC

One study evaluated clinically approved second line therapies for non-small cell lung cancer, which often is associated with poor outcomes with a progression free survival usually under 4 months, and an overall survival estimated around 7-9 months (23). Ramucirumab and docetaxel was compared with a placebo and docetaxel; median overall survival in the ramucirumab treatment arm was 10.5 months compared to 9.1 months for the placebo. Also, median progression free survival was greater for the treatment arm; however, adverse events were more prevalent, including neutropenia and leucopenia.

A study by Paz-Ares investigated a therapy consisting of pemetrexed and supportive care was compared against a placebo with supportive care intended for non-squamous NSCLC. Median progression free survival for pemetrexed was 4.1 months versus 2.8 months for the placebo. However, grade 3-4 toxicities were slightly more prevalent in the treatment arm, including anemia, neutropenia and fatigue (24).

Hepatocellular carcinoma

A single study compared FOLFOX4 (flouorouracil, leucovorin, and oxaliplatin) against the then current standard of treatment (doxorubicin) for hepatocellular carcinoma in Asian patients (25). It should be noted that sorafenib was still undergoing trials while this study was being designed; this was the only drug to have shown increased overall survival. Increased overall survival was found for FOLFOX4 compared to Doxorubicin, however, it was not statistically significant. It was significant in improving overall survival in patients (by 1.47 months) with a prognosis for survival of 3 to 4 months. A significant increase in progression free survival and response rate were noted for FOLFOX4 as well. Compared with sorafenib, this drug had showed average survival benefits in the Asian cohort of patients, and response rates were low; adverse events with sorafenib were high, including bleeding events and hand-foot-skin reactions.

Glioblastoma

A study by Malmstrom et al. compared the efficacy of temozolomide against 6-week standard radiotherapy, and against hypofractionated radiotherapy in elderly glioblastoma patients (26). Overall survival was significantly improved with temozolomide treatment over standard radiotherapy, but did not differ between hypofractionated and standard radiotherapy. Temozolomide and hypofractionated radiotherapy provided a good survival benefit in those over 70, and both provided similar overall median survival advantages. Toxicities were noted across all treatments, including seizures, fatigue, and thrombo-embolic disease.

Head and neck carcinoma

Machiels et al. examined the efficacy of zalutumumab and the current supportive care measures against supportive care alone (with optional methotrexate) in patients with metastatic squamous-cell carcinoma of the head and neck (27). Supportive care included the use of anilides, glucocorticoids, benzodiazepines, proton-pump inhibitors, and opium alkaloids. Median overall survival for the treatment group was 6.7 months, compared to the control of 5.2 months. Progression free survival and tumor response rates were improved with the zalutumumab group, and QOL was not affected by the additional drug. However, the study power was not large enough to adequately define the results as statistically significant. Adverse events were mainly noted to be related to the disease, and were present in both groups; although the treatment group had greater numbers of grade 3 or 4 events of rash, pneumonia, and headaches.

Mesothelioma

In patients with malignant mesothelioma, standard chemotherapy regimens have not shown to increase long term survival, and therefore, thalidomide was investigated for efficacy in this disease. Patients had completed a treatment of pemetrexed, with or without a platinum agent, and had failed; subsequently, patients received thalidomide and active supportive care or no thalidomide and supportive care. Median time to progression was 3.6 months in the thalidomide group and 3.5 months in the supportive care only group. Toxicities reported were similar in both groups, and were likely due to the previous therapy. Overall, thalidomide did not show any benefits to the control group, and further treatment strategies need to be investigated (28).

DISCUSSION

The integration of palliative care as a standard of care in cancer treatment has grown due to its efficacy in extending survival, improving QOL, as well as reducing symptom burden (29). As patients undergo non-curative care, and their prognosis is limited to months, attempting to extending survival as much as possible becomes a priority. This care is provided as a means to improve survival, as well as QOL.

The current paper notes a variety of developments in survival prolongation for palliative care, as well as developments in improving QOL and progression free survival. There was an increasing trend in the use of combination chemotherapy of two or three drugs over single-agent treatments or a combination of chemotherapy and radiotherapy (9, 13, 23, 25). These studies often found an increased amount of treatment related adverse effects, despite potential benefits in overall survival. Whether this cost-to-benefit ratio is worthwhile may be further investigated. Moreover, the use of intermittent therapy in certain cases provided survival benefits similar to continuous treatment, while reducing the amount of adverse events (8). The HER2 signaling inhibitor, trastuzumab, showed plenty of promise for survival prolongation in not only breast cancer patients (20), but also gastric and gastro-oesophageal cancer patients (21). This treatment should be further explored in other over expressed HER2 receptor cancers, such as ovarian, testicular, and uterine cancers. Single drug therapies, often in combination with corticosteroids, or other supportive care therapies, were found to also aid in prolonging survival (11, 12, 26, 27).

Several studies have shown the potential benefits of the use of drugs and radiotherapy in palliative care. It is important to also examine other factors involved in this multidisciplinary care system, including the early integration of palliative care, how to communicate with patients their prognosis, the impact of depression on survival, and estimating patient prognosis. These issues are potentially able to improve overall survival, progression free survival, as well as QOL.

The integration of treatment early in disease stage for patients with incurable cancer has been studied by Greer et al. They previously reported a survival advantage in early palliative care; however, their recent study did not show this when treating patients with metastatic NSCLC. Rather, the study noted a reduced use of chemotherapy towards patients' end-of-life care. This did not reduce survival, but improved QOL and mood in patients as the cohort of patients assigned to early treatment were able to enter hospice care earlier; which is considered to be clinically meaningful (29). Pirl et al. investigated the impact of depression and survival in metastatic NSCLC in an early palliative care setting (31). This randomized trial providing early palliative care showed a significant increase in survival of 3 months, producing a cohort of patients with a median survival of usually 8 to 10 months. This involved managing co-morbidities, early chemotherapy, and removing chemotherapy during near end-of-life care, subsequently improving the management of depression. A correlation between survival and depression cannot be made, although improved depression was associated with improved survival at baseline and follow-up. As depression is a modifiable outcome, this may be targeted as an important outcome in improving QOL and possibly survival.

Table 1. A summary of selected studies reflecting a clinically significant increase in overall survival, progression free survival, or QOL

Author	Total patient sample size	Cancer type	Control (survival -months)	Treatment 1 (survival - months)	Treatment 2 (survival - months)
Adams et al. 2011. (8)	1630	Advanced colorectal cancer	Continuous Oxaliplatin and Fluoropyrimidine (15.8)	Intermittent chemotherapy (14.4)	n/a
**Seymour et al. 2007. (9)	2135	Advanced colorectal cancer	Fluorouracil to failure, then Irinotecan (13.9)	Fluorouracil until failure, then combination chemotherapy (ir-15.0, ox- 15.2)	Combination chemotherapy (ir-16.7, ox- 15.4)
de Bono et al. 2010. (11)	755	Metastatic castration-resistant prostate cancer	Prednisone and Mitoxantrone (12.7)	Prednisone and Cabazitaxel (15.1)	n/a
de Bono et al. 2011. (12)	1195	Metastatic prostate cancer	Placebo-prednisone (10.9)	Prednisone and Abiraterone (14.8)	n/a
***Widmark et al. 2009. (13)	875	Locally advanced prostate cancer	Endocrine treatment (23.9%)	Endocrine and Radiotherapy (11.9%)	n/a
Fransson et al. 2009. (14)****	872	Prostate Cancer	Endocrine Treatment (QOL)	Endocrine and Radiotherapy (QOL)	n/a
Logothetis et al. 2012. (15)*****	797	Metastatic castration-resistant prostate cancer	Prednisone (13.7)	Abiraterone acetate and Prednisone (5.7)	n/a
Scher et al. 2012. (16)	1199	Castration resistant chemotherapy	Placebo (13.6)	Enzalutamide (18.4)	n/a
Parker et al. 2013. (17	921	Metastatic prostate cancer	Placebo (11.3)	Radium-223 (14.9)	n/a
*Smith et al. 2007. (20)	5102	HER2-positive breast cancer	Observation after adjuvant chemotherapy	1 year of Trastuzumab after adjuvant chemotherapy	2 years of Trastuzumab after adjuvant chemotherapy

Table 1. (Continued).

Author	Total patient sample size	Cancer type	Control (survival -months)	Treatment 1 (survival - months)	Treatment 2 (survival - months)
Bang et al. 2010. (21)	594	HER2-positive advanced gastric or gastro-oesophageal junction cancer	Chemotherapy alone (11.1)	Chemotherapy and Trastuzumab (13.8)	n/a
Garon et al. 2014. (23)	1253	Non-small-cell lung cancer	Placebo and Docetaxel (9.1)	Ramucirumab and Docetaxel (10.5)	n/a
Qin et al. 2013. (25)	371	Hepatocellular carcinoma	Doxorubicin (4.97)	FOLFOX4 - infusional flurouracil, leucovorin, oxaliplatin (6.40)	n/a
Malmstrom et al. 2012. (26)	342	Glioblastoma	Standard 6 week radiotherapy (6.0)	Temozolomide (8.3)	Hypofractionated radiotherapy (7.5)
Machiels 2011. (27)	286	Metastatic squamous-cell carcinoma of the head and neck	Supportive care with optional methotrexate (5.2)	Supportive care with Zalutumumab (6.7)	n/a

*After 1 year of treatment with trastuzumab, overall survival was 97% compared to 95% in the observational group. 2 year results were not released.

**Combination therapy could either consist of: ir, fluorouracil and irinotecan, ox - fluorouracil and oxaliplatin.

***Survival measured in percentage of men who died of prostate cancer.

****Examines QOL as a primary endpoint.

*****This study examines time to pain palliation.

Table 2. A summary of selected studies showing no improvements in overall survival, progression free survival, or QOL

Author	Sample size	Cancer type	Treatment A	Treatment B	Treatment C	Treatment D
Seymour et al. 2011. (10)	459	Colorectal	Fluorouracil with levofolinate (10.1)	Oxaliplatin and Fluorouracil (10.7)	Capecitabine (11.0)	Oxaliplatin and capecitabine (12.4)
Tannock et al. 2013. (18)	1224	Prostate	Placebo (21.2)	Aflibercept (22.1)	n/a	n/a
Quinn et al. 2013. (19)	498	Prostate	Placebo (9.1)	Atrasentan (9.2)	n/a	n/a
Dutton et al. 2014. (22)	450	Oesophageal	Placebo (3.67)	Gefitinib (3.73)	n/a	n/a
Paz-Ares et al. 2012. (24)	1022	Lung	Supportive Care (2.8)	Pemetrexed and Supportive Care (4.1)	n/a	n/a
Buikhuisen et al. 2013. (28)	222	Mesothelioma	Placebo and Supportive Care (3.5)	Thalidomide and Supportive Care (3.6)	n/a	n/a

Patients in past studies entertained false beliefs that their treatment would be curative in intent, even when presented with accurate information in chemotherapy or radiotherapy treatment (4, 30). Clear communication of the diagnosis and the corresponding treatment is a priority. This lack of understanding on treatment and prognosis can hamper clinical decision-making as patients may want rigorous therapy despite entering end-of-life care, leading to a depreciation of QOL; this may often include a large increase in fatigue, which may be a large burden for the family and patient. It is recommended by the American Society of Clinical Oncology Quality Oncology Practice Initiative to stop chemotherapy for the last couple weeks of life, as well as stop utilization of hospice care a week before death (32). The study by Chen et al. noted that this misunderstanding and lack of communication about treatment may be due to an underlying misconception about the nature of the disease itself (30). They suggest that patient education on not only the treatment modality, but also a general discussion regarding the disease, may be helpful. This was found to be more common in the elderly and non-white population in the study, suggesting that cultural factors may be a strong influence as well. A study by Temel et al. noted the benefits of early palliative care in metastatic NSCLC (33). This study demonstrated that continually discussing with patients their disease and prognosis allowed for a significant improvement in understanding their prognosis (33). Plenty of literature has been published to aid physicians in effectively working with these difficult end-of-life care discussions, however, limited articles have been published on how to assert to patients that treatment is not curative (4).

Furthering the topic of effective communication, Mack et al. examined how physicians communicate with patients with poor prognosis, and how this can be improved (34). Physicians are hesitant to explain the harsh reality of a poor prognosis, and it is evident that this can be quite detrimental to the patients' health and survival. Providing proper prognostic information is important to allow the patients and their families to make clear and informed decisions. These decisions include involvement in hospice care, allowing the patient to cope with disease in a friendlier environment, and minimizing the burden of grief or depression.

Prognostic estimates in advanced cancer settings may be very difficult to predict. In current practice, oncologists often over-estimate this timeline, which may adversely affect treatment decision and the patient's and family's decision-making and planning (5, 7, 35). Examination of prognostic factors may be useful such as stage, grade, receptor status, or histology; however non-specific complications may arise in end-stage disease such as when presenting with cachexia, thrombo-embolism, and bleeding. A study by Gripp et al. was able to accurately estimate survival through physician estimates in 61% (by pooled physicians), 55% (a physician), and 63% (by tumor board) of three separate cohorts in a variety of cancer types, while patients who died within 1 month faced a survival prediction correctly only 4.4% to 29% of the time (5). These estimates by physicians were unreliable; 63% of estimates were optimistic and 17% were pessimistic, while prognostic error correlated inversely with survival. Other studies have tried to improve on simple physician estimates by creating predictive models to estimate this (7, 35). Chow et al. investigated factors considered to markedly impact survival: primary cancer site, sites of metastasis, and Karnofsky Performance Status (8). This simplified model of a previous model was shown to provide similar responses to the validated six factor model. This could be useful in that patients would not have to complete other questionnaires, therefore lowering the burden on advanced cancer patients (7). Blanchon et al. investigated the development of a prognostic index in NSCLC patients by using prognostic factors, including age, tumor-node-metastasis, sex, performance status, and histology to determine 4-year mortality. It was found to be appropriate in predicting the 1 and 2 year risks of death. This index may also be useful in predicting risks of NSCLC patients in a clinical trial setting, as well as aiding in management of patients and resource use; however, its use in separate cohorts and different cohorts has yet to be validated.

Conclusion

This review represents a few of the major developments in palliative care within the last 8 years in terms of survival prolongation, QOL improvements, as well as minimizing toxicity. Clinicians should also note non-pharmacological considerations when managing advanced cancer patients.

Acknowledgments

We thank the generous support of Bratty Family Fund, Michael and Karyn Goldstein Cancer Research Fund, Pulenzas Cancer Research Fund, Joseph and Silvana Melara Cancer Research Fund, and Ofelia Cancer Research Fund.

References

[1] Kelley AS, Meier DE. Palliative care - a shifting paradigm. N Engl J Med 2010;363(8):781-2.

[2] Portenoy RK. Treatment of cancer pain. Lancet 2011;377:2236-47.

[3] Ferris FD, Bruera E, Cherny N, Cummings C, Currow D, Dudgeon D, et al. Palliative cancer care a decade later: accomplishments, the need, next steps - from the American Society of Clinical Oncology. J Clin Oncol 2009;27(18):3052-8.

[4] Weeks JC, Catalano PJ, Cronin A, Finkelman MD, Mack JW, Keating NL, et al. Patient's expectations about effects of chemotherapy for advanced cancer. N Engl J Med 2012;367:1616-25.

[5] Gripp S, Moeller S, Bolke E, Schmitt G, Matuschek C, Asgari S, et al. Survival prediction in terminally ill cancer patients by clinical estimates, laboratory tests, and self-rated anxiety and depression. J Clin Oncol 2007;25(22):3313-20.

[6] Temel JS, Greer JA, Muzikansky A, Gallagher ER, Admane S, Jackson VA, et al. Early palliative care for patients with metastatic non-small-cell lung cancer. N Engl J Med 2010;363(8):733-42.

[7] Chow E, Abdolell M, Panzarella T, Harris K, Bezjak A, Warde P, et al. Predictive model for survival in patients with advanced cancer. J Clin Oncol 2008;26(36):5863-9.

[8] Adams RA, Meade AM, Seymour MT, Wilson RH, Madi A, Fisher D, et al. Intermittent versus continuous oxaliplatin and fluoropyrimidine combination chemotherapy for first-line treatment of advanced colorectal cancer: results of the randomised phase 3 MRC COIN trial. Lancet Oncol 2011;12:642-53.

[9] Seymour MT, Maughan TS, Edermann JA, Topham C, James R, Gwyther SJ, et al. Different strategies of sequential and combination chemotherapy for patients with poor prognosis advanced colorectal cancer (MRC FOCUS): a randomised controlled trial. Lancet 2007;370:143-52.

[10] Seymour MT, Thompson L, Wasan HS, Middleton G, Brewster AE, Shepherd SF, et al. Chemotherapy options in elderly and frail patients with metastatic colorectal cancer (MRC FOCUS2): an open-label, randomised factorial trial. Lancet 2011;377:1749-59.

[11] de Bono JS, Oudard S, Ozguroglu M, Hansen S, Machiels JP, Kocak I, et al. Prednisone plus cabazitaxel or mitoxantrone for metastatic castration-resistant prostate cancer progressing after docetaxel treatment: a randomised open-label trial. Lancet 2010;376:1147-54.

[12] de Bono JS, Logothetis CJ, Molina A, Fizazi K, North S, Chu L, et al. N Engl J Med 2011;364(21):1995-2005.

[13] Widmark A, Klepp O, Solberg A, Angelsen A, Fransson P, Lund JA, et al. Endocrine treatment, with or without radiotherapy, in locally advanced prostate cancer (SPCG-7/SFUO-3): an open randomised phase III trial. Lancet 2009;373:301-8.

[14] Fransson P, Lund JA, Damber JE, Klepp O, Wiklund F, Fossa S, et al. Quality of life in patients with locally advanced prostate cancer given endocrine treatment with or without radiotherapy: 4-year follow-up of SPCG-7/SFUO-3, an open-label, randomised, phase III trial. Lancet Oncol 2009;10:370-80.

[15] Logothetis CJ, Basch E, Molina A, Fizazi K, North SA, Chi KN, et al. Effect of abiraterone acetate and prednisone compared with placebo and prednisone on pain control and skeletal-related events in patients with metastatic castration-resistant prostate cancer: exploratory analysis of data from the COU-AA-301 randomised trial. Lancet Oncol 2012;13:1210-7.

[16] Scher HI, Fizazi K, Saad F, Taplin M, Sternberg CN, Miller K, et al. Increased survival with enzalutamide in prostate cancer after chemotherapy. N Engl J Med 2012;367:1187-97.

[17] Parker C, Nilson S, Heinrich D, Helle SI, O'Sullivan JM, Fossa SD, et al. Alpha emitter radium-223 and survival in metastatic prostate cancer. N Engl J Med 2013;369:213-223.

[18] Tannock IF, Fizazi K, Ivanov S, Karlsson CT, Flechon A, Skoneczna I, et al. Aflibercept versus placebo in combination with docetaxel and prednisone for treatment of men with metastatic castration-resistant prostate cancer (VENICE): a phase 3, double-blind randomised trial. Lancet Oncol 2013;14:760-68.

[19] Quinn DI, Tangen CM, Hussain M, Lara Jr PN, Goldkorn A, Moinpour CM, et al. Docetaxel and atrasentan versus docetaxel and placebo for men with advanced castration-resistant prostate cancer (SWOG S0421): a randomised phase 3 trial. Lancet Oncol 2013;14:893-900.

[20] Smith I, Procter M, Gelber RD, Guillaume S, Feyereislova A, Dowsett M, et al. 2-year follow-up of trastuzumab after adjuvant chemotherapy in HER2-positive breast cancer: a randomised controlled trial. Lancet 2007;369:29-36.

[21] Bang YJ, Cutsem EV, Feyereislova A, Chung HC, Shen L, Sawaki A, et al. Trastuzumab in combination with chemotherapy versus alone for treatment of HER2-positive advanced gastric or gastro-oesophageal junction cancer (ToGA): a phase 3, open-label, randomised controlled trial. Lancet 2010;376 (9742):687-97.

[22] Dutton SJ, Ferry DR, Blazeby JM, Abbas H, Dahle-Smith A, Mansoor W, et al. Gefitinib for oesophageal cancer progressing after chemotherapy (COG): a phase 3, multicentre, double-blind placebo-controlled randomised trial. Lancet Oncol 2014;15:894-904.

[23] Garon EB, Ciuleanu TE, Arrieta O, Prabhash K, Syrigos KN, Goskel T, et al. Ramucirumab plus docetaxel versus placebo plus docetaxel for second-line treatment of stage IV non-small-cell lung cancer after disease progression on platinum-based therapy (REVEL): a multicentre, double-blind, randomised phase 3 trial. Lancet 2014. doi: 10.1016/s0140-6736(14)60845-x.

[24] Paz-Ares L, de Marinis F, Dediu M, Thomas M, Pujol JL, Bidoli P, et al. Maintenance therapy with pemetrexed plus best supportive care versus placebo plus best supportive care after induction therapy with pemetrexed plus cisplatin for advanced non-squamous non-small-cell lung cancer (PARAMOUNT): a double-blind, phase 3, randomised controlled trial. Lancet Oncol 2012;13:247-55.

[25] Qin S, Bai Y, Lim HY, Thongprasert S, Chao Y, Fan J, et al. Randomized, multicenter, open-label study of oxaliplatin plus fluorouracil/leucovorin versus doxorubicin as palliative chemotherapy in patients with advanced hepatocellular carcinoma from Asia. J Clin Oncol 2013; 31(28):3501-8.

[26] Malmstrom A, Gronbeg BH, Marosi C, Stupp R, Frappaz D, Schultz H, et al. Temozolomide versus standard 6-week radiotherapy versus hypofractionated radiotherapy in patients older than 60 years with glioblastoma: the Nordic randomised, phase 3 trial. Lancet Oncol 2012;12:916-26.

[27] Machiels JP, Subramanian S, Ruzsa A, Repassy G, Lifirenko I, Flygare A, et al. Zalutumumab plus best supportive care versus best supportive care alone in patients with recurrent or metastatic

squamous-cell carcinoma of the head and neck after failure of platinum-based chemotherapy: an open-label, randomised phase 3 trial. Lancet Oncol 2011;12:333-43.

[28] Buikhuisen WA, Burgers JA, Vincent AD, Korse CM, van Klaveren RJ, Schramel F MNH, et al. Thalidomide versus active supportive care for maintenance in patients with malignant mesothelioma after first-line chemotherapy (NVALT 5): an open-label, multicentre, randomised phase 3 study. Lancet 2013;14:543-51.

[29] Greer JA, Pril WF, Jackson VA, Muzikansky A, Lennes IT, Heist RS, et al. Effect of early palliative care on chemotherapy use and end-of-ife care in patients with metastatic non-small-cell lung cancer. J Clin Oncol 2012;30(4):394-400.

[30] Chen AB, Cronin A, Weeks JC, Chrischilles EA, Malin J, Hayman JA, et al. Expectations about the effectiveness of radiation therapy among patients with incurable lung cancer. J Clin Oncol 2013. doi:10.1200/JCO.2012.48.5748.

[31] Pirl WF, Greer JA, Traeger L, Jackson V, Lennes IT, Gallagher ER, et al. Depression and survival in metastatic non-small-cell lung cancer: effects of early palliative care. J Clin Oncol 2012;30(12):1310-5.

[32] American society of Clinical Oncology Quality Oncology Practice Initiative: (ASCO QOPI) ASCO QOPI Summary of Measures, Fall 2009. [Accessed August 15, 2014]. Available at http://qopi.asco.org /Documents/QOPIFall2009Measures Summary8-18-09.

[33] Temel JS, Greer JA, Admane S, Gallagher ER, Jackson VA, Lynch TJ, et al. Longitudinal perceptions of prognosis and goals of therapy in patients with metastatic non-small-cell lung cancer: results of a randomized study of early palliative care. J Clin Oncol 2011;29(17):2319-26.

[34] Mack JW, Smith TJ. Reasons why physicians do not have discussions about poor prognosis, why it matters, and what can be improved. J Clin Oncol 2012;30(22): 2715-7.

[35] Blanchon F, Grivaux M, Asselain B, Lebas FX, Orlando JP, Pieuqet J, et al. 4-year mortality in patients with non-small-cell lung cancer: development and validation of a prognostic index. Lancet Oncol 2006;7:829-36.

Submitted: December 19, 2014. *Revised:* January 19, 2015. *Accepted:* January 30, 2015.

In: Pain Management Yearbook 2015
Editor: Joav Merrick

ISBN: 978-1-63484-515-1

Chapter 11

COMPARISON OF THE EORTC QLQ-LC13 AND THE FACT-L FOR ASSESSMENT OF QUALITY OF LIFE IN PATIENTS WITH LUNG CANCER

Julia DiGiovanni[1], MBBCh(C), Marko Popovic[1], BHSc(C), Edward Chow[1,*], MBBS, David Cella[2], PhD, Jennifer L Beaumont[2], MS, Jasmine Nguyen[1], MBBCh(C), Dominic Chu[1], MBBCh(C), Anthony Adili[1], MBBCh(C), Natalie Pulenzas[1], BSc(C), Breanne Lechner[1], BSc(C), Henry Lam[1], MLS and Andrew Bottomley[3], PhD

[1]Rapid Response Radiotherapy Program,
Department of Radiation Oncology, Odette Cancer Centre,
Sunnybrook Health Sciences Centre, University of Toronto,
Toronto, Ontario, Canada
[2]Department of Medical Social Sciences,
Northwestern University Feinberg, IL, US
[3]European Organisation for Research and Treatment
of Cancer Headquarters, Brussels, Belgium

This review aimed to compare the development, characteristics, validity and reliability of two widely used quality of life (QOL) assessment tools in lung cancer: the EORTC QLQ-LC13 and the FACT-L. The authors found that both questionnaires were developed from input of patients and health care professionals. The QLQ-LC13 is a 13-item instrument that assesses coughing, hemoptysis, dyspnea and pain and the side effects of treatment. Two international field studies have concluded that the QLQ-LC13 is clinically valid and useful. Conversely, the FACT-L assesses general QOL and seven lung cancer-specific items, such as shortness of breath, weight loss, cough, and appetite. In a study of 116

* Correspondence: Professor Edward Chow, MBBS, MSc, PhD, FRCPC, Department of Radiation Oncology, Odette Cancer Centre, Sunnybrook Health Sciences Centre, 2075 Bayview Avenue, Toronto, ON, Canada. E-mail: Edward.Chow@sunnybrook.ca.

lung cancer patients, the FACT-L was found to have a good internal consistency, reliability, and sensitivity to changes in performance status. Ultimately, both the EORTC QLQ-LC13 and the FACT-L have been sufficiently validated; as such, decision-making should depend on the needs of the investigation.

Keywords: EORTC QLQ-LC13, FACT-L, quality of Life, lung cancer, FACT-G, EORTC QLQ-C30, oncology

INTRODUCTION

In 2012, 160,340 Americans were expected to die from lung cancer; this accounted for 28 percent of all cancer deaths (1). In this patient population, treatment can depend on the stage of the cancer, the age of the patient, possible side effects of treatment, the patient's preferences and overall health. Treatment choices may include chemotherapy, radiation therapy and surgery (2).

Quality of life (QOL) is defined as the personal satisfaction of a patient with how he or she feels and lives (3). In general, QOL aspects consist of physical, social/family, emotional, and functional well-being (4). In cancer patients, QOL is regularly assessed through quantitative questionnaires. These assessments are typically completed by the patient themselves or occasionally via a proxy (5). In general, QOL assessment has the potential to impact clinical decision-making by evaluating the effectiveness of treatment (6).

Particularly in the advanced cancer setting, assessment of patient-reported outcomes such as QOL can be used to evaluate treatment efficacy or be part of a composite endpoint to demonstrate clinical benefit (4).

Two widely utilized QOL questionnaires for cancer patients are the European Organisation for Research and Treatment of Cancer (EORTC) Quality of Life Questionnaire C30 (QLQ-C30) and the Functional Assessment of Cancer Therapy-General (FACT-G). It is important to compare the various features of these two questionnaires, as they are two of the most widely used and well-validated tools in the assessment of QOL in lung cancer patients.

The FACT-G (now version 4) is a 27-item compilation of general questions divided into four primary QOL domains: physical (PWB), social/family (SWB), emotional (EWB), and functional well-being (FWB). The EORTC QLQ-C30 comprises several solitary items and nine multi-item scales: five functional scales, three symptom scales, a global health and quality-of-life scale and an additional six single items.

These questionnaires can be completed by any cancer patient irrespective of primary cancer site. Different cancer-specific modules have been developed to supplement these core questionnaires in addressing the most relevant issues pertaining to each subset of the cancer population (7).

Lung cancer-specific questionnaires are available to supplement both the EORTC QLQ-C30 and the FACT-G. The EORTC QLQ-Lung Cancer 13 (LC13) questionnaire is a 13-item assessment tool that is coupled with the EORTC QLQ-C30, whereas the FACT-Lung (FACT-L) questionnaire combines the general FACT-G tool with an additional seven-item lung cancer-specific subscale (LCS). A third questionnaire that is sometimes used is the Lung Cancer Symptom Scale, which focuses on symptom assessment exclusively (8).

A review by Salvo et al. investigated the use of QOL instrument tools in primary lung cancer or lung metastases patients receiving palliative radiotherapy (9). The EORTC QLQ-C30 survey was the most commonly used QOL questionnaire (13 of 19 trials). Conversely, the FACT-L was used in two of the nineteen trials. Salvo et al. concluded that it is imperative that clinical trials with palliative patients also focus on QOL assessment specific to patients with lung cancer or lung metastases, especially when a cure is unattainable. When a health care professional makes the decision to evaluate QOL, the next step becomes discerning which assessment tool is most appropriate to use. In this patient population, Salvo et al. concluded that the QLQ-LC13 and the FACT-L are two recommended instruments (9).

In response to the growing recognition of the importance of QOL evaluation, knowledge of the characteristics of common tools may assist investigators and clinicians in choosing the most suitable assessment tool. The purpose of this review was to compare and contrast the development, validity, and reliability of the EORTC QLQ-LC13 and the FACT-L for the assessment of QOL in lung cancer patients.

METHODS

A literature search was conducted using Ovid MEDLINE and OLDMEDLINE (1946 to July 2013), Ovid EMBASE and EMBASE Classic (1980 to 2013 Week 28), and the Cochrane Central Register of Controlled Trials (June 2013) to identify studies that detailed the development, validity, reliability, and use of the EORTC QLQ-LC13 and the FACT-L. Search terms included subject headings and natural language keywords such as "quality of life," "questionnaire," "EORTC QLQ-LC13," "FACT-L" "survey," "instrument," "assess," "evaluation," "evaluate," "QLQ," "FACT L," "lung," "cancer," "neoplasm," and "tumor." Articles that discussed the development and/or use of at least one of these tools were included.

Only English articles were selected for potential inclusion. The following information was extracted from included studies: development, questionnaire characteristics, intended use, and reliability and validity testing (e.g., known group comparison, internal consistency, etc.).

RESULTS

Overall, there were 48 studies that were included in the search. Of these, 13 studies were included in the review.

Development

EORTC QLQ-LC13

The Quality of Life Group was first formed in 1980 by the EORTC, however it was not until 1986 that a research program was created to develop an integrated, modular approach for evaluating the QOL of patients participating in cancer clinical trials. While the long-term objective was to develop an instrument with applicability across a broad range of cancer diagnoses, it was considered appropriate to initially employ a more homogeneous patient sample for field-testing of the questionnaire. The EORTC Study Group developed a system that was focused on two basic components: 1) a core QOL questionnaire focusing on a general aspect of health-related QOL, and 2) additional lung cancer-specific modules. Over time (1987–1989 and 1990–1991), two different samples of patients with lung cancer were recruited from participating institutions in Europe, North America, Australia and Japan. In order to be eligible for both studies (hereafter referred to as studies 1 and 2) patients needed to be newly diagnosed with non-resectable lung cancer, had to plan treatment involving either chemotherapy or radiotherapy, and had to provide their informed consent (4). There were no restrictions implemented in terms of age, performance status, histological type or stage of disease. The Eastern Cooperative Oncology Group (ECOG) scale was used to measure performance status. The patients were requested to fill out the core QOL questionnaire (the EORTC QLQ-Core 36 or the QLQ-C30), which was complemented by a 13-item lung cancer-specific questionnaire module, the QLQ-LC13, at two points in time: 1. prior to the start of treatment ('pretreatment'); and 2. following the first course of radiotherapy or the second course of chemotherapy ('on-treatment'). Of 537 and 346 patients entering studies 1 and 2, respectively, 430 and 305 completed both pretreatment and on-treatment questionnaires. Thus, 17% of all patients were lost to follow-up for various reasons, including early death, disease progression and administrative failure. Withdrawal of consent was also a common reason for not completing the second questionnaire. Pretreatment performance status was significantly worse among the subgroup of patients who were lost to follow-up as compared to patients who subsequently completed the on-treatment questionnaire ($p<0.01$), which further points to poor health status as a major reason for patient attrition from the study (4).

This lung cancer-specific module was constructed in parallel with the core QLQ-C30, before the standard EORTC guidelines on module development had been established (17). It was field tested together with the previous versions of the core questionnaire (QLQ-C36 or QLQ-C30 (Version 1)) (10). Two international field studies conducted by Bergman et al. evaluated the practicality, reliability and validity of the core questionnaire supplemented by the 13-item EORTC QLQ-LC13 (4). Both questionnaires were administered to patients with non-resectable lung cancer recruited from 17 countries. In total, 883 and 735 patients, respectively, completed the questionnaire prior to and once during treatment. The symptom measures discriminated clearly between patients differing in performance status. All observed item scores changed as expected (i.e., lung cancer symptoms decreased and treatment toxicities increased) during treatment, except for one item (problems with a sore mouth). Toxicity measures changed over time, which was directly related to chemotherapy or radiotherapy. However, the single item on neuropathy, which was reported by relatively few patients, did not measure the full range of symptoms adequately (4). As this symptom typically emerges only over a longer period of time, it probably had not reached its maximum prevalence at the time of the on-treatment assessment. Despite its low prevalence, peripheral neuropathy explained a significant amount of the variance in global quality of life ratings. This is all the more striking given that the QLQ-LC13 assesses only mild complaints (i.e., tingling hands or feet). In future versions of the questionnaire, it may be useful to include additional items reflecting moderate to severe grades of neuropathy. The resulting impairment in terms of loss of feeling and strength could be expected to have even greater impact on patients' level of functioning and overall quality of life ratings.

The hypothesized scale structure of the questionnaire was partially supported by the data. The multi-item dyspnea scale met the EORTC standard for reliability testing (Cronbach's α > 0 70), while items relating to pain did not form a scale with reliability estimates acceptable for group comparisons.

In summary, the results from international field testing lend support to the EORTC QLQ-LC13 as a clinically valid and useful tool for assessing disease- and treatment-specific symptoms in lung cancer patients participating in clinical trials when combined with a core QOL questionnaire. In a few areas, however, the questionnaire could benefit from further refinements; in addition, its performance over a longer period of time still needs to be investigated (4).

FACT-L

One of the most widely used and well-validated tools developed specifically to measure the QOL of patients with lung cancer before, during, and after cancer therapy is the FACT-L questionnaire, which consists of general questions for patients with cancer (FACT-G) plus items specific to lung cancer and its associated symptoms (i.e., the LCS) (6).

The FACT-L (Version 4) is one of the newer and more comprehensive lung cancer questionnaires that has been translated to multiple languages and rigorously validated. It is widely used in clinical trials involving lung neoplasms and has high validity, reliability, internal consistency, content validity and responsiveness (11). The FACT-L estimates five concepts, four general and one lung cancer symptom-specific subscale. General subscales include PWB, SWB, EWB, and FWB. The seven-item LCS assesses symptoms commonly reported by lung cancer patients (e.g., shortness of breath; loss of weight; tightness in chest). The TOI, a measure of physical QOL in clinical trials, is derived by adding scores on the PWB and FWB subscales to the LCS.

The development of the FACT-L was first documented by Cella et al. (6). This study reported further validation data on the FACT-G with a subsample of lung cancer patients from the original publication by Cella et al. (12) and, more importantly, presented data on the Lung Cancer Subscale (LCS), which, when combined with the FACT-G, resulted in the FACT-L QOL tool (6). Patients were eligible to participate if they presented with advanced cancer, or were currently receiving chemotherapy and/or radiation. Patients unable to speak English or cognitively impaired due to CNS metastasis were not eligible for inclusion. The interview with 30 FACT-naïve lung cancer patients resulted in the generation of a 107-item pool of lung cancer items. After the 107 item pool was generated, a four-point rating of the relative importance of each potential question was obtained from 30 FACT-naïve lung cancer patients. These results were analyzed and the 107 lung questions were then further decreased to 47 which included 38 items from the first version of the FACT-G in addition to nine lung cancer-specific items of the preliminary LCS. This 47-item questionnaire became the FACT-L version 1.

Version 2 of the FACT-L was developed after reliability and validity testing of 854 patients was performed on the 38-item FACT-G version 1 (6). This process yielded a 43-item FACT-L version 2, which comprised 33 items from the FACT-G and an additional 10 items from the LCS. Version 2 of the FACT-L was then updated to a third version, which comprised 44 items (6). Although minor, changes that were performed from version 2 to version 3 included the rewording of some items to improve clarity and the addition of one item. Also important in the development of version 3 was that the FACT-G showed extensive cross-cultural endorsement after being tested on 92 Spanish-speaking patients from the United States and Puerto Rico.

Questionnaire characteristics

A direct comparison of the two questionnaires in terms of characteristics can be seen in Table 1. The EORTC QLQ-LC13 is to be used alongside the EORTC QLQ-C30, whereas the FACT-L incorporates both the core FACT-G as well as a LCS. The EORTC QLQ-C30 is a 30-item questionnaire, while the QLQ-LC13 + C30 are a total of 43 items. Conversely, the FACT-G is a 27-item questionnaire, and the FACT-L contains 36 items (6).

The QLQ-LC13 is meant for use among a wide range of lung cancer patients who often vary in disease stage and treatment modality (4).

Table 1. Comparison of the European Organization for Research and Treatment of Cancer Quality of Life Questionnaire for Patients with Lung Cancer and the Functional Assessment of the Cancer Therapy Quality of Life Measurement in Patients with Lung Cancer

Characteristic	EORTC QLQ-LC13	FACT-L
Purpose	Measure the QOL of lung cancer patients	Measure the QOL of lung cancer patients
Number of items on core questionnaire + number of items on supplement	With QLQ-C30: 30+13	27+9
Response options	Likert Scale (1–4 inclusive)	Likert Scale (0–4 inclusive)
Recall period	Past 7 days	Past 7 days
Item format	Questions	Statements
Item organization	Grouped into subscales	Not grouped
Assessed subscales	Dyspnea, Pain (Chest, Arm/Shoulder, Other), Coughing, Sore Mouth, Dysphagia, Peripheral Neuropathy, Alopecia, Hemoptysis	Physical Well-Being; Social Well-Being; Emotional Well-Being; Functional Well-Being; and Lung Cancer Subscales
Subscale components	Multi-item subscales only	No subscales
Scoring	All scaled scores are converted to a 0–100 scale with higher scores representing worse symptoms	A summed score of all items ranging from 0–28 with higher scores representing better QOL

EORTC: European Organisation for Research and Treatment of Cancer; FACT-L: Functional Assessment of Cancer Therapy Quality of Life Measurement in Patients with Lung Cancer; FACT-G: Functional Assessment of Quality of Life Measurement-General; QLQ; Quality of Life Questionnaire; QLQ LC-13: Quality of Life Questionnaire for patients with lung cancer; QOL: Quality of life.

The lung cancer module comprises both multi-item and single-item measures of lung cancer-associated symptoms (i.e., coughing, hemoptysis, dyspnea and pain) and side effects from conventional chemotherapy and radiotherapy (i.e., hair loss, neuropathy, sore mouth and dysphagia). All EORTC questionnaires have a recall period of the previous week and use a Likert scale from 1 ("not at all") to 4 ("very much") for the patients' response. Along with the functional scales assessed by the core instrument, the QLQ-LC13 allows for assessment of dyspnea and pain, coughing, sore mouth, peripheral neuropathy, alopecia and hemoptysis via single-item scales. Total scores are then converted to a 0-100 scale, with higher scores representing greater severity for symptom scales or better functioning in functional scales (4).

The FACT-L is currently in version 4 and contains a 7-item lung-cancer specific subscale and the 27-item core FACT-G questionnaire which assesses physical well-being, social well-being, emotional well-being, functional well-being, and lung cancer-specific items including shortness of breath and breathing, weight loss, cough, and appetite. All items are scored from 0 ("not at all") to 4 ("very much"). The FACT-L subscale is reported as a composite score of the FACT-G plus the LCS. The items are formatted in statements and, while they are grouped into subscales for the FACT-G, items of the LCS are not grouped. The recall period for the questionnaire is the past week.

Validity and reliability

EORTC QLQ-LC13

The EORTC-QLQ-LC13 has proven to be a valid and reliable psychometric instrument to assess health-related QOL as an outcome measure in clinical trials of patients with lung cancer. Besides a range of detailed items, it includes two Likert scales (questions 29 and 30) to capture a patient's assessment of physical condition and overall quality of life (13).

A study was conducted to investigate the information the instrument elicits to obtain a meaningful overall QOL measure useful for economic evaluations and which may be more sensitive than the original Likert scales. The principal data set for model development comprised 330 EORTC QLQ-C30 + QLQ-LC13 responses completed by 91 small-cell lung cancer patients as part of the MRC LU-16 trial of palliative chemotherapy (13). The clinical characteristics of patients at randomization were similar to those for the whole trial: 34 patients (38%) were classified with limited disease, and 55 (62%) with extensive disease (2 unknown); initial performance status was rated as moderate in 56 patients (62%), poor in 33 (36%) or very poor in 2 (2%). In the completed forms, questions in the common core (numbers 1–31) exhibited very high response rates, averaging 99.2% with no question achieving less than 97.9%. The supplementary lung cancer section (LC13), was slightly less successful with an average completion rate of 96.1% and the worst question answered on only 90% of forms (question 42: 'pain in other parts of body') (13).

Bergman et al. (4) tested the validity of the EORTC QLQ-LC13 in two studies (n=883 and 735 patients) through several methods. Clinical validity was evaluated by known group comparison, with internal consistency estimates using Cronbach's α ≥0.70 considered acceptable. This examined the questionnaire's ability to distinguish between subgroups of patients formed on the basis of clinical measures, including ECOG performance status, stage of disease, World Health Organization toxicity ratings, and treatment modality. It was found that the four-item dyspnea scale met minimal standards for reliability (Cronbach's alpha coefficient = 0.85), while items related to pain did not form a scale with reliability estimates acceptable for group comparisons. However, when pain items were assessed after combination with QLQ-C30 items relating to pain, the alpha coefficient improved, indicating that the QLQ-LC13 items on pain were correlated better to the general questionnaire pain items as opposed to each other.

Factorial analysis of variance (ANOVA) was employed to test for statistical significance of group differences. Repeated measures ANOVA was used to test for the statistical significance of QLQ-LC13 score changes as a function of observed changes in performance status. Changes in QLQ-LC13 scores over time were calculated and tested for statistical significance by means of repeated ANOVA. Consistent with both studies, poorer performance status was significantly related to increased symptom score levels for dyspnea. At the same time, there were statistically significant differences in pain scores in different groups of performance status. In one study, patients with metastases reported higher scores on pain items when compared with patients with local disease.

The responsiveness of the questionnaire to changes in health status over time was also evaluated. While there is no 'objective' clinical measure of global health status, performance status was considered as a reasonable substitute for such a measure (4).

When comparing pre-treatment QLQ-LC13 scores to on-treatment results, all symptom scores significantly decreased, as expected. As hypothesized, QLQ-LC13 scores concerned with treatment-related side effects, such as trouble swallowing, neuropathy and hair loss, increased significantly from pre-treatment to on-treatment assessment.

The relationship between treatment and side-effect scores over time was evaluated similarly, employing a repeated measures ANOVA with treatment modality as the grouping factor (chemotherapy versus radiotherapy; 19 patients with combined treatment were excluded from this analysis). Significant increases in hair loss and peripheral neuropathy were noted for those patients undergoing chemotherapy, while increasing difficulties with swallowing were reported primarily by patients receiving radiotherapy ($P < 0.001$ for both analyses). Self-reported on-treatment QLQ-LC13 side-effects were also compared with the corresponding physicians' ratings on the WHO toxicity scales. Correlations ranged from 0.19 for oral toxicity to 0.73 for hair loss, all statistically significant $P < 0.001$) (4).

As measured by the QLQ-LC13, the relative contribution of various disease and treatment-related symptoms towards explaining the variance in global QOL ratings derived from the core EORTC QLQ-C30 was examined by a stepwise multiple regression analysis (4). Twenty-five percent of the variance in pre-treatment QOL scores were explained by hemoptysis, effort dyspnea, trouble with swallowing, and pain in various sites (multiple $R = 0.50$).

In summary, the EORTC QLQ-LC13 has proven to be a valid and reliable psychometric instrument in the assessment of health-related QOL as an outcome measure in clinical trials of lung cancer (4).

FACT-L

Validation of the FACT-L was documented in a study conducted by Cella et al. (6). The FACT-L was administered to 116 patients with lung cancer and the samples were pooled for reliability and correlation analysis to derive the most stable coefficients possible. Coefficient alpha of the 9-item subscale, an indicator of uni-dimensionality, was found to be a dissatisfying 0.53. Internal consistency testing was performed, which is important for scale reliability and homogeneity of the questionnaire. Internal consistency was improved from 0.53 to 0.68 by dropping the hair loss and regret about smoking items of the LCS, resulting in a 7-item subscale. A subset of 41 patients was tested again at 2 months to evaluate sensitivity to change in Performance Status Rating (PSR) and to obtain estimates of a clinically meaningful change score for the FACT-G and the 7-item LCS. In the study, the correlation of the PSR was obtained as it is a well-known indicator of functionality status. The FACT-G and the 7-item LCS were able to classify patients according to their functional impairment (p=0.03). For the PSR, the physical well-being subscale (P = 0.02) and the LCS (P = 0.03) were statistically significant, while the functional well-being was statistically non-significant (P = 0.05). A 21-item TOI, combining scores on PWB, FWB and LCS, was highly reliable (coefficient α = 0.89) and sensitive to change in PSR (P = 0.01). This TOI is probably the most relevant and precise indicator of patient-reported QOL available for lung cancer patients who complete the FACT-L while participating in an oncology clinical trial.

To determine whether a correlation exists between changes in LCS and TOI scores and clinical response, LCS and TOI changes from baseline to 12 weeks were compared across best overall response to treatment (complete or partial response, stable disease, progressive disease). One-way ANCOVAs were performed with baseline PSR, weight loss, and number of primary metastatic symptoms as covariates. It was found that patients showing a complete or partial response had more positive changes than patients showing progressive disease (P <0 .01).

Numerous clinical trials have used the FACT-L to analyze the relationships between changes in QOL and symptoms and their correlation with tumor response and survival. In a phase II trial, 63 patients with advanced NSCLC were treated with carboplatin and paclitaxel (14). The FACT-L questionnaire was administered at baseline and at cycles 1/2, 3/4, and 5/6 in 44 (70%), 33 (52%), 34 (54%), and 18 (29%) patients, respectively. Pretreatment FACT-L scores failed to predict survival but were strongly predictive of both objective tumor response and disease control for all of the subscales (including the TOI; *P* =0 .0004), with the exception of functional well-being. The efficacy of therapy was the main determinant of FACT-L scores, which were minimally affected by the neurotoxic side effects associated with this chemotherapy regimen.

In another phase II study of 54 patients with advanced NSCLC who were treated with carboplatin/paclitaxel, the FACT-L questionnaire was completed before each cycle of chemotherapy (14). Patients who responded to treatment had higher baseline TOI scores compared with those who did not respond (64.9 versus 59.0, respectively). Between chemotherapy cycles 1 and 4, responders had a mean increase of 4.7 points in TOI score, whereas non-responders had a mean decrease of 5.6 points. Furthermore, the baseline mean

FACT-L score appeared to correlate with survival: 61.7 points for those patients who exceeded the median survival time, and 56.1 points for those who did not. However, QOL scores fluctuated throughout treatment as sample size decreased because of treatment failure, making it difficult to determine the relationship between survival and baseline QOL on the FACT-L. In addition to the relationship with treatment response, QOL as measured by the FACT-L also had a significant correlation with anemia (r = 0.38; *P* ≤0 .02).

A study by Tester et al. found that baseline FACT-L scores were valuable in predicting the likelihood of a tumor response but not in predicting disease progression (15). Furthermore, in this small phase II trial of paclitaxel monotherapy for 20 patients with advanced NSCLC, QOL improvements appeared to correlate with tumor responses. As expected, non-responding patients generally had deteriorating FACT-L scores as their disease worsened. However, improved scores were recorded for four patients with SD and two patients with disease progression, suggesting that in some cases chemotherapy can lead to symptom relief and QOL improvement in the absence of an objective tumor response.

In 2002, Cella et al. aimed to determine an accurate estimate of the point change on the LCS and TOI that was required to constitute a clinically meaningful change (16). The LCS and the TOI of the FACT-L were chosen because they depicted more clinically relevant QOL endpoints in lung cancer trials. Data was extracted from an ECOG randomized trial analyzing various chemotherapy regimens in 599 non-small cell lung cancer patients. Baseline differences in clinical parameters were used to identify upper limits for clinically meaningful change. Their analyses suggested that a two- to three-point difference on the LCS and a five- to seven-point difference on the TOI approximated clinically meaningful changes.

The LCS has been rigorously tested for clinical relevance and validity in patients with advanced lung cancer. When tested for construct validity, the LCS had a high correlation with closely related instruments, such as the Functional Living Index–Cancer, and the physical well-being and functional well-being subscales of the FACT-L. In addition, the LCS is sensitive to change in disease status over time. When tested for its sensitivity to change in patient clinical status, change in LCS was significantly related to change in PS ($P < 0.03$). The mean change in the LCS was a 2 point increase for patients with improved PS, a 0.5 point decrease for those with no change, and a 2.8 point decrease for those with a decline in PS. The TOI was also found to be highly reliable and sensitive to change in PS ($P < 0 .01$). These encouraging results have led to the inclusion of the LCS and FACT-L in many clinical trials as one of the instruments of choice for measuring symptoms and HRQOL as an endpoint.

DISCUSSION

QOL is often a factor that is overlooked by physicians in severe diseases such as lung cancer. The common focus of eliminating patients' physical symptoms and on tracing the source of the problem has the potential to sometimes neglect other aspects of patients' lives. When illness is life threatening, as in cancer, then most attention is focused on the physical condition of the patient. However, in the case of lung cancer, the effectiveness of radical treatment of the disease remains dramatically limited and expected survival is still short. Therefore, in this case, there is urgent need to improve the QOL of these patients (9).

Clinical trials in lung cancer patients have historically focused on survival and/or disease progression. However, QOL is an increasingly meaningful endpoint in this patient population. In addition to general QOL questionnaires, disease-specific questionnaires have been developed and are frequently used to provide more targeted assessments of QOL in a spectrum of lung cancer patients. Namely, the EORTC QLQ-LC13 and the FACT-L are two widely used instruments. At present, the EORTC QLQ-LC13 seems to be the more often used instrument in randomized controlled NSCLC trials (4). Since 2002, 57% of trials have used this tool, while 36% of use the questionnaires from the FACT group (4).

The EORTC QLQ-C30 along with its 13-item lung cancer module is a comprehensive assessment for QOL in lung cancer. However, its length (43 items) can sometimes be a burden for patients to complete. This becomes particularly important over time on a study, as burden of the questionnaire length may be increased. The FACT-L, which was derived from the more general cancer QOL instrument, the FACT-G, is a 36-item, lung cancer-specific QOL instrument that also includes the symptom-based LCS. The FACT-L is self-reported, and has been thoroughly tested for translational accuracy in many languages and modified for language-based cultural differences (8).

For the EORTC questionnaires, the number of items on the core questionnaire plus the number of items on the EORTC QLQ-LC13 is 43; in comparison, the FACT-L only has 36 items (Table 1). In terms of questionnaire characteristics, there are some subtle differences between the two sets of modules. The two questionnaires differ in response options: the EORTC QLQ-LC13 has a Likert scale of 1–4, compared to the FACT-L, which uses a Likert scale of 0–4. In both questionnaires, the recall period is the past 7 days. However, in the EORTC QLQ-LC13 the item format is in questions and is grouped into subscales whereas in the FACT-L the item format is in statements and items are not grouped. In both questionnaires, there are multi-item subscales only. The scoring is different in the two questionnaires: in the EORTC QLQ-LC13, all scale scores are converted to a 0–100 scale with higher scores representing worse symptoms; conversely, a simple summation is used for the FACT-L with higher scores representing better QOL (4, 6).

The development of the QLQ-LC13 was performed in two studies with two different samples of patients with lung cancer from participating institutions in Europe, North America, Australia and Japan. It was field tested together with the previous versions of the core questionnaire (QLQ-C36, QLQ-C30 (V1)) and according to strict EORTC procedures and review from the EORTC executive committee (4). Two international field studies conducted by Bergman et al. evaluated the practicality, reliability and validity of the QLQ-C30 questionnaire supplemented by the 13-item EORTC QLQ-LC13. The questionnaire was administered to patients with non-resectable lung cancer recruited from 17 countries. In total, 883 and 735 patients, respectively, completed the questionnaire prior to and once during treatment. The symptom measures discriminated clearly between patients differing in performance status. In comparison, version 1 of the FACT-L was developed in a study consisting of 45 patients and 15 health professionals. These individuals were given an in-depth interview to develop a large pool of questions (6). Testing for reliability and validity were also conducted for the FACT-L version 1 with 854 patients and a 33-item version 2 was created (6). The FACT-L (version 2) was updated to version 3, a 44-item version in 1994. The seven LCS questions were administered along with the FACT-G to 116 patients with lung cancer (6). Both questionnaires are currently in version 4.

Additionally, both instruments have acceptable validity. Clinical validity of the QLQ-LC13 was evaluated by known groups comparison. Change in QLQ-LC13 scores over time was calculated and tested for statistical significance by means of repeated ANOVA. The responsiveness of the questionnaire to changes in health status over time was also evaluated. In both EORTC questionnaires, the way in which they are validated is through changes of the questions and content through experience.

For the FACT-L, internal consistency testing was performed. Internal consistency had to be improved from 0.53 to 0.68 by dropping two questions, which boosted the alpha coefficient. PSR was also obtained because it is a well-known indicator of patient functionality status. The 21-item TOI, which combined scores on PWB, FWB and LCS, was highly reliable (coefficient $\alpha=0.89$) and sensitive to change in PSR ($P = 0.01$) (6). The use of the FACT-L in numerous clinical trials has validated its ability to measure symptoms (using the LCS) and QOL (from TOI and full FACT-L scores) in patients with lung cancer and to provide a valuable endpoint for clinical trials. The different FACT-L subscales allow QOL to be broken down into its various components for analysis. The FACT-L scores have been reproducible and sensitive to change, and they correlate with type and severity of treatment-related toxicities. With few exceptions, pretreatment scores, as well as changing scores during and after therapy, have been independently predictive of survival and objective response to treatment. The choice of FACT-L as a tool for evaluation in clinical trials of targeted agents in lung cancer allows for informative comparisons to be made between treatment regimens. It also assures a reliable and proven format for measurement of patient-reported outcomes. In addition to objective tumor response, QOL and symptom improvement are important goals in the treatment of patients with lung cancer (9).

Based upon their respective studies, both the EORTC QLQ-LC13 and the FACT-L have been found to be valid and reliable in assessing the QOL of lung cancer patients. The EORTC QLQ-LC13 has been found to have a larger body of evidence than the FACT-L. The literature pertaining to both the EORTC QLQ-LC13 and the FACT-L in lung cancer English-speaking populations has shown good psychometric properties. Both questionnaires have undergone extensive development and validation, and both questionnaires have been proven to be valid internationally (4, 6).

Clinical trials in lung cancer should continue to assess QOL to determine clinical benefits through analyzing patient-reported outcomes. Both the EORTC QLQ-LC13 and FACT-L allow this type of study which is very important in order for physicians and other health-care professionals to accurately assess the improvement or deterioration of a patient based upon their change in QOL. Currently, the EORTC QLQ-LC13 is being revised to ensure it captures all new therapies and treatments, given that these have changed to some degree in the last two decades.

This revision process will require complete review of the module and will follow specified EORTC module development procedures for updating a module (18). Relevance to thoracic surgery and new targeted therapies and applicability in both non-metastatic and metastatic patients are some areas currently being explored by the EORTC in their revisions. Further, any changes that will be made to the module will ensure that a sufficient level of comparability exists so that the results can be generalizable between the existing module and any future revised tools.

Conclusion

In closing, the choice between instruments ultimately remains on the design and goals of the study. However, it is the hope that the current article will provide healthcare professionals with a comparison of the QLQ-LC13 and the FACT-L in order to assist with clinical decision-making. The EORTC QLQ-LC13 is currently undergoing phase III testing to ensure applicability of the module to diverse patient populations in lung cancer. To our knowledge, authors of the FACT-L have not disclosed any intention to update the FACT-L from its current version. Once the QLQ-LC13 has finalized its update process according to EORTC procedures, an updated comparative review of both modules will be warranted.

ACKNOWLEDGMENTS

We thank the generous support of Bratty Family Fund, Michael and Karyn Goldstein Cancer Research Fund, Pulenzas Cancer Research Fund, Joseph and Silvana Melara Cancer Research Fund, and Ofelia Cancer Research Fund.

REFERENCES

[1] American Lung Association. Lung cancer fact sheet [Internet]. Chicago: American Lung Association; 2013. URL: http://www.lung.org/lung-disease/lung-cancer/resources/facts-figures/lung-cancer-fact-sheet.html.

[2] Aaronson NK, Ahmedzai S, Bergman B, Bullinger M, Cull A, Duez NJ, et al. The European Organization for Research and Treatment of Cancer QLQ-C30: a quality-of-life Instrument for use in international clinical trials in oncology. J Natl Cancer Inst 1993;85:365-76.

[3] Wong J, Hird A, Kirou–Mauro A, Napolskikh J, Chow E. Quality of life in brain metastases radiation trials: a literature review. Curr Oncol 2008;15(5):25-45.

[4] Bergman B, Aaronson NK, Ahmedzai S, Kaasa S, Sullivan M. The EORTC QLQ-LC13: a modular supplement to the EORTC core quality of life questionnaire (QLQ-C30) for use in lung cancer clinical trials. Eur J Cancer 1994;30A(5):635-42.

[5] National Institutes of Health. Lung cancer [Internet]. Bethesda: U.S. National Library of Medicine 2013. URL: http://www.nlm.nih.gov/medlineplus/lungcancer.html.

[6] Cella DF, Bonomi AE, Lloyd SR, Tulsky DS, Kaplan E, Bonomi P. Reliability and validity of the Functional Assessment of Cancer Therapy-Lung (FACT-L) quality of life instrument. Lung Cancer 1995;12(3):199-220.

[7] Kemmler G, Holzner B, Kopp M, Dunser M, Margreiter R, Greil R, et al. Comparison of two quality-of-life instruments for cancer patients: the Functional Assessment of Cancer Therapy-General and the European Organization for Research and Treatment of Cancer Quality of Life Questionnaire-C30. J Clin Oncol 1999;17:2932-40.

[8] Cella D. The Functional Assessment of Cancer Therapy–Lung and Lung Cancer Subscale assess quality of life and meaningful symptom improvement in lung cancer Semin Oncol 2004;31(suppl 9):11-5.

[9] Salvo N, Hadi S, Napolskikh J, Goh P, Sinclair E, Chow E. Quality of life measurement in cancer patients receiving palliative radiotherapy for symptomatic lung cancer: a literature review. Curr Oncol 2009;16(2):16-28.

[10] Chie WC, Yang CH, Hsu C, Yang PC. Quality of life of lung cancer patients: validation of the Taiwan Chinese version of the EORTC QLQ-C30 and QLQ-LC13. Qual Life Res 2004;13(1):257-62.

[11] Butt Z, Webster K, Eisenstein AR, Beaumont J, Eton D, Masters GA, et al. Quality of life in lung cancer: the validity and cross-cultural applicability of the Functional Assessment of Cancer Therapy-Lung scale. Hematol Oncol Clin North Am 2005;19:389-420.

[12] Cella DF, Tulsky DS, Gray G, Sarafian B, Linn E, Bonomi A, et al. The Functional Assessment of Cancer Therapy (FACT) scale: development and validation of the general measure. J Clin Oncol 1993;11(3):570-9.

[13] Bagust A, Barraza-Llorens M, Philips Z. Deriving a compound quality of life measure from the EORTC-QLQ-C30/LC13 instrument for use in economic evaluations of lung cancer clinical trials. Eur J Cancer 2001;37(9):1081-8.

[14] Heyes A. Clinical trial experience with Functional Assessment of Cancer Therapy–Lung in conventional and targeted non–small cell lung cancer therapy. Semin Oncol 2004;31(3 Suppl 9):16-22.

[15] Tester WJ, Jin PY, Reardon DH, Cohn JB, Cohen MH. Phase II study of patients with metastatic nonsmall cell carcinoma of the lung treated with paclitaxel by 3-hour infusion. Cancer 1997;79(4):724-9.

[16] Cella D, Eton DT, Fairclough DL, Bonomi P, Heyes AE, Silberman C, et al. What is a clinically meaningful change on that functional assessment of cancer therapy-lung (FACT-L) questionnaire? J Clin Epidemiol 2002;55(3):285-95.

[17] Blazeby J, Cull A, Groenvold M, Bottomley A. Guidelines for developing quality of life questionnaires, 3rd ed. Brussels: European Organisation for Research and Treatment of Cancer Publications, 2001.

[18] Koller M. Modules in development [Internet]. Brussels: European Organisation for Research and Treatment of Cancer Quality of Life Department; 2014. URL: http://groups.eortc.be/qol/modules-development.

Submitted: January 12, 2015. *Revised:* February 06, 2015. *Accepted:* February 12, 2015.

In Pain Management Yearbook 2015
Editor: Joav Merrick

ISBN: 978-1-63484-515-1

Chapter 12

A MULTIDISCIPLINARY BONE METASTASES CLINIC AT SUNNYBROOK ODETTE CANCER CENTRE: A REVIEW OF THE EXPERIENCE FROM 2009-2014

Selina Chow, Rachel McDonald, BSc(C), Albert Yee, MD, Joel Finkelstein, MD, Michael Ford, MD, Elizabeth David, MD, Natalie Pulenzas, BSc(C), Ronald Chow, Carlo DeAngelis, DPharm, and Edward Chow*, MBBS

Bone Metastases Site Group, Odette Cancer Centre,
Sunnybrook Health Sciences Centre, University of Toronto,
Toronto, Ontario, Canada

The objective of this study was to review Sunnybrook Odette Cancer Centre's Bone Metastases Clinic (BMC) – a one-stop clinic which provides a coordinated multidisciplinary approach to the care of cancer patients with metastatic bone disease. Patients with symptomatic bone metastases are referred to the BMC and evaluated by a team of specialists in various disciplines, including orthopedic surgery, radiation therapy, radiation oncology and interventional radiology. At initial consultation, patient demographics, reasons for referral, and case disposition were recorded. From January 2009 to December 2014, a total of 431 patients with bone metastases were referred to the BMC. The median age was 66 years (range 34-94 years) and median Karnofsky Performance Score was 70 (range 30-100). The majority of patients came from home (95%), while others came from a hospital (4%). Approximately a quarter (26%) of patients had 2 or more reasons for referral, yielding a total of 542 reasons. The predominant reason for referral was bone or neuropathic pain (52%), followed by pathological fracture (18%) and impending fracture (15%). Out of 431 patients, 428 case dispositions were recorded; 20% of patients required further investigation and/or imaging, 18% received palliative radiation, 13% were offered surgery and 13% were

* Correspondence: Professor Edward Chow MBBS, MSc, PhD, FRCPC, Department of Radiation Oncology, Odette Cancer Centre, Sunnybrook Health Sciences Centre, 2075 Bayview Avenue, Toronto, Ontario, M4N 3M5, Canada. E-mail: edward.chow@sunnybrook.ca.

referred to other supportive care services. A multidisciplinary clinic is beneficial for managing patients with bone metastases to allow for comprehensive assessment and treatment.

Keywords: bone metastases, multidisciplinary approach

INTRODUCTION

In 2014, it is estimated that there will be 191,300 new cases of cancer and 76,600 deaths from cancer in Canada (1). Metastases to bone are a frequent complication of cancer; in particular, breast, lung, prostate, thyroid, and renal cancers are the most common to develop skeletal metastases (2).

In January 1999, the Division of Orthopedics at Sunnybrook Health Sciences Centre and the Rapid Response Radiotherapy Program at Sunnybrook Odette Cancer Centre established a first-of-its-kind clinic in Canada, called the Bone Metastases Clinic (BMC). The clinic aims to offer coordinated, multidisciplinary care for patients suffering from symptomatic bone metastases. This multidisciplinary service saves the patient time and effort that would otherwise be expended during separate, sequential visits to various specialists for consultation (3).

Since the inception of the BMC in 1999, two reviews have previously been reported regarding our experience during 1999 to 2005 and 2006 to 2008. From 1999 to 2005, a total of 272 patients were consulted at the BMC (4). The second review of the BMC from 2006 to 2008 recorded a total of 254 patients (5). The objective of this paper was to update our experience at the BMC in the past 6 years (from 2009 to 2014).

METHODS

The BMC is managed by a diverse team in various specialties, including orthopedic surgery, radiation therapy, radiation oncology, interventional radiology, and a research team with the on-call support from nursing and palliative specialty. The clinic occurs every second and fourth Friday each month (3). For referral to the BMC, a pathological diagnosis of cancer and documentation of bone metastatic disease either by pathological confirmation, clinical examination, or imaging are required. The referrals can come from both our own cancer centre and the community hospitals. Additionally, referrals are triaged so that urgent cases, such as new pathological fractures and spinal cord compressions, are directed to the on-call surgical team right away.

A prospective database has been established for patients referred for assessment to the BMC since January 1999. During the initial consultation, patient demographics, cancer history, disease status, and symptom profiles were collected and recorded in the database. Site of bone metastases and the risk of fractures at the first visit were also assessed and recorded. The functional status of the patient was scored as follows: normal with pain free use of the extremity and spine, normal use with pain, significant limited use (e.g., use of prosthesis, walker, cane, crutches, and sling), and nonfunctional extremity/spine (wheelchair bound, bedridden).

Patients were assessed by an orthopedic surgeon, a radiation oncologist, and a radiation therapist at the consultation. The team then made a collective recommendation based on their assessments. If the patient was regarded as a candidate for percutaneous vertebroplasty or cementoplasty, an interventional radiologist was consulted.

RESULTS

From January 2009 to December 2014, a total of 431 patients with bone metastases were referred to the BMC. One hundred and eighty-seven patients were male (43%) and 244 were female (57%). Their median age was 66 years (range 34-94 years). The three most common primary cancer sites were breast (33%), lung (20%), and prostate (16%). The median Karnofsky Performance Score (KPS) at initial consultation was 70 (range 30-100). The majority of patients arrived from home (95%) while only 4% came from a hospital. There were a total of 542 reasons for referral recorded and a quarter of patients (26%) had 2 or more reasons for referral. The top three reasons for referral were bone and neuropathic pain (52%), pathological fracture (18%), and impending fracture (15%) (see Table 1).

Assessment

During the initial consultation with the patient, the functional status of the affected extremity/spine, the presence or risk of fractures, and the severity of the risk was recorded. The report was completed in 85% of the referred patients (n = 366). The majority of patients experienced normal use with pain (43%), followed by significant limited use (31%), and normal, pain free use of extremity/spine (20%). Only 5% of patients had complete nonfunctional use of the extremity/spine.

Eighty-eight patients (24%) were referred with pathological fractures. When assessed for risk of fractures, 20% of patients had a high risk of fractures at initial consultation. The details of the fracture risks are listed in Table 2. For patients with spinal metastases, five were referred with spinal cord compression, four had either cauda equine syndrome or nerve root deficits, and 20 presented with mechanical instability.

Case dispositions and recommendations

Of the 431 patients who received assessments, 428 case dispositions were recorded. Eighty-six patients (20%) required further investigation and/or imaging, 18% received palliative radiation, 13% were offered surgery, and 13% were referred to other supportive care services, and 36% received other recommendations (see Table 3).

Table 1. Patient Characteristics (n = 431)

		n	%
Age (Years)			
Median (Range)		66 (34-94)	
Karnofsky Performance Score			
Median (Range)		70 (30-100)	
Sex			
	Male	187	43
	Female	244	57
Primary Cancer Site			
	Breast	144	33
	Lung	85	20
	Prostate	67	16
	Renal cell	40	9
	Multiple myeloma	27	6
	Unknown	12	3
	Others	56	13
Locations where Patients Came From			
	Hospital	17	4
	Home	410	95
	Nursing home	4	1
Appointment Type			
	New patient	14	3
	Special	354	82
	Follow-up	63	15
Reason(s) for Referral*			
	Pain		
	Bone pain	209	48
	Neuropathic pain	16	4
	Fracture		
	Pathological fracture	76	18
	Impending fracture	64	15
	Abnormal diagnostic Imaging	53	12
	Review recent imaging	34	8
	Assess need for more treatment	22	5
	Assess progression of disease	11	3
	Post-surgery	8	2
	Spinal cord compression	1	0.2

Note: *some patients had more than one reason for referral.

Table 2. Orthopedic Assessment (n = 366)

		n	%
Functional Status of Extremity/Spine			
	Normal, pain-free use	75	20
	Normal use with pain	157	43
	Significant limited use	114	31
	Nonfunctional	20	5
Presence of Fracture			
	Compression	5	1
	Pathological	88	24
	Wedge	12	3
	Impending	1	0.3
Fracture Risk Assessment (Limbs)			
	Low risk	117	32
	Medium risk	1	0.3
	High risk	75	20
Extremities Risks (Weight Bearing Limbs)			
	50-74% cortex involved	13	4
	≥75% cortex involved	2	0.5
	Lytic lesion 2.5 to 5 cm in size	11	3
	Lytic lesion ≥ 5 cm in size	11	3
	Sub-trochanteric region of femur	9	2
Spinal Risks			
	Spinal cord compression	5	1
	Cauda equine syndrome OR ≥ 2 nerve root deficits	4	1
	Mechanical instability	20	5

Table 3. Case Disposition and Treatment Recommendation(s) (n = 428)

	n	%
Further investigation and imaging	86	20
Inappropriate referral	8	2
No action	123	29
Offered surgery	54	13
Palliative radiation	79	18
Referred for vertebroplasty	17	4
Referred to palliative care	4	0.9
Other supportive care services	57	13

DISCUSSION

From the initial set up of the BMC in 1999 until 2005, a total of 272 patients were seen (4). The median age was 65 years (range 28-95) and median KPS score at initial consultation was

60 (range 30-90 years) (4). During the years of 2006 to 2008, 254 patients with bone metastases were referred to the BMC. The median age was 64 years (range 29-94 years) and median KPS score was 70 (range 10-100) (5). These figures from the previous reviews of the BMC were very similar to the current review. The most common primary cancer sites in patients have been very consistent throughout the years as well; the most common and second most common primary sites during all time periods were breast and lung cancer, respectively. Prostate cancer was the third most common primary site from 1999-2005 (11%) and 2009-2014 (16%), while renal cell carcinoma was the third most common primary site from 2006-2008 (17%).

The percentage of patients seen who had two or more reasons for referral in this review (26%) was fairly similar to that throughout 1999 to 2005 (28%). In contrast, only 16% of patients from 2006 to 2008 had two or more reasons for referral. The most common reasons for referral in the first review were bone pain (42%), bone metastases (21%), high risk for pathological fracture (12%), and pathological fracture (10%) (4). In the second review, they were bone pain (69%), pathological fracture (10%), and impending fracture (8%) (5). Bone pain has remained as the prevalent reason for referral to the BMC in the past six years (52%), as well as pathological fracture (18%), and impending fracture (15%).

Of the 272 patients consulted at the BMC during the initial seven years, 40% of patients received palliative radiotherapy, 19% underwent surgery, 7% were referred to other support services such as palliative care and physiotherapy, and 7% required further investigation and/or imaging (4). In the following three years, 28% of the 254 patients who were assessed in BMC received palliative radiation, 15% were offered surgery, 20% needed further investigation and/or imaging, and 17% were referred to other support services (5). Our latest current review had 18% referred for palliative radiotherapy, 13% for surgery, 4% for interventional radiology, 20% for further investigation and 13% for other supportive care services.

When the total patient population examined from 1999 to 2005 (n=272), 2006 to 2008 (n=254), and 2009 to 2014 (n=431) are compared, it is apparent that the BMC has significantly increased in the amount of work in the most recent six years than its initial seven years. This is indicative of the continual awareness and need for multidisciplinary care in this group of patients. It is probable that the number of referrals to the BMC will remain constant.

The Odette Cancer Centre BMC clearly reveals that its integrated approach to the care of bone metastases patients enables more streamlined care, along with the elimination of inconveniences associated with separate visits to a variety of specialists for consultation. Patients seen at the BMC experience a multidisciplinary assessment to determine the best course of action in order to maximize the benefits and palliate present symptoms. This structure not only facilitates communication between the patient and multiple specialists in a one stop shopping scenario but it also allows for enhanced communication among the specialists themselves. The increased awareness of different technologies is then easily passed onto our patients.

The ultimate goal of the BMC is to enhance the overall quality of life for patients with bone metastatic disease through maintaining and expanding this one-stop clinic approach for more patients who require this support. This is crucial given that as the population ages, the burden of cancer and bone metastases may also escalate. Patient satisfaction and cost-effectiveness of the clinic should be examined, in order to confirm that it continues to offer efficient multidisciplinary care to its patients.

ACKNOWLEDGMENTS

We thank the generous support of the Bratty Family Fund, Michael and Karyn Goldstein Cancer Research Fund, Pulenzas Cancer Research Fund, Joseph and Silvana Melara Cancer Research Fund, and Ofelia Cancer Research Fund.

REFERENCES

[1] Canadian Cancer Society. Cancer statistics at a glance. URL: https://www.cancer.ca/en/cancer-information /cancer-101/cancer-statistics-at-a-glance/?region=nl.

[2] Coleman RE. Skeletal complications of malignancy. Cancer 1997;80(8 Suppl): 1588-94.

[3] Andersson L, Chow E, Finkelstein J, Connolly R, Danjoux C, Szumacher E, et al. The ultimate one-stop for cancer patients with bone metastases: New combined bone metastases clinic. Can Oncol Nurs J 1999;9(2):103-4.

[4] Li KK, Sinclair E, Pope J, Farhadian M, Harris K, Napolskikh J, et al. A multidisciplinary bone metastases clinic at Toronto Sunnybrook Regional Cancer Centre – A review of the experience from 1999 to 2005. J Pain Res 2008:1;43-8

[5] Nguyen J, Sinclair E, Yee A, Finkelstein J, Ford M, Chakraborty A, et al. A multidisciplinary bone metastases clinic at Sunnybrook Odette Cancer Centre: a review of the experience from 2006-2008. J Pain Manage 2009:2(4):435-44.

Submitted: January 02, 2015. *Revised:* February 02, 2015. *Accepted:* February 08, 2015.

In: Pain Management Yearbook 2015
Editor: Joav Merrick

ISBN: 978-1-63484-515-1

Chapter 13

CHANGE IN OVERALL SURVIVAL ASSOCIATED WITH KARNOFSKY PERFORMANCE STATUS OVER TIME

Rachel McDonald, BSc(C), Liying Zhang, PhD, Gillian Bedard, BSc(C), Erin Wong, BSc(C), Henry Lam, MLS, Marko Popovic, BHSc(C), Danielle Rodin, MD, Lori Holden, MRTT, May Tsao, MD, Elizabeth Barnes, MD, Cyril Danjoux, MD, Christine Ecclestone, BSc(C), Leigha Rowbottom, BSc(C), and Edward Chow*, MBBS

Rapid Response Radiotherapy Program,
Department of Radiation Oncology, Odette Cancer Centre,
Sunnybrook Health Sciences Centre, University of Toronto,
Toronto, Ontario, Canada

The Karnofsky Performance Status (KPS) scale is used to assess functional impairment. KPS scores have been shown to be one of the most crucial predictive factors in the survival of cancer patients. The objective was to determine whether overall survival predicted by KPS scores in patients receiving palliative radiation has increased from 2007-2012. A retrospective chart review was conducted to collect demographic information, including primary cancer site, clinic date, KPS score, and date of death. Overall survival (OS) was calculated. Kaplan-Meier survival curves and univariate Cox proportional hazard model were conducted for all patients and within KPS subgroups. A p-value <0.05 was considered statistically significant. All patients who were seen at an outpatient radiotherapy clinic in Toronto, Canada, from 2007-2012 were included in the study. Of a total 2,690 patients, 2257 (84%) were deceased. The median OS time was 2.9 months (95% CI: 2.7-3.1). All patients seen from 2007-2008 ($p < 0.0001$) and 2009-2010

* Correspondence: Professor Edward Chow, MBBS, MSc, PhD, FRCPC, Department of Radiation Oncology, Odette Cancer Centre, Sunnybrook Health Sciences Centre, 2075 Bayview Avenue, Toronto, ON, Canada. E-mail: Edward.Chow@sunnybrook.ca.

(p = 0.03) had shorter survival than those seen from 2011-2012. Survival was shorter for patients with KPS of 50-70 seen in 2007-2008 (p = 0.007) and 2009-2010 (p = 0.049) compared to 2011-2012. Survival of patients with KPS 80-100 nearly doubled from 6.6 to 12.1 months (p = 0.005) for those seen in 2007-2008 compared to those seen in 2011-2012. Survival has increased for patients within the same KPS categories from 2007-2012. Survival prognostic models that incorporate KPS may need to be temporally validated, taking into consideration latest systemic therapies with survival benefits.

Keywords: Karnofsky Performance Status, overall survival, prognostic models, advanced cancer, palliative radiation therapy

INTRODUCTION

Health care professionals are constantly faced with the challenge of predicting prognosis in order to help patients and their families make end-of-life and treatment decisions (1, 2). In the advanced cancer population, this is increasingly difficult due the heterogeneity in functional ability and level of care required for activities of daily living (1). Currently, the Karnofsky Performance Status (KPS) is one of the most commonly used tools in clinical oncology to predict prognosis (2-4).

This scale was introduced in the 1940s with the advent of cancer chemotherapy in order to describe patients' functional ability and amount of care they require in a meaningful way (3, 5). It is assessed on an 11-point scale increasing by increments of 10, with scores ranging from 0, meaning dead, to 100, meaning normal with no complaints and no evidence of disease (5). Since its introduction, the KPS has been widely validated and used in many studies, both as an independent prognostic factor, as well as a component of various prognostic models (1, 3, 6, 7).

Investigating the validity of the KPS as a prognostic marker in patients with advanced cancer, Yates et al. (3) showed a strong positive correlation between physical functioning and survival. A systematic review of twenty-two cohort studies investigating bedside prognostic factors (2) found that the KPS was a valid factor in all thirteen of the studies in which it was used. Further studies (1, 6, 7) have validated prognostic models that have included KPS as one of the strongest prognostic factors.

Although patients with advanced cancer often have goals of care centered on stabilizing or improving quality of life, recent developments and the use of systemic therapies in this patient population have been shown to increase life expectancy (8). Furthermore, advancements in palliative radiation therapy techniques, such as stereotactic radiosurgery (SRS) for brain metastases (9), may have led to improved survival as well.

Commonly, KPS is used as an objective tool to measure response to cancer treatments, with an increase in KPS representing a positive response (3). The objective of this study was to determine whether or not survival has increased over the past six years for advanced cancer patients with the same performance status.

We hypothesized that improvements in palliative cancer treatment will result in increased overall survival.

Methods

The Rapid Response Radiotherapy Program (RRRP) is an outpatient clinic at the Sunnybrook Odette Cancer Centre that provides palliative radiation for advanced cancer patients with the goal of managing symptoms and improving quality of life. All patients assessed in the RRRP between January 2007 and December 2012, regardless of whether or not they were treated with radiation therapy, were included in the study.

Data collection and patient stratification

Basic demographic information, including age, primary cancer site, clinic date, and KPS score, was collected prospectively as part of clinic procedures. Dates of death were in collected from patients' medical records in February 2014. For patients who were still alive, the date of last contact with the hospital was recorded. The study was approved by the Research Ethics Board at Sunnybrook Health Sciences Centre.

Patients were stratified into groups of two years: January 2007 to December 2008, January 2009 to December 2010, and January 2011 to December 2012. As this subset of palliative patients tend to have poor prognoses, most of these patients were likely to have died by the time of data analysis. KPS was divided into three ranges (10-40, 50-70, and 80-100) that are commonly used to categorize functional impairment (10-12). Those with a KPS of 10-40 are unable to care for themselves, often require institutional or hospital care, and may have rapidly progressing disease. Patients with a KPS 50-70 are considered able to live at home, to care for most of their personal needs with varying amounts of assistance, but unable to work. Finally, those with a KPS of 80-100 have the ability to engage in normal activity and work, and require no extra care (10-12).

Statistical analysis

Descriptive analyses were conducted in all patients using mean, standard deviation (SD), median, inter-quartiles, and ranges for age, and proportions for categorical variables. Overall survival (OS) was calculated from the first clinic date to the recorded date of death, or censored at the last follow-up date. Actuarial median survival in months with 95% confidence intervals (CIs) were calculated for all patients and for patients with breast, lung, genitourinary (GU) or gastrointestinal (GI) cancer site at each time period (Jan 2007 to Dec 2008, Jan 2009 to Dec 2010, and Jan 2011 to Dec 2012). Kaplan-Meier OS curves at different time periods were plotted in all patients and compared using log-rank test. Furthermore, Kaplan-Meier OS curves and log-rank test were also used for each KPS range (10-40, 50-70, and 80-100) to compare three different time periods in patients with a specific primary cancer site (e.g., breast or lung).

To search for significant association with KPS ranges and time periods, univariate Cox proportional hazard (PH) model of OS was used in all patients as well as within each subgroup of patients with time period. Hazard ratio (HR) and 95% CI were also calculated.

All analyses were conducted using Statistical Analysis Software (SAS version 9.3). A p-value <0.05 was statistically significant.

Table 1. Patient characteristics (n = 2688)

Age (years)		
n	2688	
Median (range)	64 (20 – 95)	
Gender		
Female	1221	(45.4%)
Male	1469	(54.6%)
KPS		
n	2567	
Median (range)	60 (10–100)	
KPS Categories		
10-40	544	(21.2%)
50-70	1485	(57.8%)
80-100	538	(21.0%)
Primary cancer site		
Lung	968	(36.0%)
Breast	457	(17.0%)
Genitourinary	658	(24.5%)
Gastrointestinal	254	(9.4%)
Other	173	(6.4%)
Unknown	180	(6.7%)
Alive Status		
Alive	433	(16.1%)
Dead	2257	(83.9%)
Time Period		
Jan2007 - Dec2008	1005	(37.4%)
Jan2009-Dec2010	893	(33.2%)
Jan2011-Dec2012	792	(29.4%)

RESULTS

A total of 2690 patients were included in the study. The median age was 64 years and there were more males (54.6%) than females (45.4%). The most common primary cancer sites were lung (36.0%), breast (17.0%), GU (24.5%), and GI (9.4%). Of the total number of patients, 433 were still alive at the time of analysis. The median KPS observed was 60 (10-100), with ranges of 10-40 in 21.2% of patients, 50-70 in 57.8% of patients, and 80-100 in 21.0% of patients.

The number of patients slightly declined over time; 1005 patients were seen between 2007 and 2008, 893 between 2009 and 2010, and 792 between 2011 and 2012. In all patients, the median survival time was 2.86 months (95% CI of 2.66-3.09 months). Patient characteristics can be found in Table 1.

Survival in all patients over time period

As shown in Table 2, different KPS categories significantly predicted survival in all patients ($p < 0.0001$); those with a greater KPS value also had greater OS (10-40 vs. 80-100: HR = 4.10; 50-70 vs. 80-100: HR = 2.06; 10-40 vs. 50-70: HR = 1.99). In addition, statistical significance was found when analyzing time period and OS ($p = 0.0003$). In all patients, those seen from 2007-2008 ($p < 0.0001$; HR = 1.24) and 2009-2010 ($p = 0.027$; HR = 1.13) had significant greater risk of death when compared to patients seen from 2011-2012. However, no significant difference ($p = 0.06$) was seen when comparing the first two time periods (Figure 1).

Table 2. Univariate Cox PH model of OS over three time periods in all patients and in patients with KPS categories

	p-value	Hazard Ratio	95% CI of HR	
In All Patients				
KPS categories	**<.0001**			
10-40 vs. 80-100	**<.0001**	4.101	3.574	4.707
50-70 vs. 80-100	**<.0001**	2.058	1.832	2.312
10-40 vs. 50-70	**<.0001**	1.993	1.795	2.213
Time Period	**0.0003**			
Jan2007 - Dec2008 vs. Jan2011-Dec2012	**<.0001**	1.243	1.117	1.383
Jan2009-Dec2010 vs. Jan2011-Dec2012	**0.0273**	1.133	1.014	1.265
Jan2007 - Dec2008 vs. Jan2009-Dec2010	0.0552	1.097	0.998	1.207
In Patients with KPS 10-40				
Time Period	0.8457			
Jan2007 - Dec2008 vs. Jan2011-Dec2012	0.5913	0.940	0.750	1.178
Jan2009-Dec2010 vs. Jan2011-Dec2012	0.8807	0.982	0.778	1.240
Jan2007 - Dec2008 vs. Jan2009-Dec2010	0.6744	0.957	0.780	1.175
In Patients with KPS 50-70				
Time Period	**0.0256**			
Jan2007 - Dec2008 vs. Jan2011-Dec2012	**0.0074**	1.212	1.053	1.396
Jan2009-Dec2010 vs. Jan2011-Dec2012	**0.0496**	1.157	1.000	1.337
Jan2007 - Dec2008 vs. Jan2009-Dec2010	0.4656	1.048	0.924	1.189
In Patients with KPS 80-100				
Time Period	**0.0200**			
Jan2007 - Dec2008 vs. Jan2011-Dec2012	**0.0052**	1.488	1.126	1.966
Jan2009-Dec2010 vs. Jan2011-Dec2012	0.0620	1.306	0.987	1.729
Jan2007 - Dec2008 vs. Jan2009-Dec2010	0.2624	1.139	0.907	1.431

Survival by time period across KPS categories

Significant differences were also found when investigating OS for patients within different KPS groups with respect to time period. Patients with a KPS 50-70 who were seen in 2007-2008 ($p = 0.007$; HR = 1.21) or 2009-2010 ($p = 0.0496$; HR = 1.16) had significantly greater risk of death when compared to those of the same KPS who were seen in 2011-2012 (median OS of 2.73, 2.96, and 3.02 months, respectively). In patients with a KPS 80-100, only those seen from 2007-2008 had a greater risk of death in comparison to those of the same KPS in 2011-2012 ($p = 0.005$; HR = 1.49). In fact, median survival between these two time periods doubled from 6.6 months in 2007-2008 to 12.1 months in 2011-2012. No significant difference was seen in OS between time periods for patients with KPS 10-40 (p = 0.85).

Overall survival of patients with specific primary cancer sites

Lung, breast, GU, and GI (927, 442, 630, and 239 patients with available KPS data, respectively) were the four most common primary cancer sites in patients who were seen in the RRRP between 2007 and 2012. In patients with breast cancer who had a KPS of 50-70, significantly higher risk of death (p = 0.0089; HR = 1.50) was associated with the time period of 2007-2008 compared to that of 2009-2010, with median OS of 3.25 and 7.36 months respectively (Figure 2). Median survival decreased for the time period of 2011-2012 to 4.27 months, but this was not statistically significant when compared to the 2007-2008 time period (p = 0.11) or to the 2009-2010 time period (p = 0.63).

Table 3. Median OS in patients with various primary sites over three time periods

	Median (95% CI) Survival Months			
Patients with KPS category	**Jan 2007 – Dec 2008**	**Jan 2009 – Dec 2010**	**Jan 2011 – Dec 2012**	**Log-rank test p-value**
Patients with Breast Cancer Site				
10-40	2.30 (1.05-3.19)	1.42 (0.69-3.55)	4.50 (0.79-9.95)	0.2975
50-70	3.25 (2.23-4.70)	7.36 (4.83-8.21)	4.27 (2.92-7.59)	**0.0246**
80-100	5.49 (2.63-22.77)	20.53 (10.41-33.91)	>34.04 months*	**0.0153**
Patients with Lung Cancer Site				
10-40	1.12 (0.85-1.38)	0.92 (0.53-1.87)	0.69 (0.53-1.12)	0.1324
50-70	2.20 (1.74-2.66)	1.84 (1.64-2.20)	2.92 (2.23-3.71)	**0.0006**
80-100	5.75 (3.78-7.72)	4.01 (2.86-5.72)	6.54 (3.25-13.90)	**0.0283**
Patients with GI Cancer Site				
10-40	1.10 (0.43 -1.87)	1.26 (0.76-2.20)	0.76 (0.33-1.77)	0.4873
50-70	2.20 (1.25-2.76)	2.20 (1.45-3.19)	1.81 (1.15-2.53)	0.9774
80-100	6.23 (2.00-32.59)	6.67 (2.40-23.59)	3.75 (2.96-14.06)	0.5364
Patients with GU Cancer Site				
10-40	1.53 (0.95-2.50)	1.40 (0.92-2.33)	0.89 (0.46-1.31)	0.1979
50-70	4.40 (3.06-4.73)	3.45 (2.60-4.34)	4.57 (3.02-6.64)	0.1282
80-100	13.44 (7.49-18.76)	15.08 (6.41-20.17)	17.35 (7.85-26.51)	0.3665

* All patients' survival probabilities were above 50%, therefore the median OS for this subgroup >34 months when the survival was reached to 55%.

Among breast cancer patients with a KPS 80-100, 2007-2008 had significantly higher probability of death compared to the latter two time periods ($p = 0.0376$, HR = 1.81; and $p = 0.0101$, HR = 2.67 when compared to 2009-2010 and 2011-2012, respectively). Median OS for patients with breast cancer with this KPS range increased from 5.49 months during 2007-2008 to 20.53 months in 2009-2010, and to greater than 34.04 months during 2011-2012 (see Figure 2).

Lung cancer patients with KPS 50-70 had greater risk of death during 2007-2008 ($p = 0.0082$; HR = 1.37) and 2009-2010 ($p = 0.0001$; HR = 1.60) when compared to 2011-2012 (median OS of 2.20 months, 1.84 months, and 2.92 months, respectively). For patients with a KPS 80-100, the time period of 2009-2010 had greater probability of death ($p = 0.0086$; HR = 1.84) compared to 2011-2012. OS during this interval increased from 4.01 months to 6.54 months (Figure 3).

Among patients with GI or GU primary cancer sites, no significant time period difference was seen between KPS categories. Median OS for each patient within each time period is shown in Table 3.

Discussion

Although the association of OS has been shown frequently in previous literature, this is the first study to our knowledge that examines how this association has changed over time with our database. Specifically, we aimed to use KPS to analyze whether or not life expectancy in advanced cancer patients has increased over the past five years. We found that the KPS is significantly related to survival and that survival in patients with the same KPS increased over the period of study. Most impressively, survival time in 2011-2012 was double that of 2007-2008 for patients with a KPS 80-100, increasing from 6.6 months to 12.06 months. Although statistical significance was not seen when comparing OS in patients with a KPS 80-100 in 2009-2010 (8.15 months) to OS in 2011-2012 (12.06 months), the increase in median survival of four months is clinically significant. Both statistical and clinical significance was found for breast cancer patients with a KPS 80-100, for whom survival was more than six times greater in 2010-2011 compared to 2007-2008 (34.04 and 5.49 months, respectively). Lung cancer patients also showed increased survival, albeit less so than breast cancer patients. Those with a KPS 50-70 had greater probability of death if they were seen in the first two time periods compared to that of 2011-2012 ($p = 0.0007$). The same was true for those with a KPS 80-100 when comparing 2009-2010 to 2011-2012 ($p = 0.0086$, median OS was 4.01 and 6.54 months, respectively).

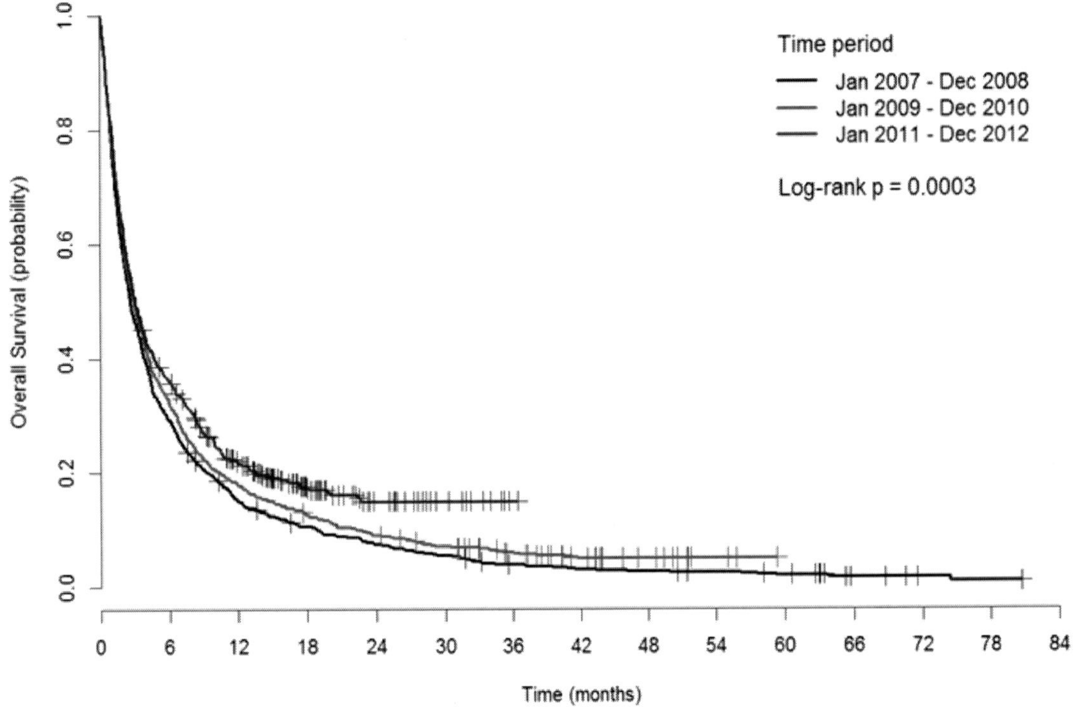

Figure 1. Kaplan-Meier OS curve in all patients over different time periods (Log-rank p = 0.0003).

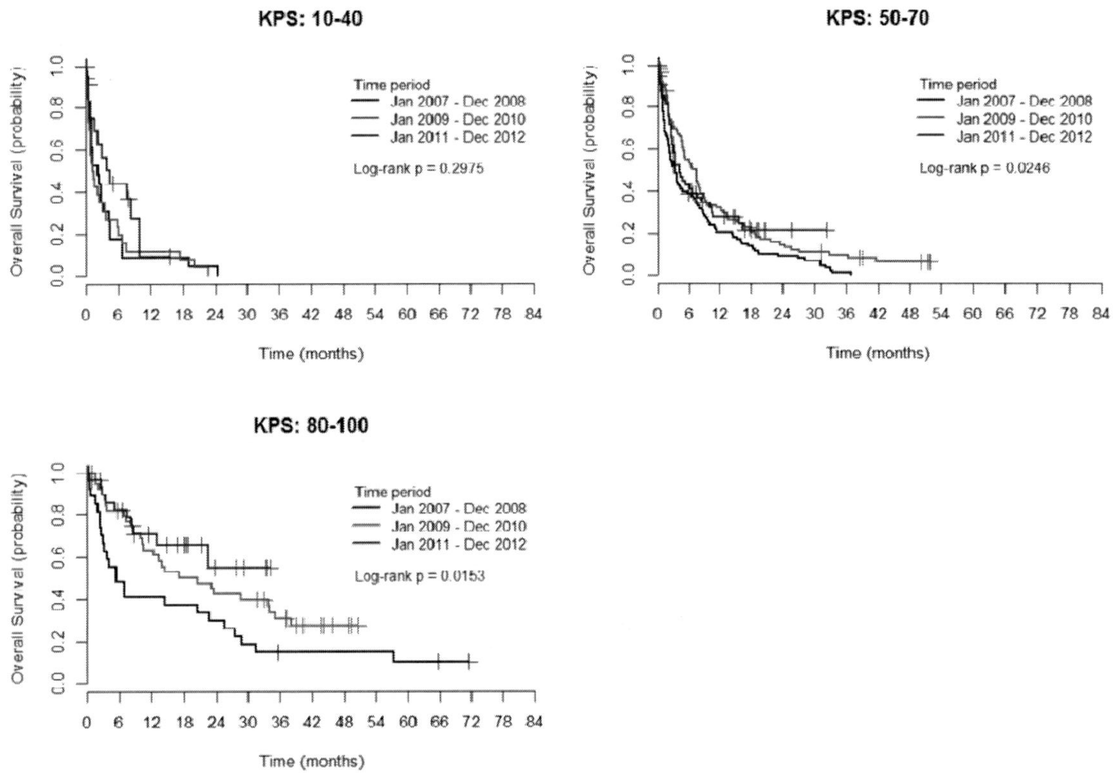

Figure 2. Kaplan-Meier OS curves for patients with breast cancer.

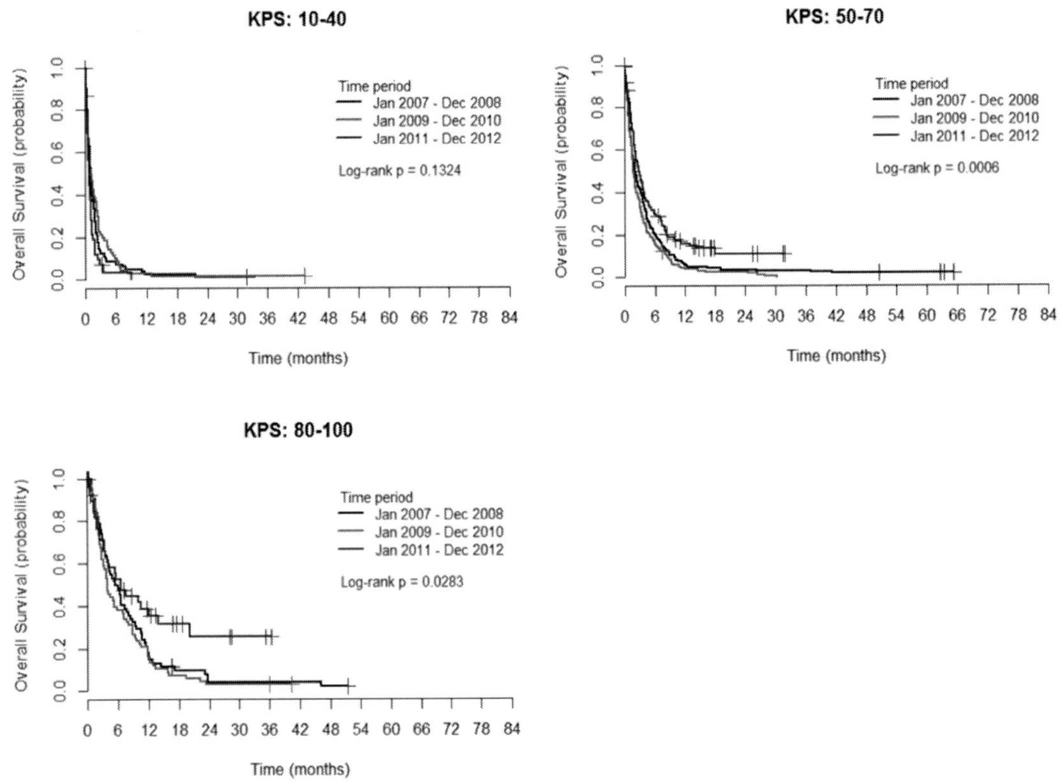

Figure 3. Kaplan-Meier OS curves for patients with lung cancer.

Accurate information about prognosis is crucial for advanced cancer patients and their physicians in order for them to appropriately weigh the costs and benefits of possible treatment (1). In addition, palliative patients and their families must be aware of prognosis in order to make advanced care plans and to resolve issues related to end-of-life. Patients and their families often ask physicians about estimated survival time. Although various factors are taken into account at arriving at such an estimate, the KPS is one of the main factors shown to be consistently used by physicians for this purpose (2-4).

The increased survival that we observed over the period of the study could be due to an improvement in systemic therapy. In a recent review of treatments for non-small-cell lung cancer, Ramalingam et al. (8) found that platinum-based combination chemotherapy has recently become the standard treatment for those with stage IV lung cancer. When comparing these treatments to supportive care on its own, patients receiving the platinum-based combination chemo-therapy experienced increased OS as well as quality of life (8). Furthermore, investigations into the molecular basis of non-small cell lung cancer (NSCLC) has allowed for the development of inhibitors that target these pathways. For example, Erlotinib is now a standard EGFR inhibitor used in maintenance therapy, and has led to an increase in progression free survival when compared to placebo (13).

Similar to lung cancer, research into the molecular basis of breast cancer has allowed for the development of targeted therapies. Many therapies now intervene in specific receptor pathways known to play a role in cancer development, including the estrogen receptor (ER), progesterone receptor (PR), and the human epidermal growth factor receptor (HER2) (14). Trastuzumab, for example, targets the HER2 pathway and was approved for use in conjunction with cisplatin and a fluoropyrimidine by the Food and Drug Administration (FDA) in 2010. The approval was based on a randomized control trial in which patients who received Trastuzumab in conjunction with chemotherapy had an OS of 2 months greater than patients who received chemotherapy alone (15). Many other targeted therapies have been developed in addition to Trastuzumab, one of which is Lapatinib. Lapatinib was approved after a phase-three trial demonstrated longer median time to progression when it was used in conjunction with standard therapy (14). These two pharmaceuticals have paved the way for further research into receptor pathways and many clinical trials are now underway.

Another factor that could account for this increased survival is the increased use of more aggressive treatments for palliative patients, such as stereotactic radiosurgery (SRS) for brain metastases. A study conducted by El Gantery and colleagues investigated the efficacy of SRS alone versus whole brain radiation therapy (WBRT) alone, versus the two modalities together. Overall, the authors observed median survival of 8, 5.5, and 12 months, respectively (16). Hyun et al. concluded similar results in their 2013 meta-analysis; patients treated with SRS+WBRT had greater survival (10.7 months) when compared to WBRT alone (6.0 months) and SRS alone (7.9 months) (17).

In recent years, a paradigm shift regarding the introduction of palliative care early in disease trajectory has commenced. This was largely influenced by the work of the American Society of Clinical Oncology which, in 1998, published an article and recommendations regarding palliative care (18). Many palliative care models have been developed and implemented as a result of this work, and many institutions are beginning to incorporate palliative care physicians as part of their service (18). Furthermore, the early integration of palliative care in disease trajectory has been shown to increase OS. For example, a study conducted by Temel et al. (19) randomized patients diagnosed with NSCLC to receive early palliative care in conjunction with standard care, or standard care alone. Results showed patients in the early palliative care group experienced greater survival. Similar results were shown by Otsuka et al. (20) who compared early versus late referral to outpatient palliative care, also for patients with NSCLC. Median survival in patients referred early to palliative care was 13.6 months, compared to 2.7 months in the late referral group.

Our results greatly impact the interpretation of previously developed prognostic models, as they show a significant increase in prognosis over time for all patients, and especially in those with lung or breast primaries. Therefore, prognostic models currently employed in practice that include KPS as a factor may underestimate survival. Our results draw attention to the need to temporally validate prognostic models incorporating KPS in order to ensure their accuracy and relevancy to current patient populations. In addition, with recent developments in palliative chemo and radiation therapy resulting in greater overall survival, the inclusion of treatment as a factor in future prognostic model should be investigated.

Limitations

Dates of death for patients were obtained from electronic medical records (EMR). These records were updated shortly before data analysis to include dates of death from the National Cancer Registry. However, if the death did not occur at Sunnybrook Health Sciences Centre, it is possible that patients could have died between the EMR update and the date of data analysis. In that case, they were censored at their last follow up.

Our data includes palliative patients with a variety of primary cancer sites, although it is limited to patients referred for palliative radiotherapy. Future research is needed to externally validate these findings in other centres.

Conclusion

Our results show that KPS is predictive of overall survival and that OS has improved for patients stratified to different KPS groups from 2007-2012. The most significant increase in OS was seen in patients with breast and lung cancer with a KPS 80-100, but no significant change was identified in patients with GI or GU cancer. These results may reflect improvements in palliative treatments including chemotherapy and radiation, as well as an earlier integration of palliative care into the treatment of advanced cancer. Furthermore, our results impact the validity of current prognostic models that include KPS as a factor. These prognostic models require temporal validation in order to retain their usefulness in palliative practice. Future studies investigating systemic treatment as a factor in prognosis are likely to improve the accuracy of prognostic models.

ACKNOWLEDGMENTS

We thank the generous support of Bratty Family Fund, Michael and Karyn Goldstein Cancer Research Fund, Pulenzas Cancer Research Fund, Joseph and Silvana Melara Cancer Research Fund, and Ofelia Cancer Research Fund. The authors have no conflicts of interest to disclose. We have full control of all primary data.

REFERENCES

[1] Chow E, Fung K, Panzarella T, Bezjak A, Danjoux C, Tannock I. A predictive model for survival in metastatic cancer patients attending an outpatient palliative radiotherapy clinic. Int J Radiat Oncol Biol Phys 2002;53(5):1291-302.

[2] Vigano A, Dorgan M, Buckingham J, Bruera E, Suarez-Almazor ME. Survival prediction in terminal cancer patients: a systematic review of the medical literature. Palliat Med 2000;14(5):363-74.

[3] Yates JW, Chalmer B, McKegney FP. Evaluation of patients with advanced cancer using the Karnofsky performance status. Cancer 1980;45(8):2220-4.

[4] Culleton S, Dennis K, Koo K, Zhang L, Zeng L, Kwong J, et al. Correlation of the palliative performance scale with the Karnofsky performance status in an outpatient palliative radiotherapy clinic. J Pain Manage 2011;4(4):427-33.

[5] de Kock I, Mirhosseini M, Lau F, Thai V, Downing M, Quan H, et al. Conversion of Karnofsky Performance Status (KPS) and Eastern Cooperative Oncology Group Performance Status (ECOG) to Palliative Performance Scale (PPS), and the interchangeability of PPS and KPS in prognostic tools. J Palliat Care 2013;29(3):163-9.

[6] Hwang SS, Scott CB, Chang VT, Cogswell J, Srinivas S, Kasimis B. Prediction of survival for advanced cancer patients by recursive partitioning analysis: role of Karnofsky performance status, quality of life, and symptom distress. Cancer Invest 2004;22(5):678-87.

[7] Lam PT, Leung MW, Tse CY. Identifying prognostic factors for survival in advanced cancer patients: a prospective study. Hong Kong Med J 2007;13(6):453-9.

[8] Ramalingam SS, Owonikoko TK, Khuri FR. Lung cancer: New biological insights and ecent therapeutic advances. CA Cancer J Clin 2011;61(2):91-112.

[9] Linskey ME, Andrews DW, Asher AL, Burri SH, Kondziolka D, Robinson PD, et al. The role of stereotactic radiosurgery in the management of patients with newly diagnosed brain metastases: a systematic review and evidence-based clinical practice guideline. J Neurooncol 2010;96(1):45-68.

[10] Mor V, Laliberte L, Morris JN, Wiemann M. The Karnofsky Performance Status Scale. An examination of its reliability and validity in a research setting. Cancer 1984;53(9):2002-7.

[11] Peus D, Newcomb N, Hofer S. Appraisal of the Karnofsky Performance Status and proposal of a simple algorithmic system for its evaluation. BMC Med Inform Decis Mak 2013;13(1):72.

[12] Schag CC, Heinrich RL, Ganz PA. Karnofsky performance status revisited: reliability, validity, and guidelines. J Clin Oncol 1984;2(3):187-93.

[13] Cappuzzo F, Ciuleanu T, Stelmakh L, Cicenas S, Szczesna A, Juhasz E, et al. Erlotinib as maintenance treatment in advanced non-small-cell lung cancer: a multicentre, randomized, placebo-controlled phase 3 study. Lancet Oncol 2010;11(6):521-9.

[14] Perez EA, Spano JP. Current and emerging targeted therapies for metastatic breast cancer. Cancer 2012;118(12):3014-25.

[15] National CI. FDA Approval for Trastuzumab. 2013. URL: http://www.cancer.gov/cancertopics/druginfo/fda-trastuzumab. Accessed 04/10, 2014.

[16] El Gantery MM, Abd El Baky HM, El Hossieny HA, Mahmoud M, Youssef O. Management of brain metastases with stereotactic radiosurgery alone versus whole brain irradiation alone versus both. Radiat Oncol 2014;9:116-717X-9-116.

[17] Hyun MK, Hwang JS, Kim JH, Choi JE, Jung SY, Bae JM. Survival outcomes after whole brain radiation therapy and/or stereotactic radiosurgery for cancer patients with metastatic brain tumors in Korea: a systematic review. Asian Pac J Cancer Prev 2013;14(12):7401-77.

[18] Ferris FD, Bruera E, Cherny N, Cummings C, Currow D, Dudgeon D, et al. Palliative cancer care a decade later: accomplishments, the need, next steps -- from the American Society of Clinical Oncology. J Clin Oncol 2009;27(18):3052-8.

[19] Temel JS, Greer JA, Muzikansky A, Gallagher ER, Admane S, Jackson VA, et al. Early Palliative Care for Patients with Metastatic Non Small-Cell Lung Cancer. N Engl J Med 2010;363(8):733-42.

[20] Otsuka M, Koyama A, Matsuoka H, Niki M, Makimura C, Sakamoto R, et al. Early palliative intervention for patients with advanced cancer. Jpn J Clin Oncol 2013;43(8):788-94.

Submitted: January 15, 2015. *Revised:* February 20, 2015. *Accepted:* February 27, 2015.

In: Pain Management Yearbook 2015
Editor: Joav Merrick

ISBN: 978-1-63484-515-1

Chapter 14

ANALYSIS OF SYMPTOM CLUSTERS IN PATIENTS WITH BRAIN METASTASES WITH THREE DIFFERENT STATISTICAL METHODS

Erin Wong[1], BSc(C), Liying Zhang[1], PhD, Marc Kerba[2], MD, Palmira Foro[3], MD, Brita Danielson[4], MD, May Tsao, MD[1], Nemica Thavarajah[1], BSc, Paul Cheon[1], MD(C), Cyril Danjoux[1], MD, Natalie Pulenzas[1], BSc(C), and Edward Chow[1,*], MBBS

[1]Rapid Response Radiotherapy Program,
Department of Radiation Oncology, Odette Cancer Centre,
Sunnybrook Health Sciences Centre, University of Toronto,
Toronto, Ontario, Canada
[2]Department of Radiation Oncology, Tom Baker Cancer Centre,
Calgary, Alberta, Canada
[3]Parc de Salut Mar Hospital de l'Esperanc, Barcelona, Spain
[4]Department of Radiation Oncology, Cross Cancer Institute,
Edmonton, Alberta, Canada

Common symptoms that occur together are described as symptom clusters (SCs). Determining SCs is therapeutically important as treating one symptom in a cluster may serve to alleviate other symptoms and improve quality of life. Our goal is to describe SC profiles for patients at baseline and at follow-up after radiotherapy treatment for brain metastases using three different statistical techniques. A review of a prospective database included 155 patients at baseline and 100 patients at 1-month follow-up who completed the EORTC QLQ-BN20 or BN20+2. Three different statistical methods: principal component analysis (PCA), exploratory factor analysis (EFA), and hierarchical cluster analysis (HCA) were applied. Cronbach's alpha was used to assess internal consistency

[*] Correspondence: Professor Edward Chow MBBS, MSc, PhD, FRCPC Department of Radiation Oncology, Odette Cancer Centre, Sunnybrook Health Sciences Centre, 2075 Bayview Avenue, Toronto, Ontario, Canada. E-mail: Edward.Chow@sunnybrook.ca.

and reliability of the derived clusters. At baseline, HCA and EFA identified two clusters while PCA identified three clusters associated with brain metastases. 1) 'concentrating difficulty,' 'motor dysfunction,' 'seizures,' 'drowsiness' and 'remembering difficulty,' 2) 'future uncertainty,' 'headaches,' 'hair loss' and 'bladder control,' 3) 'itchy skin,' and 'weakness of legs' were also consistently grouped in the same cluster. Post-radiation, PCA and EFA identified the exact same cluster while HCA identified 4 clusters. 1) 'future uncertainty,' 'drowsiness' and 'hair loss,' 2) 'communication difficulty,' 'remembering difficulty,' 3) 'concentrating difficulty,' 'visual disorder,' 4) 'motor dysfunction' 'weakness of legs,' 'bladder control,' and 5) 'headaches' and 'seizures' were consistently grouped in the same cluster. Consistency of grouping indicates higher correlation between symptoms. Our results suggest that SCs are modified by radiation treatment for brain metastases. No single statistical technique was best to describe SCs in our population.

Keywords: symptom clusters, brain metastases, whole brain radiotherapy

INTRODUCTION

Brain metastases are the most common type of brain neoplasms occurring in approximately 20-40% of patients. Brain metastases commonly originate from primary breast, lung, melanoma, kidney and colorectal cancer (1). They are associated with a variety of symptoms including headaches and focal weakness, which are the most common, but also motor weakness, balance problems, seizures, visual problems and altered mental status (2-4).

For advanced cancer patients, such as brain metastases patients, symptom palliation is of upmost concern. This stems from symptom alleviation in the improvement of quality of life. For many advanced cancer patients, they present with a multitude of concurrent symptoms, an average of 11-13, which may be due to the cancer itself or its treatments (5). Due to the quantity and possible interaction of concurrent symptoms, the palliation of one symptom may not lead to a direct positive effect on the patient's quality of life. This suggests the need of further research on relationships between symptoms and understand its effect on patients with advanced cancer (6).

Symptom clusters were first reported by Dodd et al. in 2001. Symptoms clusters were defined as three or more symptoms occurring together that are related, although etiology may not concur (7). Later, Kim et al. redefined symptoms clusters as two or more symptoms that occur together, are related and act as a stable group, independent of other clusters (8). The knowledge of symptom clusters may aid health care professionals in the improvement of quality of life in brain metastases patients.

In the research of symptoms clusters, there currently lacks a universal method of analysis. There are three commonly used analytical methods which are effective in extracting symptoms clusters: principal cluster analysis (PCA), hierarchical cluster analysis (HCA) and exploratory factor analysis (EFA) (9). As such, the purpose of our study was to explore the presence of SCs using three different statistical analyses at both baseline and follow-up after radiotherapy treatment for brain metastases.

METHODS

This analysis includes pooled data from two previous data sets. From October 2009 to July 2010, patients with brain metastases referred for whole brain radiotherapy (WBRT) at three Canadian centers and one center in Spain were included in this study. All research was conducted with institutional REB approval.

From March 2010 to November 2010, patients with brain metastases referred to Sunnybrook Odette Cancer Center for WBRT, radiosurgery/gamma knife or neurosurgical resection were approached for study. Patients over the age of 18 years with histologically or radiologically documented brain metastases were included. The Sunnybrook Health Sciences Centre Research Ethics Board approved this research.

Data collection

At baseline consultation, patients enrolled from October 2009 to July 2010 completed the EORTC QLQ-BN20 and the EORTC QLQ-C30 at baseline and 1 month follow up. Patients enrolled from March 2010 to November 2010, completed the EORTC QLQ-BN20+2 and the EORTC QLQ-C15PAL at baseline and 1-month follow-up. Demographic information was also collected from both patient cohorts. This included age, gender, primary cancer site, Karnofsky Performance Status (KPS) and treatments.

Quality of life instrument and scoring

The EORTC QLQ-BN20 is the brain cancer supplementary module to the EORTC QLQ-C30, the general "core" questionnaire. It contains 20 items with 4 multi-item scales (13 items) and 7 singular items. The four subscales of the BN20 are: future uncertainty (FU) (four items), visual disorder (VD) (three items), communication deficit (CM) (three items), and motor dysfunction (MD) (three items). The remaining 7 items assess symptoms of disease such as headaches (H), seizures (S), drowsiness (Dr), weakness of legs (WL), bladder control (BC) and treatment toxic effects such as hair loss (HL), itchy skin (IS). Each item is rated on a Likert scale from 1 to 4 (1 = 'not at all', 2 = 'a little,' 3 = 'quite a bit,' and 4 = 'very much'). All items were scored based on EORTC scoring procedure. Raw scores were standardized using linear transformation so that scores ranged from 0 to 100. For the four scales and seven single items, a higher score represents poorer quality of life (see Appendix 1).

The EORTC QLQ-BN20+2 is an in-development brain cancer supplementary module to the EORTC QLQ-C15PAL, the shortened "general" questionnaire. It contains 22 items, similar to the EORTC QLQ-BN20 with two additional questions. As such, it included the same four subscales and seven symptoms and treatment toxicity as the EORTC QLQ-BN20, however two additional questions gauging concentrating difficulty (CD) and remembering difficulty (RD) were added. Items were scored based on EORTC scoring procedure. Raw scores were standardized using linear transformation so that scores ranged from 0 to 100. For the four scales and nine single items, a higher score represents worse quality of life (see Appendix 2).

Statistical analysis

The statistical methods used to analyze symptom clusters were principal component analysis (PCA), exploratory factor analysis (EFA) and hierarchical cluster analysis (HCA).

Principal component analysis (PCA)

PCA with varimax rotation was performed on the EORTC QLQ-BN20 and the EORTC QLQ-BN20+2 domains and single items to examine whether interrelationships existed between symptoms. PCA is an appropriate procedure that transforms a number of observed variables into a smaller number of variables (called principal components). The number of significant principal components was selected for with an Eigenvalue >1.0 and having each component accounting for at least 10% of total variation. The highest factor loading score predicted the assignment of individual symptoms to an independent factor. The internal consistency and reliability of the derived clusters was assessed with Cronbach's alpha. Among the identified significant components, a varimax rotation was performed to simplify interpretation of the solution. A varimax rotation is an orthogonal rotation; it tends to maximize the variance of a column of the factor pattern matrix. A robust relationship and correlation among variables can be seen from the biplot graphs. On the biplot graphs, the longer length of arrow, the larger the correlation. While the closer distance between arrows, the higher correlation between these variables.

Exploratory factor analysis (EFA)

To identify unknown groupings from a range of symptoms, the exploratory factor analysis (EFA) is the most commonly applied method of cancer symptom cluster identification (8, 10). Applied to symptom cluster research in oncology, factor analysis is a statistical approach used for finding the common factors that explain the correlation between symptoms and, extending this conceptually, finding the commonality that "binds" 2 (or more) symptoms together into a common concept (11). Factor analysis is used to predict a set of latent factors that are responsible for covariance among a group of symptoms. Symptoms due to this latent factor would co-vary more strongly with each other than they would with symptoms that are affected by a different latent factor (10). EFA was applied to the EORTC QLQ-BN20 or BN20+2. The maximum likelihood methods were applied for approximately multivariate normal data, and the varimax orthogonal rotation method was also used. The numbers of factors were also selected by the eigenvalue >1.0. The PROC FACTOR procedure in Statistical Analysis Software (SAS) was conducted for this analysis.

Hierarchical cluster analysis (HCA)

Hierarchical Cluster Analysis (HCA) is another procedure that can be used to define a symptom cluster. Cluster analysis is an exploratory technique that it is used to discover underlying groups of individuals who are similar in their symptom experience or symptom profile (10). Therefore, this method is focused on classification and trying to put similar entities together into a cluster and separate this cluster from other clusters. The PROC VARCLUS in SAS ran clusters on the basis of *centroid* components. R^2 values of each symptom with its own cluster and with its nearest cluster were calculated. The $1\text{-}R^2$ ratio is the ratio of one minus the value in the "Own Cluster" column to one minus the value in the "Next Closest" column. Low ratios indicate well-separated clusters. The proportion of variation explained by clusters was also reported. The PROC TREE procedure in SAS was applied to generate a graphical display of the clusters and demonstrate cluster hierarchy. All calculations were carried out using SAS (version 9.3, SAS Institute, Cary, NC) statistical software.

RESULTS

Between October 2009 to November 2010, 155 patients completed the EORTC QLQ-BN20 or EORTC QLQ-BN20+2 at baseline (Table 1) while 100 patients completed it at follow-up. Mean age of patients was 60 years, ranging from 22 to 86 years and 54% of patients were female. The most common primary cancer sites are lung (52%), breast (23%), colon (6%) and melanoma (6%). Most patients underwent WBRT (61%), radiosurgery/gamma knife with or without WBRT (34%), neurosurgery (5%) and symptom management (1%).

Table 1. Patients characteristics (n = 155)

Age (years)		
n	155	
Mean ± SD	60.1 ± 11.3	
Median (range)	61 (22–86)	
Karnofsky Performance Status		
n	152	
Mean ± SD	75.7 ± 14.3	
Median (range)	80 (40–100)	
KPS > 80		
No	106	(69.74%)
Yes	46	(30.26%)
Sex		
Female	83	(53.55%)
Male	72	(46.45%)
Education		
High School	64	(42.67%)
University	49	(32.67%)
Elementary School	14	(9.33%)
Masters Or PhD	5	(3.33%)
Others	18	(12.00%)
Employment status		
Retired	71	(47.02%)
Employed	48	(31.79%)
Unemployed	32	(21.19%)
Cohabitant		
Spouse	64	(41.56%)
Spouse and child(ren)	42	(27.27%)
Alone	23	(14.94%)
Child(ren)	13	(8.44%)
Other	12	(7.79%)

Table 1. (Continued).

Married Status		
Married	104	(67.53%)
Single	18	(11.69%)
Age (years)		
Widowed	10	(6.49%)
Partner	1	(0.65%)
Other	21	(13.64%)
Primary Cancer Site		
Lung	80	(51.61%)
Breast	35	(22.58%)
Colon	10	(6.45%)
Melanoma	9	(5.81%)
Renal Cell/Kidney	5	(3.23%)
Others	14	(9.03%)
Unknown	2	(1.29%)
Patients Group		
Neurosurgery	8	(5.16%)
Radiosurgery/Gamma knife with or without whole brain radiotherapy	52	(33.55%)
Whole Brain Radiotherapy	94	(60.65%)
Symptom Management (e.g., Steroids)	1	(0.65%)
No. of Brain metastases		
1	42	(28.57%)
2 to 3	54	(36.73%)
>3	51	(34.70%)
Previous Systemic Treatment		
No	55	(35.95%)
Yes	98	(64.05%)

Symptom clusters at baseline

At baseline, of the four scales, patients scored most highly on the future uncertainty scale with a mean score of 38.4 and the motor dysfunction scale with a mean score of 24.2. Of the nine symptoms/toxicity items, the most prevalent items were drowsiness, headache, and remembering difficulty with a mean score of 32.0, 24.0, and 22.3, respectively.

Principal component analysis (PCA)

PCA derived three clusters at baseline with eigenvalue >1.0 and each component accounting for at least 10% of the total variation. Cluster 1 consisted of future uncertainty, visual disorder, headaches, hair loss, bladder control and communication deficit and accounted for 26% of the total variance. Cluster 2 consisted of concentrating difficulty, motor dysfunction, seizures, drowsiness and remembering difficulty and accounted for 15% of the total variance. The final cluster consisted of itchy skin and weakness of legs and accounted for 10% of the total variance (see Table 2). The internal reliability of the clusters was represented by a Cronbach's alpha of 0.70, 0.71, and 0.44, respectively. As such, this indicated that the first two clusters had good internal consistencies however the third cluster had weak internal consistency (see Table 2).

The final communality refers to the percent of variance in an observed variable that was accounted for by the retained components. It shows that all the variables are well accounted for by 3 components, with final communality estimates ranging from 0.33 for future uncertainty to 0.78 for motor dysfunction, except for remembering difficulty, which was 0.17. Figure 1a shows the biplot among the first 3 principal components. The three clusters were clearly evident in the biplot between components 2 and 3.

Table 2. PCA, EFA and HCA of the four scales and nine symptom/toxicity items on the EORTC QLQ-BN20/BN20+2 at Baseline

	Item	Component 1	Component 2	Component 3	Final communality
PCA	future uncertainty	**0.55**	0.04	0.16	0.33
	visual disorder	**0.67**	0.17	-0.16	0.51
	headaches	**0.53**	0.13	0.27	0.37
	hair loss	**0.59**	-0.04	0.44	0.54
	bladder control	**0.61**	0.26	0.24	0.49
	communication deficit	**0.59**	0.32	-0.34	0.56
	concentrating difficulty	0.22	**0.82**	-0.11	0.73
	motor dysfunction	0.39	**0.71**	0.34	0.78
	seizures	-0.43	**0.63**	0.07	0.59
	drowsiness	0.15	**0.66**	-0.08	0.47
	remembering difficulty	0.22	**0.32**	-0.14	0.17
	itchy skin	0.16	-0.03	**0.79**	0.65
	weakness of legs	0.03	-0.06	**0.74**	0.60
	% of variance	26%	15%	10%	
	Cronbach's alpha	0.70	0.71	0.44	
EFA	concentrating difficulty	**0.81**	0.04		0.66
	motor dysfunction	**0.65**	0.51		0.68
	drowsiness	**0.60**	0.06		0.37
	communication deficit	**0.49**	0.12		0.25
	visual disorder	**0.36**	0.30		0.22
	seizures	**0.33**	-0.17		0.14
	remembering difficulty	**0.31**	0.03		0.10
	itchy skin	-0.13	**0.61**		0.39
	hair loss	0.06	**0.59**		0.35
	bladder control	0.34	**0.54**		0.41
	weakness of legs	-0.16	**0.46**		0.24
	headaches	0.18	**0.44**		0.23
	future uncertainty	0.16	**0.40**		0.18
	% of variance	72%	28%		
	Cronbach's alpha	0.78	0.63		

Table 2. (Continued).

			R^2		
		Item	Own Cluster	Next Cluster	$\frac{1 - R^2_{Own\ cluster}}{1 - R^2_{Next\ cluster}}$
HCA	Cluster 1	concentrating difficulty	0.66	0.02	0.35
		visual disorder	0.28	0.07	0.77
		motor dysfunction	0.57	0.25	0.58
		seizures	0.13	0.01	0.88
		drowsiness	0.38	0.006	0.62
		communication deficit	0.38	0.03	0.64
		remembering difficulty	0.24	0.01	0.77
	Cluster 2	future uncertainty	0.33	0.04	0.70
		headaches	0.38	0.09	0.68
		hair loss	0.54	0.03	0.48
		itchy skin	0.39	0.0000	0.61
		weakness of legs	0.28	0.002	0.72
		bladder control	0.38	0.14	0.73

Exploratory Factor Analysis (EFA)

From the eigenvalues and proportions of variance for the scales and symptoms of the EORTC QLQ-BN20/BN20+2 at baseline, EFA derived two factors, which were retained (eigenvalue >1.0), and the cumulative variance showed as 100%. The first cluster included concentrating difficulty, motor dysfunction, drowsiness, communication deficit, visual disorder, seizures and remembering difficulty. The second cluster included itchy skin, hair loss, bladder control, weakness of legs, headaches and future uncertainty.

The internal consistency as determined by the Cronbach's alpha was 78% for the first cluster and 63% for the second cluster (see Table 2).

Hierarchical cluster analysis (HCA)

Using the HCA method, the centroid cluster algorithm split the variables into the two clusters (see Table 2). The first cluster contains difficulty concentrating, visual disorder, motor dysfunction, seizures, drowsiness, communication deficit and remembering difficulty. The second cluster contains future uncertainty, headaches, hair loss, itchy skin, weakness of legs and bladder control. The first cluster explained 36% of the total variation of the cluster. The second cluster explained 38% of the total variation. If cluster 1 were split into additional clusters due to the smallest proportion of variation (36%), only the symptom of seizure would have been split out. Since a symptom cluster must contain more than one symptom, the two symptom clusters were maintained. The tree diagram in Figure 2a visually represents the two clusters as identified using HCA. From the diagram, it demonstrated that one cluster explained 23.4% of variation, while two clusters explained up to 36.7% of the total variation. Additionally, the smallest correlation between the items and their own cluster component was 0.13 (seizure in Cluster 1). The inter-cluster correlation between Cluster 1 and Cluster 2 was 0.27 (very small).

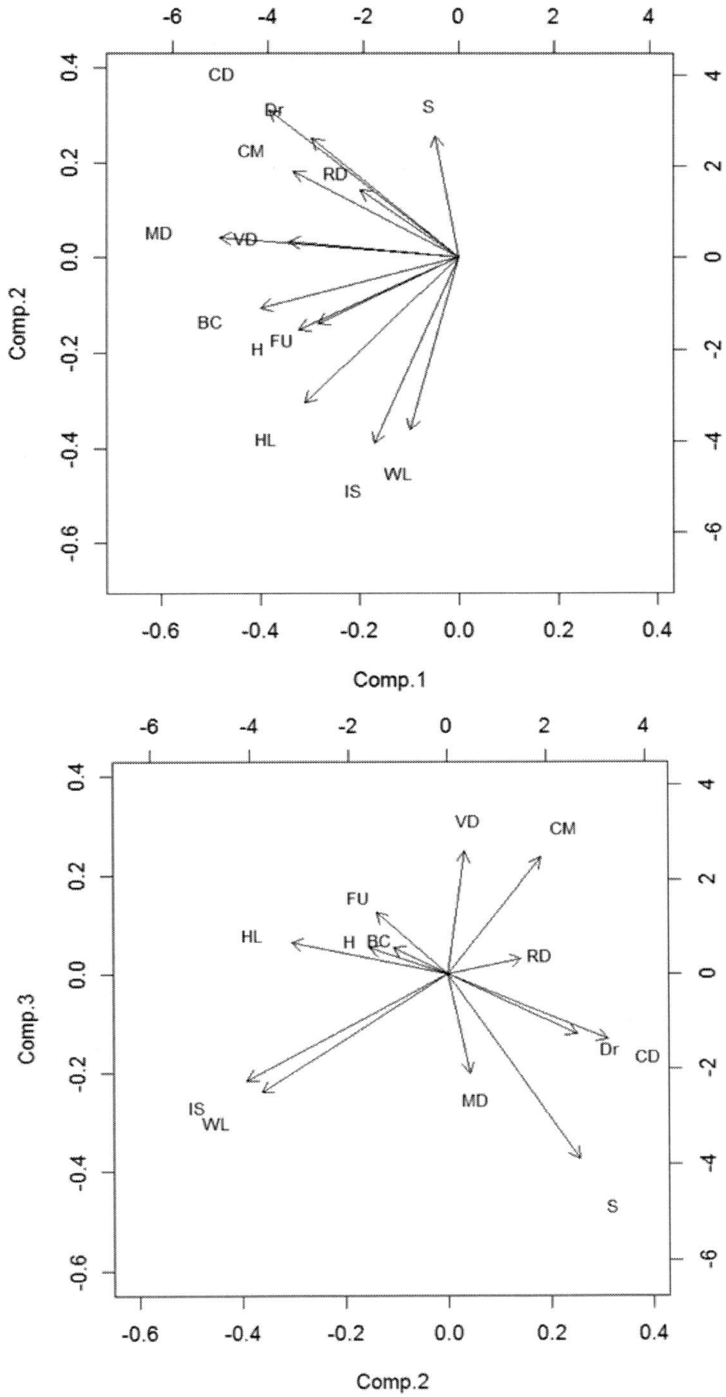

Figure 1a. (Continued).

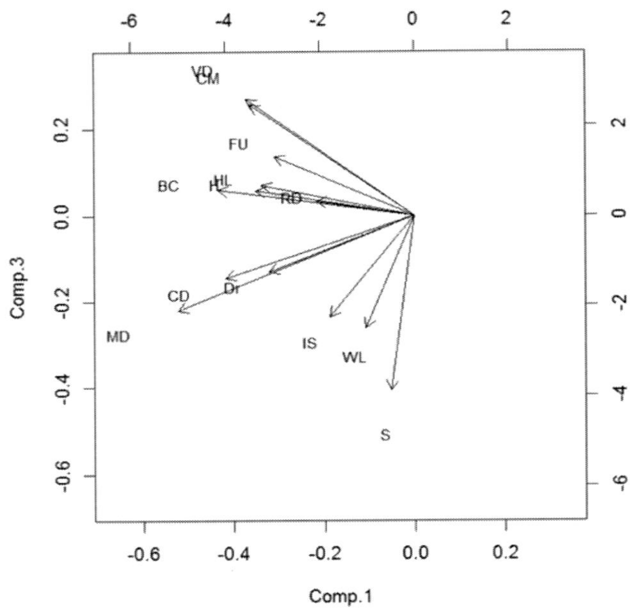

Figure 1a. Biplot among three principal components or clusters at baseline.

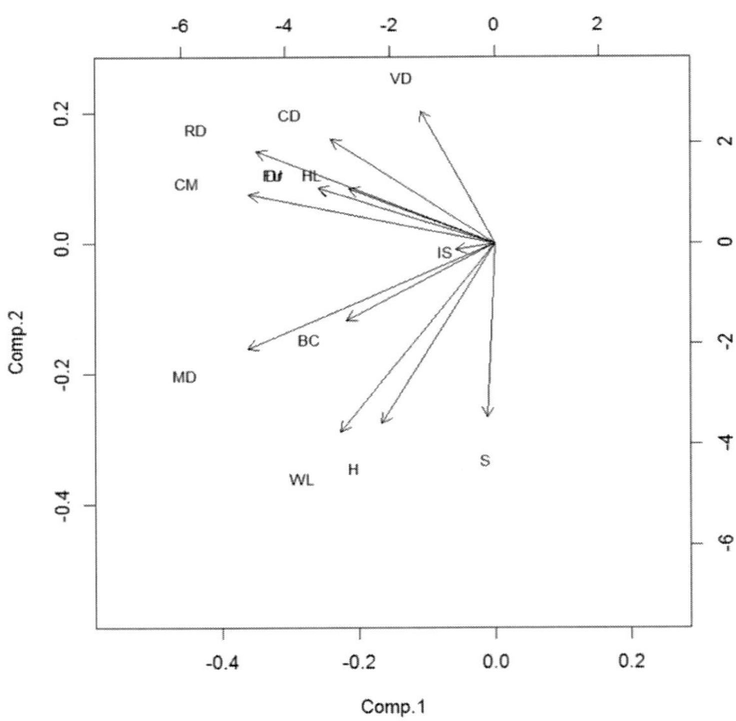

Figure 1b. Biplot between First Two Principal Clusters at Follow-Up.

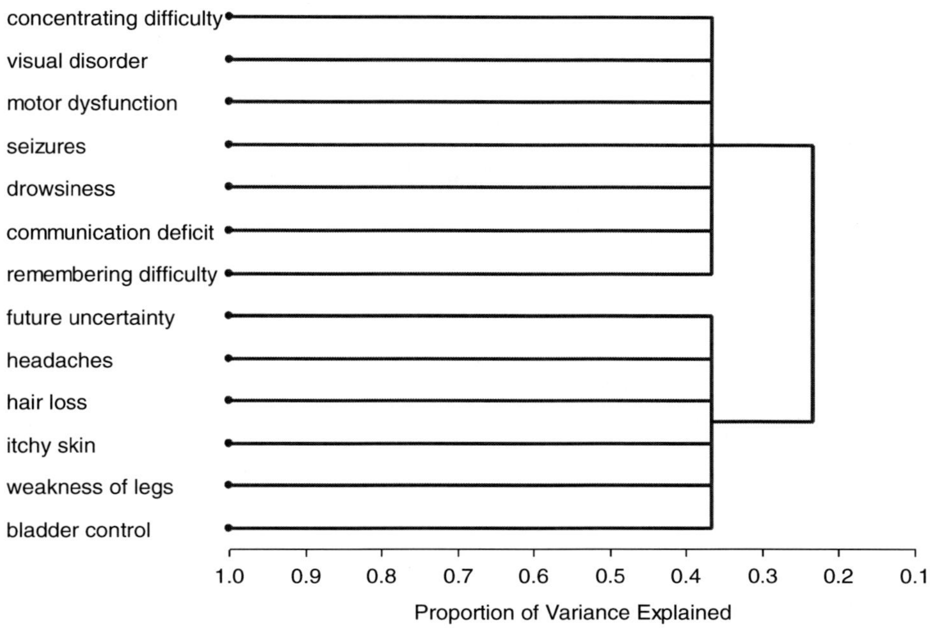

Figure 2a. PROC TREE procedure-generated diagram displaying two cluster solution and cluster hierarchy at baseline.

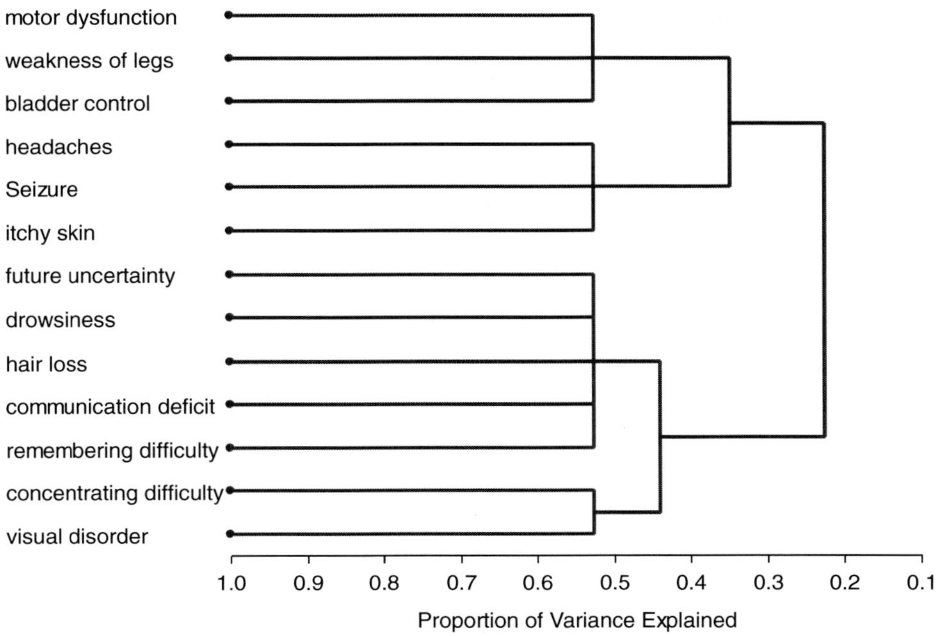

Figure 2b. PROC TREE procedure-generated diagram displaying two cluster solution and cluster hierarchy at follow-up.

Comparison among the three different analytical methods

From these three analyses (PCA, EFA, and HCA), we obtained the exact same two clusters using the HCA and EFA analyses, while PCA resulted in three clusters for this study. Using these three methods, concentrating difficulty, motor dysfunction, seizures, drowsiness and remembering difficulty were always grouped in the same cluster; future uncertainty, headaches, hair loss and bladder control were grouped in the same cluster; and itchy skin and weakness of legs were always grouped in the same cluster.

This indicates higher correlation among those items (Table 3).

Symptom clusters at follow-up

At follow-up, of the four scales, patients scored most highly on the future uncertainty scale with a mean score of 38.4 then followed by the motor dysfunction scale with a mean score of 24.2. Of the nine symptoms/toxicity items, patients reported worse drowsiness, remembering difficulty and weakness of legs with a mean score of 36.7, 21.3 and 20.9 respectively.

Table 3. Symptom Clusters from the EORTC QLQ-BN20 identified at Baseline and 1-month Follow-up using Three Statistical Methods

Symptoms	Baseline (n = 155)			1-Month Follow-Up (n = 100)		
	PCA	EFA	HCA	PCA	EFA	HCA
Future uncertainty	□	□	□	□	□	□
Visual disorder	□	○	○	□	□	□
Headaches	□	□	□	○	○	❖
Hair loss	□	□	□	□	□	□
Bladder control	□	□	□	○	○	○
Communication deficit	□	○	○	□	□	□
Concentrating difficulty	○	○	○	□	□	□
Motor dysfunction	○	○	○	○	○	○
Seizures	○	○	○	○	○	❖
Drowsiness	○	○	○	□	□	□
Remembering difficulty	○	○	○	□	□	□
Itchy skin	□	□	□	□	□	❖
Weakness of legs	□	□	□	○	○	○

* Corresponding symbols indicate symptoms/subscale were in the same cluster.

FU: follow-up, PCA–Principal component analysis, EFA–exploratory factor analysis, HCA–hierarchical cluster analysis.

PCA

PCA derived two clusters with eigenvalues greater than 1.0 and accounting for at least 10% of total variation. The first cluster consisted of remembering difficulty, communication deficit, concentrating difficulty, future uncertainty, drowsiness, hair loss, visual disorder and itchy skin and accounts for 26% of total variance. The second cluster consisted of weakness of legs, headaches, motor dysfunction, seizure, and bladder control and accounts for 13% of total variance (Table 4). For 2 symptoms clusters, the internal reliabilities were close to 0.70, which had good internal consistency.

The final communality shows that all the variables were well accounted for by the 2 components except for itchy skin (0.015), with final communality estimates ranging from 0.235 for hair loss to 0.698 for motor dysfunction. In Figure 1b, the two clusters were easily demonstrated in the current biplot between the two clusters.

EFA

From the eigenvalues and proportions of variance for the scales and symptoms of the EORTC QLQ-BN20/BN20+2 at follow-up, EFA derived 2 factors, which were retained (eigen value > 1.0), and the cumulative variance shown as 100%. The first cluster included remembering difficulty, communication deficit, concentrating difficulty, drowsiness, future uncertainty, hair loss, visual disorder, and itchy skin. The second cluster included weakness of legs, motor dysfunction, headaches, bladder control and seizure. The internal consistency as determined by the Cronbach's alpha was 71% for the first cluster and 68% for the second cluster (Table 4).

HCA

First, the centroid cluster algorithm split the variables into the two clusters. The first cluster explained 37% of the total variation. The second cluster explained 33% of the total variation. Cluster 2 was then split because of the smallest proportion of variation (33%). After HCA split cluster 2, the new Cluster 2 explained 62% and Cluster 3 explained 43% of the total variation. HCA then split cluster 1 into two additional clusters.

As displayed in Table 4, Cluster 1 included future uncertainty, drowsiness, hair loss, and communication deficit and explained 47% of the total variation. Cluster 2 consisted of remembering difficulty and motor dysfunction and explained 62% of the total variation. Cluster 3 consisted of headaches, seizure, and itchy skin and explained 43% of the variation. Finally, Cluster 4 consisted of concentrating difficulty and visual disorder and explained 66% of the total variation. The four centroid components accounted for 53% of the variability in the 13 items, and all cluster components accounted for at least 43% of the total variation in the corresponding cluster. Additionally, the smallest correlation between the items and their own cluster component was 0.35 (hair loss in Cluster 1). The inter-cluster correlation between Cluster 1 and Cluster 2 was 0.39, between Cluster 1 and Cluster 4 was 0.32. Other correlations were very weak correlations.

The tree diagram in Figure 2b visually represents the four clusters as identified using HCA. From the diagram, it demonstrated 2 larger clusters or four smaller clusters. One cluster explained 23% of variation; two clusters explained up to 35% of variation, three clusters explained 44% of total variation, while four clusters explained 53% of total variation.

Table 4. PCA, EFA and HCA of the Four Scales and Nine Symptom/Toxicity Items on the EORTC QLQ-BN20/BN20+2 at Follow-Up

	Item	Component 1	Component 2	Final communality
PCA	remembering difficulty	**0.79**	0.09	0.63
	communication deficit	**0.74**	0.22	0.60
	concentrating difficulty	**0.60**	-0.05	0.37
	future uncertainty	**0.56**	0.10	0.33
	drowsiness	**0.56**	0.10	0.33
	hair loss	**0.48**	0.06	0.24
	visual disorder	**0.40**	-0.27	0.24
	itchy skin	**0.10**	0.08	0.02
	weakness of legs	0.13	**0.76**	0.60
	headaches	0.03	**0.68**	0.49
	motor dysfunction	0.51	**0.66**	0.70
	Seizure	-0.25	**0.50**	0.31
	bladder control	0.29	**0.43**	0.27
	% of variance	26%	13%	
	Cronbach's alpha	0.69	0.68	
EFA	remembering difficulty	**0.79**	0.09	0.63
	communication deficit	**0.74**	0.18	0.58
	concentrating difficulty	**0.48**	0.05	0.23
	drowsiness	**0.48**	0.10	0.24
	future uncertainty	**0.46**	0.13	0.23
	hair loss	**0.38**	0.09	0.15
	visual disorder	**0.27**	-0.09	0.08
	itchy skin	**0.10**	0.01	0.009
	weakness of legs	0.06	**0.80**	0.64
	motor dysfunction	0.45	**0.74**	0.7
	headaches	0.09	**0.40**	0.171
	bladder control	0.24	**0.32**	0.16
	Seizure	-0.15	**0.28**	0.10
	% of variance	72%	**28%**	
	Cronbach's alpha	0.71	**0.68**	

		Item	R^2 Own Cluster	R^2 Next Cluster	$\frac{1-R^2_{Own\ cluster}}{1-R^2_{Next\ cluster}}$
HCA	Cluster 1	future uncertainty	0.4105	0.0690	0.6332
		drowsiness	0.4267	0.0425	0.5988
		hair loss	0.3502	0.0577	0.6896
		communication deficit	0.6666	0.0952	0.3685
		remembering difficulty	0.5454	0.1427	0.5302
	Cluster 2	motor dysfunction	0.7401	0.2356	0.3401
		weakness of legs	0.6660	0.0324	0.3452
		bladder control	0.4743	0.0705	0.5655
	Cluster 3	headaches	0.4655	0.1135	0.6030
		Seizure	0.4613	0.0125	0.5456
		itchy skin	0.3744	0.0082	0.6308
	Cluster 4	concentrating difficulty	0.6570	0.1300	0.3942
		visual disorder	0.6570	0.0232	0.3511

Cluster 1 explained 47%, 2nd Cluster explained 62%, 3rd Cluster explained 43%, and 4th Cluster explained 66% of the total variation.

Comparison among the three different analytical methods

From these 3 analyses (PCA, EFA, and HCA), we derived the same clusters from PCA and EFA analyses, and HCA suggested 4 small clusters for this study. Using three methods, the following items were always grouped in the same cluster, indicating higher correlation among those items. Future uncertainty, drowsiness and hair loss were consistency grouped together. Similarly, communication deficit and remembering difficulty were grouped together. Finally, 'concentrating difficulty and visual disorder,' 'motor dysfunction, weakness of legs and bladder control,' and 'headaches and seizure' were also consistency grouped together (Table 3).

DISCUSSION

A literature search found five other studies investigating symptom clusters in patients with brain metastases in three different patient populations. The instruments used to assess symptoms and QOL in patients included the Edmonton Symptom Assessment Scale and the Spitzer Quality of Life Index (SQLI) with an additional 17-symptom questionnaire (6, 9, 12-14). One conference abstract utilized the M.D. Anderson Symptom Inventory-Brain Tumor Module (MDASI-BT) (15). Our current symptom cluster analysis using the EORTC QLQ-BN20/BN20+2 in patients with brain metastases, adds important information to the current literature.

We used three different statistical methods (PCA, EFA, HCA), which are exploratory and descriptive, to identify symptom clusters. Although all three methods are used to derived symptom cluster, their underlying methodology differ greatly. EFA explores the underlying structure of a group of symptoms. It combines symptoms in "factors" and examines the relationships of symptoms within a group (12, 16). HCA assesses the clustering of individuals with similar symptom patterns (16). Due to this type of analysis, it is most useful clinically as it distinguishes clusters with distinct profiles, therefore enabling clinicians to target treatments towards the clusters of symptoms (12). Finally, PCA, which is a data reduction technique, reduces the symptoms into few components. It does so based on variance (16). PCA determines a few components to substitute the original variable accurately, by accounting for the total variance in a variable. No assumptions are made on the underlying structure or causality (12, 16). Although there are vast differences between the methods and the symptom clusters it derives, no single method is superior over the others (12).

In our current study at baseline, HCA and EFA derived the exact same clusters while at follow-up, PCA and EFA derived the exact same clusters. Furthermore, at both baseline and follow-up certain scales and symptom/toxicity items were consistently group together, suggesting a strong correlation between those items which was confirmed through multiple types of analysis. Although there were no consistent cluster findings with the three different statistical methods, the consistency seen between two different statistical methods at both baseline and follow-up was greater than that observed in another study using the SQLI in a similar patient cohort (9). Another study by Chen et al. only found strong correlation between the clusters derived by PCA and HCA, which was not found within our current study (13).

Currently, some studies in different cancer populations have used the same three statistical methods while others have employed additional statistical methods. Examples of which include, multivariate analysis of variance employed by Chan et al. (17), hierarchical multiple regression analysis as employed by Fox et al. (18), multidimensional scaling as used by Gleason et al. (19) and also the Pearson correlation as used by Maliski et al. (20). The incongruency in the cluster findings of the current study and the different methods used by other studies, highlight a major barrier in the field of symptom cluster research: the lack of consensus on a method to derive symptom clusters. Due to this inconsistency, comparisons between patient populations are difficult.

There were two major limitations in this current study. Firstly, the patient population included a variety of primary cancer sites, which can lead to greater variations in symptoms experienced thus affecting the derived symptom clusters. Secondly, another limitation was the tool used in this assessment. The EORTC QLQ-BN20/BN20+2 assessed both quality of life aspects as well as individual symptoms/toxicity items however this may not have covered all symptoms experienced by patients with brain metastases.

CONCLUSION

This study aimed to determine symptoms clusters in patients with brain metastases using the EORTC QLQ-BN20/BN20+2 and compare three different statistical methods. Although complete agreement was not found among the three methodologies, certain scales or symptoms consistently clustered together at baseline and follow-up, which suggest association. At baseline, 'concentrating difficulty, motor dysfunction, seizures, drowsiness and remembering difficulty' were always grouped in the same cluster; 'future uncertainty, headaches, hair loss and bladder control' were grouped in the same cluster; and 'itchy skin and weakness of legs' were grouped in the same cluster. At follow-up, 'future uncertainty, drowsiness and hair loss,' 'communication deficit and remembering difficulty,' 'concentrating difficulty and visual disorder,' 'motor dysfunction, weakness of legs and bladder control,' and 'headaches and seizure' were consistently grouped together. Future studies should address the lack of consensus on the method of analysis for deriving clusters therefore allowing for future comparison.

ACKNOWLEDGMENTS

We thank the generous support of Dr. Mark Clemons, a participating investigator from the Ottawa Hospital Cancer Centre in Canada and the Bratty Family Fund, Michael and Karyn Goldstein Cancer Research Fund, Pulenzas Cancer Research Fund, Joseph and Silvana Melara Cancer Research Fund, and Ofelia Cancer Research Fund.

APPENDIX 1. EORTC QLQ–BN20

Patients sometimes report that they have the following symptoms. Please indicate the extent to which you have experienced these symptoms or problems during the past week.

During the past week:	**Not at all**	**A little**	**Quite a bit**	**Very much**
1. Did you feel uncertain about the future?	1	2	3	4
2. Did you feel you had setbacks in your condition?	1	2	3	4
3. Were you concerned about disruption of family life?	1	2	3	4
4. Did you have headaches?	1	2	3	4
5. Did your outlook on the future worsen?	1	2	3	4
6. Did you have double vision?	1	2	3	4
7. Was your vision blurred?	1	2	3	4
8. Did you have difficulty reading because of your vision?	1	2	3	4
9. Did you have seizures?	1	2	3	4
10. Did you have weakness on one side of your body?	1	2	3	4
11. Did you have trouble finding the right words to express Yourself?	1	2	3	4
12. Did you have difficulty speaking?	1	2	3	4
13. Did you have trouble communicating your thoughts?	1	2	3	4
14. Did you feel drowsy during the daytime?	1	2	3	4
15. Did you have trouble with your coordination?	1	2	3	4
16. Did hair loss bother you?	1	2	3	4
17. Did itching of your skin bother you?	1	2	3	4
18. Did you have weakness of both legs?	1	2	3	4
19. Did you feel unsteady on your feet?	1	2	3	4
20. Did you have trouble controlling your bladder?	1	2	3	4

APPENDIX 2. EORTC QLQ–BN20 + 2 COGNITIVE ITEMS

Patients sometimes report that they have the following symptoms. Please indicate the extent to which you have experienced these symptoms or problems during the past week.

During the past week:	**Not At all**	**A little**	**Quite a bit**	**Very much**
1. Did you feel uncertain about the future?	1	2	3	4
2. Did you feel you had setbacks in your condition?	1	2	3	4
3. Were you concerned about disruption of family life?	1	2	3	4
4. Did you have headaches?	1	2	3	4
5. Did your outlook on the future worsen?	1	2	3	4
6. Did you have double vision?	1	2	3	4
7. Was your vision blurred?	1	2	3	4
8. Did you have difficulty reading because of your vision?	1	2	3	4
9. Did you have seizures?	1	2	3	4
10. Did you have weakness on one side of your body?	1	2	3	4
11. Did you have trouble finding the right words to express yourself?	1	2	3	4
12. Did you have difficulty speaking?	1	2	3	4
13. Did you have trouble communicating your thoughts?	1	2	3	4
14. Did you feel drowsy during the daytime?	1	2	3	4
15. Did you have trouble with your coordination?	1	2	3	4
16. Did hair loss bother you?	1	2	3	4
17. Did itching of your skin bother you?	1	2	3	4
18. Did you have weakness of both legs?	1	2	3	4
19. Did you feel unsteady on your feet?	1	2	3	4
20. Did you have trouble controlling your bladder?	1	2	3	4
21. Have you had difficulty in concentrating on things like reading a newspaper or watching television?	1	2	3	4
22. Have you had difficulty remembering things?	1	2	3	4

REFERENCES

[1] Gavrilovic IT, Posner JB. Brain metastases: epidemiology and pathophysiology. J Neurooncol 2005;75(1):5-14.

[2] Bezjak A, Adam J, Barton R, Panzarella T, Laperriere N, Wong CS, et al. Symptom response after palliative radiotherapy for patients with brain metastases. Eur J Cancer 2002;38(4):487-96.

[3] Tsao MN, Rades D, Wirth A, Lo SS, Danielson BL, Gaspar LE, et al. Radiotherapeutic and surgical management for newly diagnosed brain metastasis(es): An American Society for Radiation Oncology evidence-based guideline. Pract Radiat Oncol 2012;2(3):210-25.

[4] Patchell RA. The management of brain metastases. Cancer Treat Rev 2003;29(6):533-40.

[5] Portenoy RK, Thaler HT, Kornblith AB, Lepore JM, Friedlander-Klar H, Coyle N, et al. Symptom prevalence, characteristics and distress in a cancer population. Qual Life Res 1994;3(3):183-9.

[6] Chow E, Fan G, Hadi S, Wong J, Kirou-Mauro A, Filipczak L. Symptom clusters in cancer patients with brain metastases. Clin Oncol (R Coll Radiol) 2008;20(1):76-82.

[7] Dodd MJ, Miaskowski C, Paul SM. Symptom clusters and their effect on the functional status of patients with cancer. Oncol Nurs Forum 2001;28(3):465-70.

[8] Kim HJ, McGuire DB, Tulman L, Barsevick AM. Symptom clusters: concept analysis and clinical implications for cancer nursing. Cancer Nurs 2005;28(4):270-82; quiz 283-4.

[9] Khan L, Cramarossa G, Lemke M, Nguyen J, Zhang L, Chen E, et al. Symptom clusters using the Spitzer quality of life index in patients with brain metastases--a reanalysis comparing different statistical methods. Support Care Cancer 2013;21(2):467-73.

[10] Barsevick AM, Whitmer K, Nail LM, Beck SL, Dudley WN. Symptom cluster research: conceptual, design, measurement, and analysis issues. J Pain Symptom Manage 2006;31(1):85-95.

[11] Kim HJ, Abraham IL. Statistical approaches to modeling symptom clusters in cancer patients. Cancer Nurs 2008;31(5):E1-10.

[12] Chen E, Khan L, Zhang L, Nguyen J, Zeng L, Bedard G, et al. Symptom clusters in patients with brain metastases-a reanalysis comparing different statistical methods. J Radiat Oncol 2013;2(1):95-102.

[13] Chen E, Nguyen J, Khan L, Zhang L, Cramarossa G, Tsao M, et al. Symptom clusters in patients with advanced cancer: A reanalysis comparing different statistical methods. J Pain Symptom Manage 2012;44(1):23-32.

[14] Hird A, Wong J, Zhang L, Tsao M, Barnes E, Danjoux C, et al. Exploration of symptoms clusters within cancer patients with brain metastases using the Spitzer Quality of Life Index. Support Care Cancer 2010;18(3):335-42.

[15] Armstrong TS, Gning I, Vera-Bolanos E. Symptom clusters in patients with brain metastases. Neuro-oncology 2009;11(5):654.

[16] Skerman HM, Yates PM, Battistutta D. Multivariate methods to identify cancer-related symptom clusters. Res Nurs Health 2009;32(3):345-60.

[17] Chan CW, Richardson A, Richardson J. A study to assess the existence of the symptom cluster of breathlessness, fatigue and anxiety in patients with advanced lung cancer. Eur J Oncol Nurs 2005;9(4):325-33.

[18] Fox SW, Lyon D. Symptom clusters and quality of life in survivors of ovarian cancer. Cancer Nurs 2007;30(5):354-61.

[19] Gleason JF Jr, Case D, Rapp SR, Ip E, Naughton M, Butler JM Jr, et al. Symptom clusters in patients with newly-diagnosed brain tumors. J Support Oncol 2007;5(9):427-33, 436.

[20] Maliski SL, Kwan L, Elashoff D, Litwin MS. Symptom clusters related to treatment for prostate cancer. Oncol Nurs Forum 2008;35(5):786-93.

Submitted: February 05, 2015. *Revised:* March 23, 2015. *Accepted:* March 29, 2015.

In: Pain Management Yearbook 2015
Editor: Joav Merrick
ISBN: 978-1-63484-515-1

Chapter 15

INITIAL PRESENTATION OF HIGH PROSTATE-SPECIFIC ANTIGEN (PSA): A CASE REPORT

Catherine Lang[1], BSc, Linda Probyn[1,2,*], MD, FRCPC, Natalie Pulenzas[3], BSc(C), Rachel McDonald[3], BSc(C), Leigha Rowbottom[3], BSc(C), and Edward Chow[3], MBBS, MSc, PhD, FRCPC

[1]Department of Medical Imaging, University of Toronto, Toronto, Ontario, Canada
[2]Department of Medical Imaging, Sunnybrook Health Sciences Centre, Toronto, Ontario, Canada
[3]Department of Radiation Oncology, Sunnybrook Health Sciences Centre, University of Toronto, Toronto, Ontario, Canada

Widespread population screening for prostate cancer using the prostate-specific antigen (PSA) test has led to a decrease in rates of both metastatic disease and cancer deaths related to prostate cancer. We present a case of extremely elevated PSA levels in an 86-year-old male patient with widespread metastatic disease. This case highlights in importance of the PSA test being used only as one component of a multivariate approach to detecting and treating prostate cancer. However, the limited specificity of the PSA test for detecting clinically significant lesions has led to the over detection of benign conditions resulting in unnecessary biopsies and treatment. We will discuss that the prostate health index (PHI) is an alternative formula for detecting prostate cancer. The PHI incorporates measurements of unbound PSA, which has been associated with benign conditions, and the PSA isoform (-2) proPSA, which has been associated with clinically significant prostate cancer. The PHI has been shown to outperform the PSA test with improved specificity for prostate cancer detection in several population screening trials.

Keywords: prostate cancer, prostate-specific antigen, prostate health index, bone metastases

[*] Correspondence: Linda Probyn, MD, FRCPC, Department of Medical Imaging, University of Toronto, 263 McCaul Street, Toronto, Ontario, M5T 1W7, Canada. E-mail: linda.probyn@sunnybrook.ca.

INTRODUCTION

In Canada, the most common cancer for males is prostate cancer, with 1 in 8 men expected to be diagnosed in their lifetime (1). The incidence rate of prostate cancer peaked in 1993 and 2001, and was followed by a decline in the subsequent years (1). These peaks can both be traced to two waves of intensified screening activity using the prostate-specific antigen (PSA) test (1). The PSA test is not currently recommended in Canada as a population-based screening test as there is ongoing uncertainty regarding its utility (1-3). The PSA test has been used to try to identify tumours at an early, curable stage (3). However, the PSA test has not been able to discriminate between benign and clinically significant tumours, resulting in an increase in prostate cancer diagnosis, but no change in the resulting mortality rates (3). In a population screening trial in Europe, it was calculated that in order to prevent one death, 1,055 men would need to be screened and 37 would be need to be treated, resulting in 36 patients receiving a cancer diagnosis and treatment without changing their survival outcome (3, 4).

The PSA, also known as kallikrein-3, was first discovered by Richard Ablin in the 1970s (3, 5). It is a glycoprotein formed by the prostate gland that functions to liquefy serum, promote sperm motility, and dissolve cervical mucus (3, 6). In 1991, Catalona et al. suggested its use to detect prostate cancer at an early, more curable stage, instead of the traditional digital rectal exam (DRE) (3, 7). In their study, men with a PSA level of equal to or greater than 4 μg/L were biopsied, and malignant lesions were identified in 33% of the 112 men tested (3, 7). Since then, it has been concluded that PSA test provides increased sensitivity over the DRE, but the PSA test lacks specificity as elevated PSA could be due to benign prostate hypertrophy, recent manipulations of the prostate due to massage or biopsy, or prostatitis (3).

We present a patient with an extremely elevated PSA level at presentation. The patient has widespread bone metastases of an unknown origin. This case demonstrates using the PSA test as an indicator of prostate cancer, and highlights the controversial utility of using the PSA test for population-based screening.

CASE REPORT

An 86 year-old man was referred to the Rapid Response Radiotherapy Program (RRRP) at Sunnybrook Health Sciences Centre for consideration of palliative radiotherapy for symptomatic bone metastases of unknown origin. The patient was known to have prostate hypertrophy and a recent transurethral resection of the prostate (TURP) and biopsy performed at an outside institution showed no evidence of carcinoma.

An enlarged prostate was initially noted on an abdominal ultrasound where it was measured at 5.7 cm x 5.6 cm x 6.5 cm for a volume of 93 cc. At this time, blood work was also completed which indicated high alkaline phosphatase (ALP) levels (227 units/liter; normal range 45-120 units/liter). High ALP, which can correspond to increased bone cell activity, indicated the likelihood of Paget's disease or cancer that had metastasized to the bone. A chest x-ray indicated that there was no evidence of Paget's disease or other bony abnormality. Subsequent blood work indicated abnormal parathyroid hormone (PTH) levels

(13.6 pmol/l; normal range 1.6-6.9 pmol/l) and insufficient vitamin D levels (32 nmol/l; insufficient range 25-74 nmol/l). Both the increased PTH levels and insufficient vitamin D levels were indicative of irregular bone growth.

After the time of referral to the RRRP, the patient had plain film imaging of the lumbosacral spine as well as the pelvis and bilateral femurs. The lumbosacral spine showed mixed lytic and sclerotic lesions in the lower lumbar spine with involvement of the visualized sacrum and ilium. The pelvic and bilateral femur radiographs revealed further diffuse mixed lytic osseous lesions in the lower lumbar spine, sacrum, ilium, and pubic rami. A pathologic fracture in the right iliac was also noted. These radiographic findings were consistent with an outside bone scan that showed diffuse abnormality compatible with marrow replacing lesions. Following these radiographs, CT scans of the lumbar spine, pelvis and both femurs were obtained. Diffuse blastic, mainly sclerotic metastases were again noted throughout the lumbar spine, sacrum, pelvis, both femurs and tibia/fibula. Perineural cysts were also noted in the sacrum.

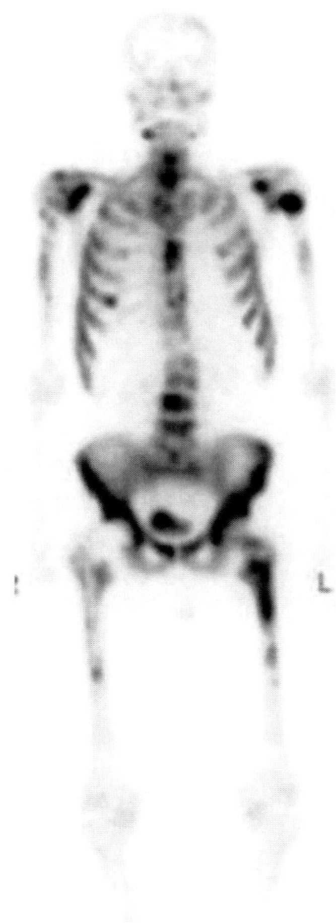

Figure 1. Whole body $Tc^{99}m$-MDP bone scan indicating widespread diffuse increased uptake in the spine, mandible, skull base, ribs, sternum, pelvis, proximal humeri, proximal femurs and scapulae.

Following these studies, another $Tc^{99}m$ diphosphate bone scan of the whole body was ordered. The bone scan again revealed increased uptake in the spine, mandible, skull base, ribs, sternum, pelvis, proximal humeri, proximal femurs and scapulae (Figure 1). These findings corresponded to the sclerotic lesions demonstrated on CT. The bone scan was noted to be a superscan of widespread osseous metastases, with associated reduced soft tissue and kidney visualizations.

The patient returned to the RRRP and further blood work was ordered. The blood work came back abnormal with extremely elevated PSA levels (2462 ng/ml; normal range <4.0ng/ml), elevated aspartate tranferase (AST) levels (88 units/l; normal 10-40 units/l), and grossly elevated ALP levels (3383 units/l; normal range 45-120 units/l).

The patient was then referred to a genitourinary radiation oncologist. It was concluded that the extremely elevated PSA and imaging results were indicative of widespread bony metastatic disease of prostate origin even though the outside TURP had reported a benign pathology. The patient was prescribed hormonal treatment of Zoladex (goserelin) injections and an LHRH agonist for treatment of high PSA. The patient was also prescribed Actonel DR (risedronate delayed-release) to strengthen his bones. It was suggested to proceed with radiotherapy of an 8Gy in one fraction to the entire pelvis as the patient remained quite symptomatic.

A follow-up CT of the cervical and thoracic spine noted extensive osteolytic and osteosclerotic lesions throughout cervical spine, thoracic spine, and visualized portions of the ribs and shoulder girdle were essentially confluent. There was also prominent destruction of the skull base extending into the clivus.

Discussion

In this case report we describe a patient with extremely elevated PSA levels at presentation. The purpose of the PSA test is to try to identify early-stage prostate tumours, and widespread screening has successfully reduced the amount of metastatic disease and death rates due to prostate cancer (3, 8). However, the limited specificity of the PSA test makes population screening controversial as many clinically non-significant tumours may be detected resulting in unnecessary biopsies and cancer treatments (8).

The new Prostate Health Index (PHI) may provide a successful alternative to the traditional PSA test, and aid in distinguishing clinically significant prostate tumours from benign conditions (8). Studies have shown that PSA elevation from benign conditions is associated with a higher proportion of unbound or free PSA circulating in the blood (8-10). Test specificity has been further increased by the identification of PSA isoforms, particularly the [-2] form of proPSA, that have improved performance in detecting prostate cancer on biopsy (8, 11, 12). The PHI combines all three PSA forms using the following formula:

$$PHI = \frac{[-2]proPSA}{free\ PSA} * \sqrt{PSA}$$

A patient with both a higher total PSA and a larger ratio of (-2) proPSA to free PSA will have a high PHI score and will be more likely to have clinically significant prostate cancer. Several population-screening trials have shown the PHI to outperform the traditional PSA test by demonstrating increased sensitivity calculated in the range of 80-95%, and thereby has the potential to reduce unnecessary biopsies and the over detection of benign lesions (8, 13-15).

For the patient described in this case report, the cancer was ultimately presumed to be of prostate origin even though the preceding prostate biopsy was negative. Prostate biopsies are significantly associated with increased risk of hospitalization and a repeated biopsy is not appropriate in the context of an elderly patient with extensive metastatic disease (16). The patient received hormonal treatment to manage his reported bony pain, and will be monitored for continued pain symptoms. Subsequent biopsy confirmed prostate cancer.

Conclusion

In conclusion, we report the finding of very high PSA levels in a patient. This supports the use of the PSA blood test as only one component of a multivariate approach, including the PHI, to diagnosing prostate cancer.

Acknowledgments

We thank the generous support of the Bratty Family Fund, Michael and Karyn Goldstein Cancer Research Fund, Pulenzas Cancer Research Fund, Joseph and Silvana Melara Cancer Research Fund, and Ofelia Cancer Research Fund.

References

[1] Canadian Cancer Society's Advisory Committee on Cancer Statistics. Canadian Cancer Statistics 2014. Toronto, ON: Canadian Cancer Society, 2014.

[2] Levy I. Prostate cancer: The epidemiologic perspective. Can J Oncol 1994;4 (Suppl 1):4–7.

[3] Pezaro C, Woo HH, Davis ID. Prostate cancer: measuring PSA. Intern Med Jounral 2014.

[4] Schroder FH, Hugosson J, Roobol MJ, Tammela TL, Ciatto S, Nelen V, et al. Prostate-cancer mortality at 11 years of follow-up. N Engl J Med 2012; 366: 981–90.

[5] Ablin R. The great prostate mistake. New York Times 2010 Mar 09. URL: http://www.nytimes.com/2010/03/10/opinion/10Ablin.html?_r=0.

[6] Arneth B. Clinical significance of measuring prostate-specific antigen. Lab 2009; 40:487–91.

[7] Catalona WJ, Smith DS, Ratliff TL, Dodds KM, Coplen DE, Yuan JJ, et al. Measurement of prostate-specific antigen in serum as a screening test for prostate cancer. N Engl J Med 1991;324:1156–61.

[8] Loeb S, Catalona WJ. The Prostate Health Index: a new test for the detection of prostate cancer. Ther Adv Urol 2014;6(2):74-7.

[9] Lilja H, Christensson A, Dahlen U, Matikainen M, Nilsson O, Petterson K, et al. Prostate-specific antigen in serum occurs predominantly in complex with alpha 1-antichymotrypsin. Clin Chem 1991;37:1618-25.

[10] Stenman U, Leinonen J, Alfthan H, Rannikko S, Tuhkanen K, Alfthan O. A complex between prostate-specific antigen and alpha 1-antichymotrypsin is the major form of prostate-specific antigen in serum of pateitns with prostatic cancer: assay of the complex improves clinical sensitivity for cancer. Cancer Res 1991; 51:222-6.

[11] Catalona W, Bartsch G, Rittenhouse H, Evans C, Linton H, Amirkhan A, et al. Serum pro prostate specific antigen improves cancer detection compared to free and complexed prostate specific antigen in men with prostate specific antigen 2 to 4 ng/ml. J Urol 2003;170:2181-5.
[12] Sokoll L, Sanda M, Feng Z, Kagan J, Mizrahi I, Broyles D, et al. A prospective multicenter, National Cancer Institute Early Detection Research Network study of [-2] proPSA: improving prostate cancer detection and correlating with cancer aggressiveness. Cancer Epidemiol Biomarkers Prev 2010;19:1193-1200.
[13] Catalona W, Partin A, Sanda M, Wei J, Klee G, Bangma C, et al. A multicenter study of [-2]pro-prostate specific antigen combined with prostate specific antigen and free prostate specific antigen for prostate cancer detection in the 2.0 to 10.0 ng/ml prostate specific antigen range. J Urol 2011;185:1650-5.
[14] Sanda M, Wei J, Broyles D, Shin S, Partin A, Klee G, et al. Evaluation of the Prostate Health Index (PHI) for improving prostate cancer detection and identification of clinically significant prostate cancer in the 4 to 10 ng/ml PSA range. Proceeding of American Urological Association Annual Meeting, San Diego 2013.
[15] Lazzeri M, Haese A, Abrate A, de la Taille A, Redorta J, McNicholas T, et al. Clinical performance of serum prostate-specific antigen isoform [-2]proPSA (p2PSA) and its derivatives, % p2PSA and the prostate health index (PHI), in men with a family history of prostate cancer: results from a multicentre European study, the PROMEtheuS project. BJU Int 2013;112:313-21.
[16] Loeb S, Sokoll L, Broyles D, Bangma C, van Schaik R, Klee G, et al. Prospective multicenter evaluation of the Beckman Coulter Prostate Health Index using WHO calibration. J Urol 2013;189:1702-6.

Submitted: January 05, 2015. *Revised:* February 02, 2015. *Accepted:* February 09. 2015.

In: Pain Management Yearbook 2015
Editor: Joav Merrick

ISBN: 978-1-63484-515-1

Chapter 16

BRAIN METASTASES AS A FIRST PRESENTATION OF LUNG CANCER

Madeleine Lao, Nicholas Lao, BMSc(C), Arnav Agarwal, MD(C), Natalie Pulenzas, BSc(C), Marko Popovic, BHSc(C), Sherlyn Vuong, BSc(C), Rachel McDonald, BSc(C), Leigha Rowbottom, BSc(C) and Edward Chow*, MBBS

Rapid Response Radiotherapy Program,
Department of Radiation Oncology, Odette Cancer Centre,
Sunnybrook Health Sciences Centre, University of Toronto,
Toronto, Ontario, Canada

Lung cancer has the highest mortality rate of cancers in the world, and commonly metastasizes to the brain. Given that advanced stages of lung cancer often result in metastases that have limited viable treatment options, prognosis is often poor for these patients. This holds true, and perhaps even more so, for patients whose first presentation of lung cancer is brain metastases. We present the case of an 89 year-old female patient with brain metastasis as her first presentation of lung cancer. She was treated with palliative radiotherapy of the whole brain.

Keywords: brain metastases, non-small cell lung cancer, whole-brain radiotherapy

INTRODUCTION

Lung cancer has the highest mortality rate and third highest incidence of all cancers in the world (1). Lung cancer commonly metastasizes to the brain, which occurs in approximately 40% of all lung cancer cases (2). Given that advanced stages of lung cancer often result in

* Correspondence: Professor Edward Chow, MBBS, MSc, PhD, FRCPC, Department of Radiation Oncology, Odette Cancer Centre, Sunnybrook Health Sciences Centre, 2075 Bayview Avenue, Toronto, ON, Canada. E-mail: Edward.Chow@sunnybrook.ca.

metastases that have limited viable treatment options, prognosis is often poor for these patients. This holds true, and perhaps even more so, for patients whose first presentation of lung cancer is brain metastases.

If metastatic lung cancer to the brain is left untreated, a patient's median survival time is 3-6 months (3). Survival can be prolonged with whole-brain radiotherapy (WBRT) (4). In addition, stereotactic radiosurgery (SRS) can be used in conjunction with whole-brain radiotherapy in selected patients (5, 6). In this report, we present the case of an 89 year-old woman with brain metastasis as her first presentation of lung cancer.

CASE REPORT

An 89 year-old female presented to the Emergency Department at the Sunnybrook Health Sciences Centre in June 2014 with lower back pain from a fall. She had fallen several times in the days before because of visual disturbances. She had a previous complex medical history of atrial fibrillation, angina, hypertension, hyperlipidemia, a transient ischemic attack in 1997, right lower lobe pneumonia in 2008, and irritated seborrheic keratosis of the right leg in 2009. A computed tomography (CT) scan of the head in addition to a magnetic resonance imaging (MRI) scan confirmed four brain metastases and resulting bilateral occipital and right parietal edema, with the primary cancer likely being lung, breast or melanoma.

A CT scan of the chest in June 2014 also showed a large heterogeneous right hilar mass with a necrotic centre that was highly suspicious for a primary lung malignancy. This mass caused obstruction of the right middle lobe bronchus and subsequent complete collapse of the right middle lobe. There was also similar pleural thickening and atelectasis in the right posterior basal segment.

The patient then underwent a bronchoscopy with a transbronchial biopsy, which was suboptimal due to significant bleeding and hypoxia. The initial biopsy suggested an invasive, poorly differentiated adenocarcinoma. Upon receiving the results of a repeat biopsy, it was confirmed to be metastatic non-small cell lung cancer (NSCLC). Later that month the patient was referred to the Rapid Response Radiotherapy Program at the Sunnybrook Odette Cancer Centre for consideration of palliative radiotherapy for brain metastasis. The patient later began palliative radiotherapy of the whole brain with 20 Gy in five fractions.

DISCUSSION

Brain metastases are a common complication of NSCLC, occurring in 30-50% of patients (7). Furthermore, brain metastases are found in 10% of patients with NSCLC at the time of diagnosis, which is common for this patient population (2). In this case report, brain metastases were the first indication of cancer, which prompted further investigation for the primary source.

As radiography has become more advanced, diagnostic modalities such as contrast-enhanced MRI and CT alone scans have become more accurate in diagnosing brain metastases. However, MRI and CT may not distinguish between metastatic brain tumours and primary malignant brain tumours, and should be used in conjunction with a biopsy in order to ensure an accurate diagnosis (8).

Prognosis is poor for patients with NSCLC and brain metastases, with survival being in the order of months (3). There are several treatment options available, the most prevalent of which is WBRT. WBRT may be of use in palliating neurological symptoms caused by brain metastases, and therefore may be beneficial in increasing quality of life (3). However, there are limitations to radiotherapy. A study by Gijtenbeek et al. (9) suggests that WBRT might only be temporarily beneficial to the patient, as they may later suffer from radiation-induced toxicity. Late radiation-induced toxicity from WBRT typically occurs 90 days from the start of treatment and includes neurocognitive degeneration following a pattern of mental function decline approximately 4 months after treatment, a subsequent improvement in mental function, and finally an irreversible impairment that may occur months or years after treatment (10).

An alternative to WBRT is SRS in selected patients, which is becoming more frequently used. In contrast to WBRT, SRS focuses a single high dose of radiation on a small area. When used in conjunction with WBRT, it has shown to be more effective than WBRT alone. For instance, in a study by Minniti et al. (5), patients who received WBRT alone had a median survival of 7.2 months, while patients who received WBRT with SRS had a median survival of 10.3 months. In another randomized controlled trial by Andrews et al. (6), 167 patients with one to three newly diagnosed brain metastases were given WBRT and SRS while 164 patients were randomized to WBRT alone. Patients with a single brain metastasis in the WBRT plus SRS group had a longer survival time of 6.5 months when compared to the 4.9 months of survival following WBRT alone. Based on these findings, the study concluded that WBRT and SRS should be the standard treatment for single brain metastases and should be considered for patients with two or three brain metastases (6). Another option for treatment is SRS alone. A study by Aoyama et al. (11) included 132 patients with 1 to 4 brain metastases who were treated with either WBRT and SRS or SRS alone. There was no improvement in survival in the group with WBRT and SRS versus the group with SRS alone, though there were higher rates of brain tumour recurrence in the SRS group (76.4%) than in the WBRT and SRS group (46.8%) (11).

Another concern is misdiagnosis with first presentation of brain metastases due to the limitations of radiography. A review by Jin et al. (12) included 206 patients who first presented with brain metastases and who later were diagnosed with lung cancer. Of the initial group of patients, 20 were lost prior to follow up, leaving 186 for analysis. The patients had a median age of 57 years and a median Karnofsky performance status of 80. Jin et al. (12) concluded that there were high rates of misdiagnosis upon initial presentation (46.8%). Because the patients did not have symptoms related to their primary tumor, they were more likely to see a neurosurgeon or neurologist first, rather than an oncologist. Without detailed radiography and without further evaluation for systemic disease, the patients were misdiagnosed with non-metastatic brain lesions at the time of initial presentation (12). The operating neurosurgeon later concluded that they were in fact metastatic lesions from systemic cancer after resection or biopsy. However, Jin et al. (12) concluded that SRS with WBRT still provided the best outcome, with a median survival time of 19 months.

Ultimately, brain metastases are a common occurrence in advanced stages of lung cancer, and it is common that patients with lung cancer have brain metastases at the time of first diagnosis (2). However, without medical radiography and a tissue diagnosis by biopsy, it is difficult to accurately diagnose a patient with lung cancer from a first presentation of brain metastases. The keys to prolonging survival and increasing quality of life are rapid diagnosis and effective and appropriate treatment.

CONCLUSION

It is fairly common for patients to have brain metastases upon first diagnosis of lung cancer. Appropriate and immediate treatment of brain metastases with WBRT in conjunction with SRS has been proven to increase median survival time when compared to WBRT alone in selected patients (5, 6). However, there is potential for misdiagnosis when brain metastases present first in lung cancer (12). As a result, oncologists should thoroughly investigate and analyze MRI, CT, and biopsy findings when patients first present with brain lesions.

ACKNOWLEDGMENTS

We thank the generous support of Bratty Family Fund, Michael and Karyn Goldstein Cancer Research Fund, Pulenzas Cancer Research Fund, Joseph and Silvana Melara Cancer Research Fund, and Ofelia Cancer Research Fund.

REFERENCES

[1] Jemal A, Bray F, Center MM, Ferlay J, Ward E, Forman D. Global cancer statistics. CA Cancer J Clin 2011;61(2):69-90.

[2] Schuette W. Treatment of brain metastases from lung cancer: chemotherapy. Lung Cancer 2004;45 (Suppl 2):S253-7.

[3] Qin H, Pan F, Li J, Zhang X, Liang H, Ruan Z. Whole brain radiotherapy plus concurrent chemotherapy in non-small cell lung cancer patients with brain metastases: a meta-analysis. PLoS One 2014; 9(10):e111475.

[4] Chitapanarux I, Goss B, Vongtama R, Frighetto L, De Salles A, Selch M, Duick M, et al. Prospective study of stereotactic radiosurgery without whole brain radiotherapy in patients with four or less brain metastases: Incidence of intracranial progression and salvage radiotherapy. J Neurooncol 2003;61(2):143-9.

[5] Minniti G, Salvati M, Muni R, Lanzetta G, Osti MF, Clarke E, et al. Stereotactic radiosurgery plus whole-brain radiotherapy for treatment of multiple metastases from non-small cell lung cancer. Anticancer Res 2010;30(7):3055-61.

[6] Andrews DW, Scott CB, Sperduto PW, Flanders AE, Gaspar LE, Schell MC, et al. Whole brain radiation therapy with or without stereotactic radiosurgery boost for patients with one to three brain metastases: phase III results of the RTOG 9508 randomised trial. Lancet 2004;363(9422):1665-72.

[7] Arrieta O, Villarreal-Garza C, Zamora J, Blake-Cerda M, de la Mata MD, Zavala DG, et al. Long-term survival in patients with non-small cell lung cancer and synchronous brain metastasis treated with whole-brain radiotherapy and thoracic chemoradiation. Radiat Oncol 2011;6:166.

[8] Soffietti R, Ruda R, Mutani R. Management of brain metastases. J Neurol 2002;249(10);1357-69.

[9] Gijtenbeek JM, Ho VK, Heesters MA, Lagerwaard FJ, de Graeff A, Boogerd W. [Practice guideline 'brain metastases' (revision)]. Ned Tijdschr Geneeskd 2011;155(52):A4141.

[10] McTyre E, Scott J, Chinnaiyan P. Whole brain radiotherapy for brain metastasis. Surg Neurol Int 2013;4(Suppl 4): S236-44.

[11] Aoyama H, Shirato H, Tago M, Nakaqawa K, Toyoda T, Hatano K, et al. Stereotactic radiosurgery plus whole-brain radiation therapy vs stereotactic radiosurgery alone for treatment of brain metastases: a randomized controlled trial. JAMA 2006;295(21):2483-91.

[12] Jin J, Zhou X, Liang X, Huang R, Chu Z, Jiang J, et al. Brain metastases as the first symptom of lung cancer: a clinical study from an Asian medical center. J Cancer Res Clin Oncol 2013;139(3):403-8.

Submitted: January 10, 2015. *Revised:* February 02, 2015. *Accepted:* February 10, 2015.

In: Pain Management Yearbook 2015
Editor: Joav Merrick

ISBN: 978-1-63484-515-1

Chapter 17

SCLEROTIC HUMERAL METASTASIS AT RISK OF FRACTURE

Nicholas Lao, BMSc(C), Linda Probyn, MD, Rachel McDonald, BSc(C), Leigha Rowbottom, BSc(C), Marko Popovic, BHSc(C), Natalie Pulenzas, BSc(C), Sherlyn Vuong, BSc(C) and Edward Chow*, MBBS
Sunnybrook Health Sciences Centre,
University of Toronto, Toronto, Ontario, Canada

Bone is one of the most common sites for metastatic cancer, and complications such as pathological fracture can reduce a bone's load-bearing capabilities. When treating impending fractures, surgery can be very effective at returning the affected area to acceptable function. However, this may only be effective in patients with certain disease types and performance status. We present the case of an 81-year-old male patient who was diagnosed with prostate cancer and bone metastases. A sclerotic lesion of his humerus was found to be at risk for pathological fracture and was treated using radiotherapy and bone-strengthening agents.

Keywords: prostate cancer, radiotherapy, impending fracture, sclerotic metastasis

INTRODUCTION

Bone is one of the most common sites for metastatic cancer, affecting approximately 65-75% of prostate cancer patients (1). Bone metastases can cause considerable pain and skeletal-related events, including spinal cord compression and pathological fracture.

---

* Correspondence: Professor Edward Chow, MBBS, MSc, PhD, FRCPC, Department of Radiation Oncology, Odette Cancer Centre, Sunnybrook Health Sciences Centre, 2075 Bayview Avenue, Toronto, ON, Canada. E-mail: Edward.Chow@sunnybrook.ca.

Pathological fracture due to metastatic destruction can reduce a bone's load-bearing capabilities. Initially, trabecular disruption and microfractures form, resulting in a loss of bone integrity (1). This increases the risk of a pathological fracture, causes pain and discomfort, and decreases the patient's quality of life, especially if left untreated (2). Treatment of impending fractures aims to strengthen the area to prevent fracture, relieve pain associated with the lesion, and return acceptable functioning to the affected area (2). Treatments include surgical fixation to stabilize the area, radiotherapy to promote bone healing, and bone strengthening agents such as bisphosphonates to prevent loss of bone mass. A combination of treatments is commonly used to prevent a fracture.

Pathological fractures of long bones are a fairly common complication, and can occur in up to 40% of patients with bone metastases of long bones (3, 4). The humerus is the second most common long bone after the femur to experience a pathological fracture (2). Surgical fixation is recommended to treat fractures of the humerus because of the high re-fracture rate seen with cast bracing and radiation (5).

We present the case of a patient who was diagnosed with prostate cancer and bone metastases. A sclerotic lesion of his humerus was found to be at risk for pathological fracture. While surgical fixation can be very effective at stabilizing a long bone impending fracture and provide return of function to the area, this procedure is only well suited to patients who are in otherwise, generally good condition and with certain metastatic disease characteristics. Although this patient was experiencing pain from the humeral metastasis, the location and lesion type were such that surgical fixation was not necessary (6). Therefore, the patient was treated using radiotherapy and bone strengthening agents only.

CASE REPORT

On October 2nd of 2014, an 81 year-old male was seen in the Rapid Response Radiotherapy Program at the Sunnybrook Health Sciences Centre for increasing pain in his humerus. Despite the pain, the patient was not severely functionally impaired and presented with a Karnofsky Performance Status (KPS) of 90. The patient had been diagnosed with prostate cancer in 2010 which led to a transurethral resection in February of 2013.

A bone scan completed in September of 2014 revealed multiple foci of very intense activity throughout the axilla and proximal skeleton in keeping with bony metastasis. The bone scan also showed increased uptake in the lateral right seventh rib. An x-ray image of the humerus and right shoulder in October showed a large sclerotic lesion in the proximal mid humeral shaft extending over a distance of approximately 14 centimetres (Figure 1).

In addition, there was aggressive periosteal reaction along the proximal humeral shaft, which increased the risk of pathological fracture. A subsequent x-ray of the right ribs showed a sclerotic lesion in the right seventh rib with extension and periosteal reaction. This also placed the rib at an increased risk of pathological fracture. Lastly, an x-ray of the lumbar/sacral spine showed known sclerotic metastases at L1 with pathologic compression fracture and mild anterior wedging. Sclerotic lesions were also seen at T11, L5 and S1.

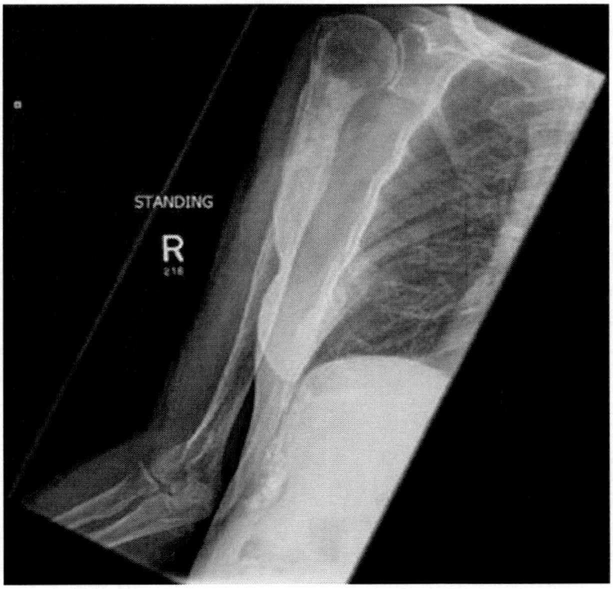

Figure 1. An x-ray of the right shoulder and humerus shows a large sclerotic lesion in the right proximal/mid humeral shaft extending over a distance of approximately 14 cm. There is aggressive periosteal reaction along the proximal humeral shaft. Sclerotic lesion is also noted in the right 7th rib with expansion and periosteal reaction.

The patient received 3000 cGy of radiation in 10 fractions for pain relief and to reduce the risk of fracture in his humerus and right rib. He received a single 8 Gy treatment to his lumbar spine for sclerotic lesions at T11, L5, and S1, and for his pain in the lower spine and pelvis. The patient was also prescribed denosumab, a bone strengthening agent.

The patient was seen in December for a follow-up appointment. At the time, the patient had experienced significant pain relief in his shoulder, ribs and spine as a result of the radiation treatment. In addition, new x-ray images of the right shoulder and right rib showed little to no change in the size and state of disease in his rib or humerus.

DISCUSSION

Some treatments, such as surgical fixation, can be very effective for the treatment of impending fracture, and can allow for the return of acceptable function to the bone (2). However, surgical intervention is not suitable for all patients, especially for those with low KPS or conditions which can make surgery dangerous or life-threatening to the patient. In addition, surgical intervention may not be suitable if it is not necessary for the well-being of a palliative patient. After review by the orthopedic surgeon, the patient of our report did not undergo surgical fixation, but proceeded with radiotherapy to the humerus and rib of 3000 cGy in 10 fractions.

A scoring system developed by Mirels et al. (6) uses several factors to determine if a bone lesion requires surgical fixation, or can be treated with radiotherapy. This system assigns a score of 1 to 3 to each category of site, pain, type, and size of the lesion. The patient presented in this report had a blastic/sclerotic lesion located in an upper limb causing moderate pain with an unclear size relative to bone diameter. Using this scoring system, the total score for the patient is calculated to be between 5 and 7, depending on the size of lesion. It is noted by Mirels et al. (6) that a score of 7 or below would not require prophylactic fixation and could be safely irradiated without risk of fracture. Conversely, a score of 8 or greater would require prophylactic fixation before irradiation (6). A sclerotic lesion may be at low risk for fracture and not require fixation because of its mechanism of mineralization and thickening of the bone, while a lytic lesion may be more prone to fracture. Therefore, pain relief through radiotherapy in addition to denosumab for bone strengthening were the treatments chosen to relieve the patient's pain.

Multiple or single fraction radiotherapy treatments are possible, with great dispute to which are optimal for this patient population. Multiple fraction treatments may not be used in patients with lower performance status as they find it more difficult to complete a multi-fraction schedule compared to receiving a single fraction. At the same time, in patients with a majority of complicated bone metastases from unfavourable histologies, a multi-fraction schedule can cause greater healing of the patient's bone metastases by allowing for a higher total dose of radiation (7). A study by Steenland et al. (8) found that the pathological fracture incidence for patients with bone metastases treated with single-fraction radiation was significantly higher when compared to multi-fraction radiotherapy. In addition, a systematic review by Sze et al. (9) indicated the risk of pathological fracture was 1.82 times greater (95% CI 1.06–3.11) in patients treated with single fraction radiotherapy compared with multiple fractions. However, a more recent systematic review (10) found there was no difference in risk of pathological fracture for patients treated with single or multiple fraction radiotherapy regimens ($P = 0.72$).

Patients experiencing impending pathological fracture due to bone metastases should receive treatment choices aimed at increasing quality of life and returning the area to normal or acceptable use with minimal delay. In addition, life expectancy should be taken into account when deciding the most appropriate treatment (3). Surgical overtreatment of patients with short life expectancy can occur and cause unnecessary morbidity and a decrease in quality of life. In select cases, other treatment options, including the use of radiotherapy and bone-strengthening agents, may be more cost-effective and provide greater benefit to the patient (11).

Conclusion

It is commonly known that patients diagnosed with bone metastases as a result of prostate cancer can also experience skeletal-related events such as pathological fracture. When treating impending fractures, surgery can be very effective at returning the affected area to acceptable function. However, depending on the patient's performance status and disease type, this may not be the best option. If treating with radiotherapy to relieve pain and allow for bone healing, a multi-fraction schedule is recommended. However, this may not be optimal depending on the patient's state of disease, histology, or life expectancy. Therefore, it is always important to examine all relevant factors before making a decision on management of an impending pathological fracture from metastatic cancer.

ACKNOWLEDGMENTS

We thank the generous support of Bratty Family Fund, Michael and Karyn Goldstein Cancer Research Fund, Pulenzas Cancer Research Fund, Joseph and Silvana Melara Cancer Research Fund, and Ofelia Cancer Research Fund.

REFERENCES

[1] Coleman RE. Skeletal complications of Malignancy. Cancer 1997;80(8):1588-94.

[2] Piccioli A, Maccauro G, Rossi B et al. Surgical treatment of pathologic fractures of humerus. Injury 2010;41:1112-6.

[3] Sarahrudi K, Hora K, Heinz T, Millington S, Vecsei V. Treatment results of pathological fractures of the long bones: a retrospective analysis of 88 patients. Int Orthop 2006;30:519-24.

[4] Fidler M. Incidence of fracture through metastases in long bones. Acta Orthop Scand 1981;52(6): 623-7.

[5] Lin JT. Bony pathology in the cancer patient. J Womens Health 2002;11(8):691-702.

[6] Mirels H. Metaswtatic disease in long bones. a proposed scoring system for diagnosing impending pathological fracture. Clin Orthop Relat Res 1989;(249):256-64.

[7] Lo SS, Holden L, Lutz ST, Liu RK, Chow E. Should all patients with uncomplicated bone metastases be treated with a single 8-Gy fraction? Expert Rev Pharmacoecon Outcomes Res 2010;10(2):95-8.

[8] Steenland E, Leer J, van Houwelingen H, Post WJ, van den Hout WB, Kievit J, et al. The effect of a single fraction compared to multiple fractions on painful bone metastases: a global analysis of the dutch bone metastasis study. Radiother Oncol 1999;52:101-9.

[9] Sze WM, Shelley MD, Held I, Wilt TJ, Mason MD. Palliation of metastatic bone pain: single fraction versus multifraction radiotherapy – A systematic review of randomised trials. Clin Oncol 2003;15:345-52.

[10] Chow E, Zeng L, Salvo N, Dennis K, Tsao M, Lutz S. Update on the systematic review of palliative radiotherapy trials for bone metastases. Clin Oncol 2012;24(2):112-24.

[11] Tatar Z, Soubrier M, Dillies AF, Verrelle P, Boisgard S, Lapeyre M. Assessment of the risk factors for impending fractures following radiotherapy for long bone metastases using CT scan-based virtual simulation: a retrospective study. Radiat Oncol 2014;9:227.

Submitted: January 10, 2015. *Revised:* February 04, 2015. *Accepted:* February 10, 2015.

In: Pain Management Yearbook 2015
Editor: Joav Merrick

ISBN: 978-1-63484-515-1

Chapter 18

RAPID PROGRESSION OF BONE METASTASES AND PSA IN PROSTATE CANCER

Jonathan Tam, MD(C), Linda Probyn, MD, Natalie Pulenzas, BSc(C), Sherlyn Vuong, BSc(C), Rachel McDonald, BSc(C), Leigha Rowbottom, BSc(C), and Edward Chow*, MBBS PhD
Sunnybrook Health Sciences Centre,
University of Toronto, Toronto, Ontario, Canada

Prostate cancer is the most commonly diagnosed neoplasm in men. While both bone metastases and development of castrate resistant cancer are indicative of advanced disease, a clear temporal relationship between the two has yet to be developed. This report presents a 74-year-old male with metastatic prostate cancer who progressed to castrate resistance within 4 months.

Keywords: castrate resistant prostate cancer, bone metastasis, prostate adenocarcinoma

INTRODUCTION

One in seven men in the United States will develop prostate cancer in their lifetime, making prostate cancer the most commonly diagnosed neoplasm in men and the second most common cause of male cancer mortality (1). While prostate cancers with localized and regional staging have a 5-year survival rate nearing 100%, the presence of distant metastases at time of diagnoses decreases the 5-year survival rate below 30% (1). The most common site of distant metastasis for prostate cancer are as follows: bone (90%), followed by lung (46%), liver (25%), and pleura (21%) (2). For patients with bone metastasis, the median survival is

* Correspondence: Professor Edward Chow, MBBS, MSc, PhD, FRCPC, Department of Radiation Oncology, Odette Cancer Centre, Sunnybrook Health Sciences Centre, 2075 Bayview Avenue, Toronto, ON, Canada. E-mail: Edward.Chow@sunnybrook.ca.

reported to be between 9 months (3) and 30-35 months (4) depending on individual presentation and factors such as age, the use of chemotherapy, or the use of radiotherapy.

Metastasis to bone is highly symptomatic and accompanied by severe bone pain as well as increased risk of fracture, spinal cord compression, and motor impairment (5). Patients are treated with hormone therapy, chemotherapy, radiation therapy, and surgery with the treatment goal of managing tumor size, maintaining bone health, and minimizing pain (4). The mainstay treatment for advanced prostate cancer continues to be androgen deprivation therapy (ADT) with the goal of chemically castrating the patient and limiting the burden of cancer (6). A systematic review by Kirby et al. reported that approximately 10-20% of prostate cancer patients develop castrate resistant prostate cancer (CRPC) within 5 years of initial diagnosis (3).

Due to advances in prostate-specific antigen (PSA) screening, the vast majority of prostate cancer cases are diagnosed prior to metastatic disease. A cohort study in Denmark (N = 23,087) reports that only 3% of patients presented with bone metastases at prostate cancer diagnosis (7). In the patient group free from metastasis at initial diagnoses, there is also a high prevalence (>84%) of bone metastases at the point of CRPC diagnosis (3). However, a clear temporal relationship between the development of metastases and the development of castrate resistance has yet to be developed (3).

This report presents the case of 74-year-old male diagnosed with metastatic prostate cancer who progressed to CRPC within 4 months.

CASE STORY

A 74-year-old male was referred to the Rapid Response Radiotherapy Program (RRRP) in August 2014 with bone pain and a recent diagnosis of metastatic prostate cancer following a positive biopsy. Pathology of the specimen was assigned a Gleason score of 4 plus 3. At the time of diagnosis, the patient had a PSA of 668 and both the bone scan and the CAT scan suggested multiple bone metastases (Figures 1, 2). At the time of presentation, the patient had chronic back pain and urination issues that were treated with Finasteride, Tamsulosin, and analgesics. The patient was started on Degarelix shortly after diagnosis.

In August of 2014 the patient received 8 Gy in one fraction of palliative radiotherapy to a sclerotic lesion at T8 and in the right rib cage with good pain response. A lab report in early September 2014 showed that PSA levels decreased to 67, indicating success of Degarelix therapy. The patient returned with multiple areas of bone pain and additional radiation of 8 Gy in one fraction was given to L2 in September 2014, and a single dose of 8 Gy to the left ribcage in October of 2014.

The patient was relatively stable with PSA levels of 39.5 and 45 in October and November, respectively. However, in December of 2014, PSA rose significantly to 126 and the patient experienced new areas of pain in the bilateral shoulders and proximal humeri. Imaging in January of 2015 also correlated with PSA testing, as there was evidence for progression (Figures 3, 4). He was then classified as having castrate-resistant prostate cancer and accordingly switched to Abiraterone in December. The PSA was 391 one month later.

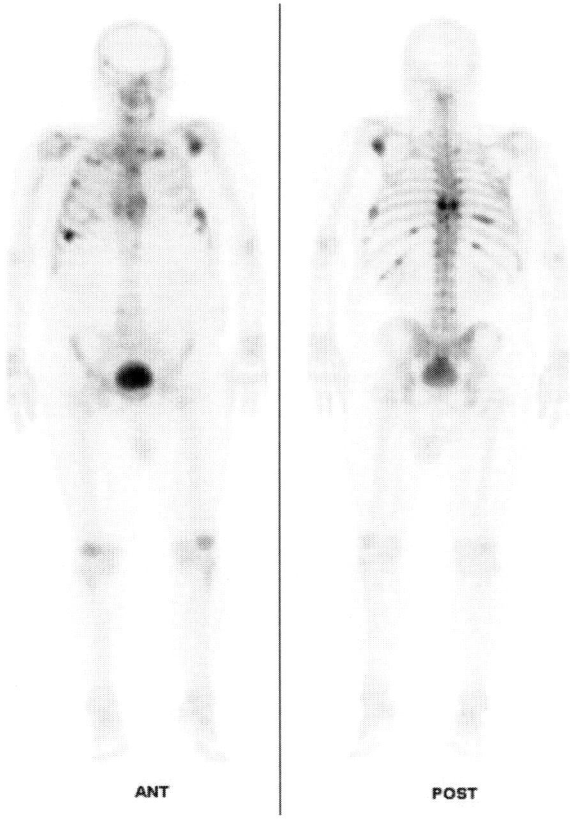

Figure 1. Bone Scan from August 2014.

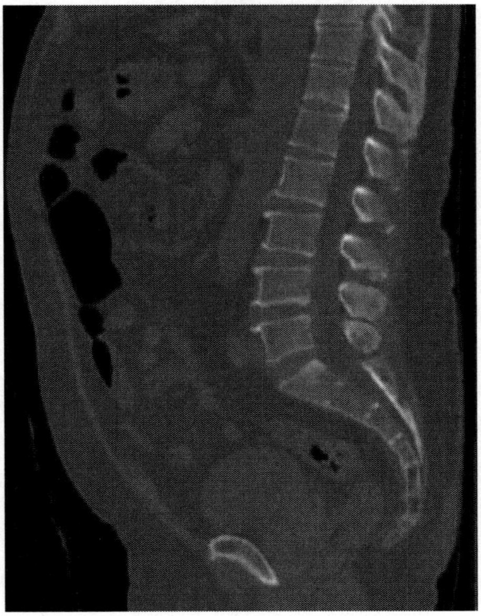

Figure 2. CAT scan from August 2014.

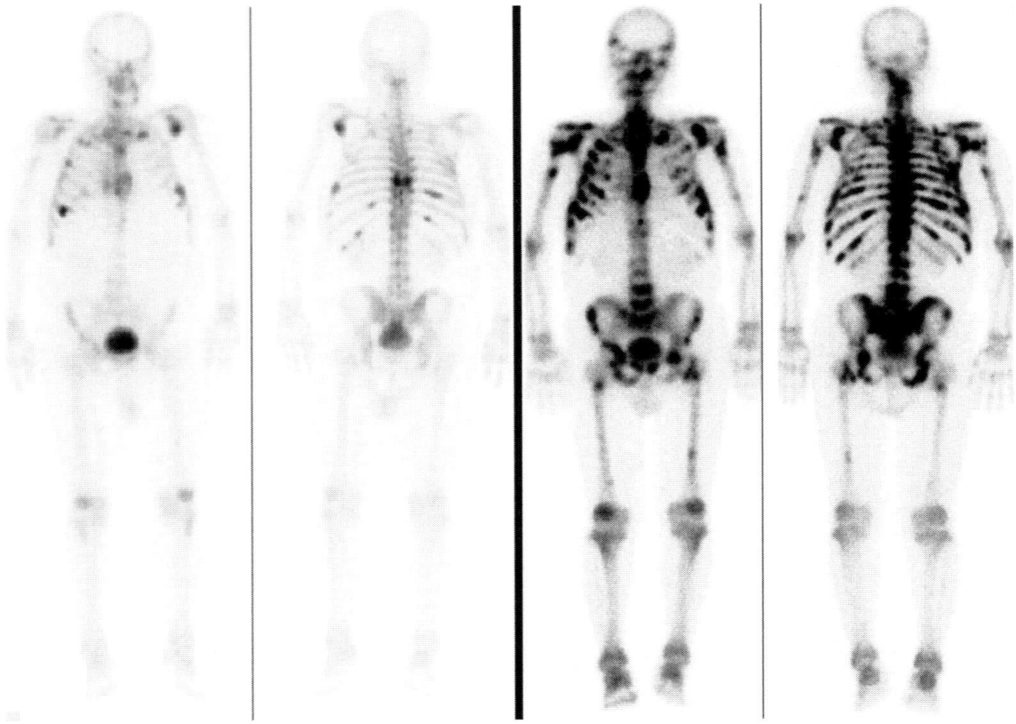

Figure 3. Bone Scan from August 2014 (left) compared to January 2015 (right) illustrating progression of bone metastases.

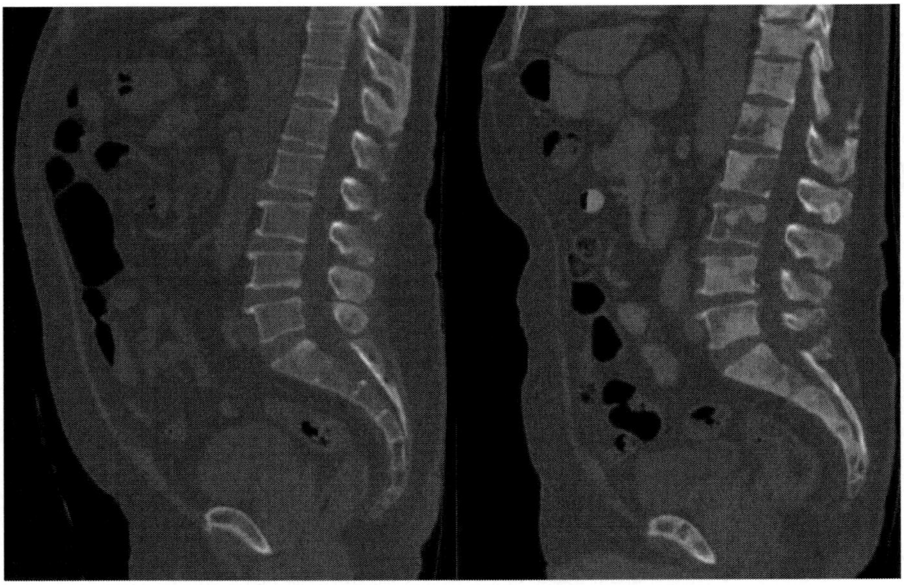

Figure 4. CAT scan from August 2014 (left) compared to January 2015 (right) illustrating progression of bone metastases.

Palliative radiation was considered for pain relief as he had multiple new areas of pain including the shoulders, lumbar spine and pelvis, which correlated with areas of bone metastases. However, due to the rapidly progressing cancer, it was determined that the patient should be started on chemotherapy and radiation would be postponed until there are gaps in the chemotherapy schedule.

DISCUSSION

The patient presented with prostate adenocarcenoma and bone metastasis and was shortly started on Degarelix. ADT worked and the patient's PSA dropped to 76 by September 2014. The PSA continued to stay low, indicating the success of ADT, throughout October and November. The PSA rose significantly to 126 in December and many new areas of bone metastases became visible on imaging (see Figure 2). The 3-4 month rapid progression to CRPC is noteworthy given that patients without metastases take years to progress to CRPC (3). The incredible growth of the metastases from first presentation (Figure 1) despite the initial success of ADT is especially striking (Figure 2).

CRPC can develop through many mechanisms, but most studies agree that androgens are supplied to the tumor through alternative means (8). While the goal of ADT is to suppress the hypothalamic-pituitary-gonadal axis production of testosterone and DHT, recent studies have shown that tumors may acquire the ability to increase the local concentration of biologically active androgens or alter the activity of tumor androgen receptors (e.g., through ligand sensitization, increased expression, or mutation) (8). Regardless of the mechanism of resistance, CRPC and metastases both correlate highly with disease progression, and patient mortality.

While no clear temporal relationship between bone metastasis and CRPC has been established, there is a very high prevalence of (>84%) of bone metastases at the point of CRPC diagnosis (3). This patient's 3-4 month rapid progression to CRPC may be related to the presence of metastasis and advanced disease at diagnosis. More research should be done to better understand the temporal correlation between the development of metastasis and CRPC to better understand disease progression and the impact on patient mortality.

ACKNOWLEDGMENTS

We thank the generous support of Bratty Family Fund, Michael and Karyn Goldstein Cancer Research Fund, Pulenzas Cancer Research Fund, Joseph and Silvana Melara Cancer Research Fund, and Ofelia Cancer Research Fund.

REFERENCES

[1] Siegel R, Ma J, Zou Z, Jemal A. Cancer Statistics, 2014. CA Cancer J Clin 2014;64(1):9-29.

[2] Bubendorf L, Schöpfer A, Wagner U, Sauter G, Moch H, Willi N, et al. Metastatic patterns of prostate cancer: an autopsy study of 1,589 patients. Hum Pathol 2000;31(5):578-83.

[3] Kirby M, Hirst C, Crawford ED. Characterising the castration-resistant prostate cancer population: a systematic review. Int J Clin Pract 2011;65(11):1180-92.
[4] Carlin BI, Andriole GL. The natural history, skeletal complications, and management of bone metastases in patients with prostate carcinoma. Cancer 2000;88 (12):2989-94.
[5] Saad F, Clarke N, Colombel M. Natural history and treatment of bone complications in prostate cancer. Eur Urol 2006;49(3):429-40.
[6] Moul JW. Utility of LHRH antagonists for advanced prostate cancer. Can J Urol 2014;21(21):22-7.
[7] Nørgaard M, Jensen AØ, Jacobsen JB, Cetin K, Fryzek JP, Sørensen HT. Skeletal related events, bone metastasis and survival of prostate cancer: a population based cohort study in Denmark (1999 to 2007). J Urol 2010;184(1):162-7.
[8] Sharifi N. Minireview: Androgen metabolism in castration-resistant prostate cancer. Mol Endocrinol 2013;27(5):708-14.

Submitted: January 12, 2015. *Revised:* February 05, 2015. *Accepted:* February 10, 2015.

In: Pain Management Yearbook 2015
Editor: Joav Merrick

ISBN: 978-1-63484-515-1

Chapter 19

INCIDENCE OF SUBTROCHANTERIC FEMUR FRACTURE DURING RADIATION THERAPY: A CASE REPORT

Sherlyn Vuong, BSc(C), Natalie Pulenzas, BSc(C), and Edward Chow*, MBBS, PhD

Rapid Response Radiotherapy Program, Department of Radiation Oncology,
Odette Cancer Centre, Sunnybrook Health Sciences Centre,
University of Toronto, Toronto, Ontario, Canada

Bone is a common structure for metastases to occur in prostate cancer patients, occurring in 90% of primary prostate cancer patients. Lytic lesions, which can weaken affected bony structures, can increase the risk of fracture in a patient, especially if it occurs in an area that is weight bearing. Radiotherapy, a treatment most commonly used to alleviate pain caused by bone metastases, and to stimulate bone growth in areas that are weakened from osteolytic lesions. We report the case of an 86-year old man who despite undergoing radiation treatment, had bone metastasis progression which later lead to a pathological fracture in the subtrochanteric femur.

Keywords: subtrochanteric femur, pathological fracture, prostate cancer, bone metastases

INTRODUCTION

Prostate cancer is the second most commonly diagnosed cancers for males in the developed world, the first being lung cancer (1). Prostate cancer can metastasize to other locations within the body, but has a higher probability in metastasizing to the bone. In one study, it was noted that 90% of the patients with primary prostate cancer had metastases to the bone, 86% of them being the only site (2). For cancerous lesions that occur in the femur, approximately

* Correspondence: Professor Edward Chow MBBS, MSc, PhD, FRCPC Department of Radiation Oncology, Odette Cancer Centre, Sunnybrook Health Sciences Centre, 2075 Bayview Avenue, Toronto, Ontario, Canada. E-mail: Edward.Chow@sunnybrook.ca.

one-third of them are located in the subtrochanteric area (3). Bone metastases may result in increased risk for fractures, especially in areas where the structural components of the bone have been compromised from osteolysis. When the osteolysis is in weight-bearing areas such as the hip, there is an increased risk for fracture, with about 60% of all hip fractures being within the femoral neck area (4).

Radiotherapy to the bone, most commonly used for relief of pain from symptomatic bony lesions, is also used to slow down tumor growth, increase osteoproliferation, and prevent fractures caused by disease (5). With an overall response rate of 60% (patients showing some extent of pain relief from radiotherapy), 70% of the cases will have bone recalcification (5). However, despite radiation, there may still be a possibility for fracture. In this case study, we report an 86-year old man who despite palliative radiation, had bone metastases that continued to progress and experienced a pathological fracture to the subtrochanteric femur.

CASE REPORT

An 86-year-old male, who was first seen due to severe hip pain, was diagnosed with prostate cancer in 2009 with a Gleason score of 9. He was also presented with osteoblastic metastases to multiple areas in the pelvis, in addition to metastatic disease throughout the axial skeleton, including the spine, ribs, and sternum. The patient had a past history of hyperlipidemia, hypothyroidism, reflux disease and bilateral knee replacement, and was symptomatic for the bone metastases in his spine and pelvis region.

The patient, placed on androgen deprivation therapy, was prescribed injections of Zoladex (Goserelin) and Casodex (Bicalutamide) pills. He was also prescribed Cyproterone Acetate 2 years after. Vitamin D and Calcium supplements were given as well. In 2012, after noting a significant elevation in the patient's PSA level, was diagnosed with castrate-resistant prostate cancer and Bicalutamide was stopped. An X-Ray done in the same year showed cortical osteolysis and permeation in the subtrochanteric left femur, which lead to a high risk for pathological fracture in that area. In the subsequent year, the bony lesions had spread to the base of the skull and both humeri, and the patient was taken off of Casodex. Xgeva (Denosumab) was also started in 2013 due to the patient's high risk for fractures, but because the patient had hypocalcemia and could no longer take Vitamin D or Calcium due to side effects, it was stopped after two doses. The patient then developed a partial fracture in the T9 vertebral body and the 7th rib.

The patient was seen in the Bone Metastases Clinic at the Sunnybrook Odette Cancer Centre in June of 2014 for their increased risk for fracture in the proximal femoral region. However, because the lesion in the left hip had not been previously radiated and the frailty of the patient, it was decided that radiation treatment would be the most prudent course of action to proceed with first, and that the potential for surgery could be re-evaluated later on. The patient was then seen in the Rapid Response Radiotherapy Program (RRRP) that same day for assessment of radiation treatment. The patient had a previous history of radiation treatments to multiple areas in varying doses and fractionations starting in 2012. These areas included the spine, ribs, and left mid shaft of the femur. In 2014, 20Gy in 5 fractions were given to the left shoulder and right hip. The left hip was then planned for 30Gy in ten fractions of radiation. However, during this course of radiation to the left hip, the patient had experienced a pathological fracture of the subtrochanteric region of the left femur with associated varus angulation and posterior displacement. Ultimately, only 9 out of the 10 fractions were received. Surgery was needed, and the patient underwent a reconstructive nailing of the left femur. A month later, another pathological fracture caused by a fall developed which was located in the humerus. The patient was then assigned non-operative pain management due to their high risk for post-operative wound infection and complications.

DISCUSSION

To assess the incidence of pathological fractures that might occur during radiation treatment or post-irradiation, it is important to analyze the risks for fractures in patients to assign appropriate preventative treatment. When radiation treatment is given, factors such as patient age, dose, field size and number of fractionations are commonly considered to reduce any serious radiation-induced changes in the bone (6). However, fractionation may be less of a factor for evaluating which radiation treatment to give. Based on a study done by Chow et al. (7), it showed no significant difference for fracture risk in patients undergoing single or multiple fractionations.

A factor that should be considered in assessing the risk for fracture is the presence of past fractures in a patient. According to a study done by Kanis et al. (8), patients with previous fractures to any bone structures have a higher chance for future fractures to occur elsewhere later in life.

In some studies, it has been said that irradiation can also have a negative effect on the ability of the bone to withstand compression. Radiation treatment, used to affect cancerous cells, can also potentially damage radiosensitive healthy bone cells such as osteoblasts, osteocytes, and osteoclasts (9), which might affect bone mineralization and thus bone strength (10). However, from another study done by Koswig and Budach (11), they note that multi-fractionated palliative irradiation shows significant recalcification of the osteolytic bone lesions, which can re-strengthen the radiated bone area weakened by lytic lesions.

Androgen deprivation therapy (ADT) medications such as Zoladex (goserelin), and Casodex (Bicalutamide) can also contribute to a higher risk for fracture (12). Commonly used to improve the overall survival of localized prostate cancer patients in conjunction with radiation (13), ADT medications can have adverse effects such as decreasing the bone mineralization density (BMD) (12). A lower BMD content affects bone strength, and with this, the risk for fracture increases.

In addition, areas that are affected by lytic lesions, which weaken bone structure, can also affect the risk for fracture to occur. Lytic lesions in weight-bearing areas such as the subtrochanteric femur will have a higher likelihood of fracture as they are exposed to greater mechanical forces on a frequent basis.

When these factors are examined during the time of assigning radiation treatment, effective treatments can be given which will maximize quality of life while minimizing the burden on patients.

Conclusion

Although the occurrence is uncommon, it is important to note that there are many underlying factors that contribute to the incidence of pathological fracture in a patient. Fracture history in patients, types of hormone therapies, as well as the location of lytic lesions should all be considered when deciding the most effective method to treat painful bone metastases. If radiation treatment were assigned, dosage and fractionations would be the next factors to consider; making sure that if there is a risk for pathological fracture, the assigned dosage and fractionation is catered towards bone recalcification in the corresponding areas. With this in mind, the next step would be to explore other options that would improve bone strength in patients that are in high risk for pathological fractures to reduce the chances of it from occurring.

Acknowledgments

We thank the generous support of Bratty Family Fund, Michael and Karyn Goldstein Cancer Research Fund, Pulenzas Cancer Research Fund, Joseph and Silvana Melara Cancer Research Fund, and Ofelia Cancer Research Fund.

References

[1] Jemal A, Bray F, Center MM, Ferlay J, Ward E, Forman D. Global cancer statistics. CA Cancer J Clin 2011;61(2):69-90.

[2] Hess KR, Varadhachary GR, Taylor SH, Wei W, Raber MN, Lenzi R, et al. Metastatic patterns in adenocarcinoma. Cancer 2006;106(7):1624-33.

[3] Weiss RJ, Ekström W, Hansen BH, Keller J, Laitinen M, Trovik C, et al. Pathological subtrochanteric fractures in 194 patients: A comparison of outcome after surgical treatment of pathological and non-pathological fractures. J Surg Oncol 2013;107(5):498-504.

[4] Basso T, Klaksvik J, Syversen U, Foss OA. Biomechanical femoral neck fracture experiments - A narrative review. Injury 2012;43(10):1633.

[5] Tatar Z, Soubrier M, Dillies A, Verrelle P, Boisgard S, Lapeyre M. Assessment of the risk factors for impending fractures following radiotherapy for long bone metastases using CT scan-based virtual simulation: a retrospective study. Radiat Oncol 2014;9(1):227.

[6] Mitchell MJ, Logan PM. Radiation-induced changes in bone. Radiographics 1998;18(5):1125-36.

[7] Chow E, Zeng L, Salvo N, Dennis K, Tsao M, Lutz S. Update on the systematic review of palliative radiotherapy trials for bone metastases. Clin Oncol 2012;24(2):112-24.

[8] Kanis JA, Johnell O, Laet CD, Johansson H, Oden A, Delmas P, et al. A meta-analysis of previous fracture and subsequent fracture risk. Bone 2004;35(2):375.

[9] Libshitz HI. Radiation changes in bone. Semin Roentgenol 1994;29(1):15-37.

[10] Bussard KM, Gay CV, Mastro AM. The bone microenvironment in metastasis; what is special about bone? Cancer Metastasis Rev 2008;27(1):41-55.

[11] Koswig S, Budach V. Remineralization and pain relief in bone metastases after different radiotherapy fractions (10 times 4 Gy vs 1 time 8 Gy). A prospective study. Strahlenther Onkol 1999;175(10): 500-8.

[12] Nguyen PL, Alibhai SMH, Basaria S, D'Amico AV, Kantoff PW, Keating NL, et al. Adverse effects of androgen deprivation therapy and strategies to mitigate them. Eur Urol 2014. pii: S0302-2838(14)00650-2. doi: 10.1016/j.eururo.2014.07.010.

[13] D'Amico AV, Chen M, Renshaw AA, Loffredo M, Kantoff PW. Androgen suppression and radiation vs radiation alone for prostate cancer: A randomized trial. JAMA 2008;299(3):289-95.

Submitted: February 01, 2015. *Revised:* March 20, 2015. *Accepted:* March 29, 2015.

SECTION THREE: POST-TRAUMATIC STRESS, BURNOUT AND CANCER

In: Pain Management Yearbook 2015
Editor: Joav Merrick

ISBN: 978-1-63484-515-1

Chapter 20

A CANADIAN SUMMARY: POST-TRAUMATIC STRESS DISORDER IN CANCER PATIENTS

Christina Crowe**, *HBSc, MA, Counselling Psych
Faculty of Behavioral Sciences, Yorkville University, Fredericton, New Brunswick, Canada

Post-traumatic stress disorder (PTSD) has been well described in the literature as it pertains to military personnel, victims of childhood abuse or trauma, violence and some chronic terminal illness. The subspecialty of psycho-oncology has also contributed a growing body of evidence around PTSD in adult and pediatric cancer patients. This summary review examines the current landscape of trauma recognition and treatment within the context of cancer care. Diagnosis, assessment, treatment and special considerations for each are reviewed.

Keywords: post-traumatic stress disorder, post-traumatic growth, cancer patients, breast cancer

INTRODUCTION

Post-traumatic stress disorder (PTSD) has been widely recognized by clinicians among veterans, current military personnel, and first responders such as police, firefighters and paramedics, as well as victims of trauma, such as violence, sexual assault or war. While the diagnosis of a life-threatening illness has been included as a potential trauma in the DSM-IV under PTSD for some time, it is still a relatively new field of research, largely found in the psycho-oncology subspecialty (1).

* Correspondence: Christina Crowe, HBSc, MACP, Faculty of Behavioral Sciences, Yorkville University, Yorkville Landing Suite 102, 100 Woodside Lane, Fredericton, New Brunswick E3C 2R9, Canada. E-mail: Christina@christinacrowe.ca.

Cancer patients are increasingly the subject of research with identification, diagnosis, interventions and outcomes being reported, for several different disease types. While the goal of cancer treatment is to cure the patient of cancer whenever possible, many patients relapse, or are only diagnosed in the advanced (terminal) stage of cancer. Further, many treatments that cannot cure patients of their disease focus on palliation: controlling or reducing pain and disease symptoms while maintaining a patients quality of life. This can result in many patients living with cancer as a chronic disease, or at least, cancer that is not immediately life threatening.

Research supports the notion that a cancer diagnosis is in fact traumatic, however not all patients will develop proven PTSD or symptoms of PTSD (PTSS). In an exploration of patients with advanced cancer who develop PTSD, 66.7% report that their cancer diagnosis was the traumatic event for them, despite other traumas, such as the death of a loved one (2). An Australian study of women with ovarian cancer found similar rates of PTSD (9-10%) among the patients as in the general population (3). The women who reported PTSD symptoms had poorer quality of life, depression, anxiety and maladaptive coping, such as avoidance, substance use and self-blame (3).

PTSD is described in the "Diagnostic and statistical manual IV" (DSM-IV), the history of which will be reviewed in more detail later, but for the purposes of this background, it's important to note its application in cancer research. Johnson (4) defined PTSD in cancer care, "as a psychiatric diagnosis indicative of a disturbance of the normal capacity to resolve cognitive and emotional responses to a traumatic event, is a chronic disorder of overlapping comorbid symptoms such as depression and anxiety" (see Figure 1).

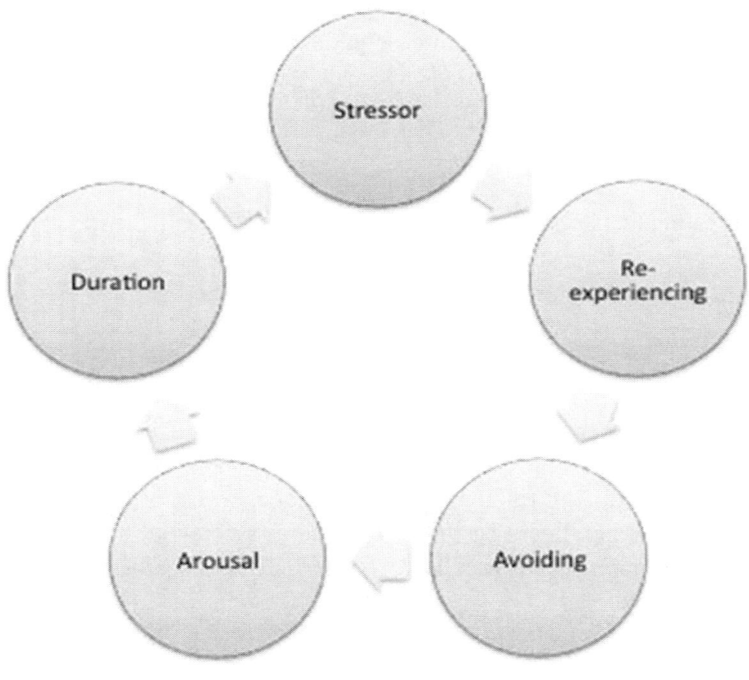

Figure 1. DSM-IV Criteria for post-traumatic stress disorder. Adapter from Bush (2010).

The field of psycho-oncology has also contributed to the understanding of post-traumatic growth (PTG), otherwise known as the deep personal growth development that can sometimes be seen in patients after PTSD, as it specifically relates to cancer (5). Sometimes cancer patients have been known to say, cancer was 'the best thing that happened to me' after it spurred them on to make major lifestyle changes, or reconnect with loved ones (5). It would be less socially appropriate to note how trauma from war or assault could have ever been a good thing, especially given the scale of impact on other victims, so the PTG phenomenon is more widely discussed and accepted in the context of cancer recovery and survivorship (5).

Most discussions of cancer treatment are logically divided into treatment settings, such as neo-adjuvant, adjuvant, advanced or metastatic, as well as further classified by the age groups childhood, young adult, adult, or elderly. This reflects different goals or strategies of treatment, as well as myriad patient and disease factors that influence treatment approaches. While oncology health care professionals, including nurses, pharmacists, radiation oncologists, surgical oncologists and medical oncologists, surround the patient to treat the cancer, many patients are left to pick up the pieces of their mental health, or psychological wellbeing, on their own. Given the complexity of disease treatment and patient factors, existing guidelines are continuously being expanded on with the research from the newer subspecialty of psycho-oncology. For example, in 2013, National Comprehensive Cancer Network (NCCN) published an update to the 2006 guidelines for distress management, giving direction to oncology professionals on how to refer for cancer patients experiencing emotional distress [6]. Although the NCCN guidelines unfortunately do not cover PTSD specifically, it sends the important message that a cancer patient's emotional state is an important treatment consideration. This guide will limit itself to issues related to those patients who are susceptible to developing PTSD, its identification and treatment, and will not cover other issues related to cancer treatment and survivorship (such as 'normal' worry, depression, anxiety, sexuality or life after cancer).

It's important to differentiate between the 'normal' worry and anxiety one might assume a patient would have about their cancer treatment and outcomes, to when more specific interventions might be indicated for depression, anxiety and PTSD symptoms. Using tools such as the Brief Cancer-Related Worry Inventory could be useful to this end (7). As a specific disease site, breast cancer yields the most research evaluating connections between emotional distress and disease outcomes. Despite the acknowledgement that fears about uncertainty of treatment might undermine an appropriate diagnosis of PTSD, an initial prospective study concludes a large number of women with an early (adjuvant) breast cancer diagnosis demonstrate the need for psychosocial counselling and support in this early treatment phase (1). A recent observational study reported that 23% of 1,139 women with newly diagnosed localized breast cancer experienced post-traumatic stress disorder (PTSD) symptoms (8). It is notable that the overall incidence of PTSD in the general population is about half of that found in the study (8). A previous study found the rate of PTSD in women with metastatic breast cancer to double at 52% (9). Another prospective study looked at neo-adjuvant and adjuvant breast cancer patients comparing assessment results post (neo-adjuvant) surgery and one year later. After one year, about half of the patients continued to suffer from symptoms of PTSD, but predictors of this result included a history of depression and traumatic experiences. This study suggests early assessment and identification could be meaningful for these patients (10).

Understanding the factors that predispose cancer patients to develop symptoms of PTSD has practice implications, and as such is also a focus of research. Links between childhood trauma and adult physical and mental health have been widely established by the groundbreaking Adverse Childhood Experiences (ACE) study (11). This group of researchers has also positively correlated smoking behaviors and risk of lung cancer with higher ACE scores (12). Another study looked at the presence of traumatic emotional, physical, and sexual abuse with breast cancer related intrusive symptoms (13). Emotional abuse was a unique predictor of intrusive symptoms; the study results suggest a breast cancer diagnosis might trigger emotional and cognitive responses that are similar to patient's prior traumatic experiences. The implications of this study affect both medical physicians as well as mental health professionals treating women with breast cancer; discussions of both subject matters, the cancer and the adverse childhood experiences might increase breast cancer related intrusive symptoms and interventions for both might be beneficial (13).

Many cancer centre programs already recognize the importance of psychosocial support for patients. Research suggests there are also socioeconomic risks associated with cancer patients developing PTSD symptoms; one study shows women with PTSD (and a history of mood and anxiety disorders) were four times more likely to be unable to work due to the emotional distress, compared to control cancer patients without PTSD (14). The research question has been asked, can psychological interventions also change the course of illness for a patient? One randomized study intervention with a stepped-care approach (increasing interventions with increasing symptoms) is currently looking at supporting patients 'where they are at' (their current coping mechanisms). In this study design authors conclude all interventions should be directed at symptoms that can directly change the course of illness for a patient, and include interventions like stress management, individual and group counselling (15).

Pérez (16) conducted a study in adjuvant breast cancer patients, evaluating symptoms of PTSD during treatment, at the end of treatment and at six to twelve months follow up. The study had specified endpoints examining the relationship between post-traumatic stress symptomology (PTSS) and Type C personality described as "A temperament seen in those who appear quiet and introspective but are actually frustrated and swallow anger, and who may have an increased risk of cancer; type Cs are the polar opposite of type As; they are non-emotional, non-assertive, and appease others to the point of self-effacement and self-sacrifice" (16). PTSS was consistent across all phases of diagnosis, treatment and follow up. The results showed feelings of hopelessness/helplessness and Type C personality were positively correlated with PTSD symptomology, followed by trait dissociation, anxious preoccupation, cognitive avoidance and symptoms of acute stress disorder. The three mediators of PTSS and Type C personality during treatment were anxious preoccupation, cognitive avoidance, and helplessness/hopelessness (17). These study results give clinicians some indication of where helpful interventions might impact the patient journey.

A patient's individual psychological approach to their cancer diagnosis and treatment can also have a clinically significant impact on their treatment outlines. A recent study examined the effects and characteristics of patients with PTSD symptoms versus those without specific PTSD symptoms. The study showed patients with PTSD symptoms had a significantly lower Karnofsky Performance Status (a scale of functional impairment), higher ratings of mood disturbance, lower ratings of functional status, and lower quality of life (QOL) than patients with no PTSD. In terms of prognostic factors, a lower Karnofsky Performance Status and presence of bone metastases predicted a higher likelihood of being classified as having PTSD. The study concluded early identification and mental health interventions may impact the onset of psychological distress and improve health outcomes (18).

Research has revealed the positive relationship between traumatic stress and increased risk for diseases like cancer in general. A 2014 study looked at the potential for increased carcinogenesis through emotional stress causing increased DNA damage and impaired DNA repair mechanisms. This study examined the effect of psychotherapy (Narrative Exposure Therapy – NET) on DNA breakage and repair in patients with and without trauma exposure. This study revealed higher levels of DNA breakage in individuals with PTSD and trauma-exposed subjects, indicating that trauma stress is associated with DNA breakage. Further, in a second pre-specified subgroup, psychotherapy reversed both DNA strand break accumulation and PTSD symptoms. This important study shows psychotherapy can demonstrate changes at the molecular level in humans, and for the first time shown an association between traumatic stress and DNA breakage (19). Striving for better outcomes is almost always the driving force behind clinical research. Therefore finding ways to positively affect these factors are incumbent upon all research clinicians.

POST-TRAUMATIC GROWTH

Is there any hope to offer patients or clients with cancer about the course of their psychological health as they move through their cancer journey? As previously mentioned, the concept of post-traumatic growth (PTG) has also been widely described in the literature and likely witnessed by many oncology professionals with their patients. A study examining the potential for PTG in breast cancer patients with PTSD symptoms found younger age and perception of cancer as their traumatic stressors were associated with greater PTG (20). Psychological interventions by all clinicians should therefore be sensitive to the potential for PTG, both in design of treatment and in outcome assessment (20). This might be of particular importance to younger adult patients with cancer, children, or those for whom survivorship will hold a long life ahead of them. In supporting the potential for PTG, clinicians are trained to look for 'teachable moments,' which include three components: "the event 1) increases perceptions of personal risk and outcome expectancies, 2) prompts as strong affective or emotional response, and 3) redefines self-concept or social role" (5). As Bell (5) pointed out, clinicians have an opportunity in cancer care, to actively create a teachable moment, rather than just wait around for one to occur, through health education and promotion.

CHILDHOOD CANCER

PTSD was first described in childhood cancer survivors in the 1980's, but was not widely researched until more than a decade later (21). While for the most part, assessment and interventions are well established in pediatric cancer, there can also be a risk for over-diagnosis. There are many factors in a child's experience with cancer that can contribute to post-traumatic stress and it is incumbent upon clinicians to take care with PTSD diagnosis and follow up (21). Particular attention should be paid to the differences between assessment measures, timing of assessment relative to diagnosis, the criteria used to define the outcome, and identification of the precipitating traumatic event. Interventions using cognitive behavioral therapy (CBT) techniques for the treatment of PTSS in adolescent and young adult cancer survivors have been empirically supported (22).

Diagnosis

The development and understanding of PTSD as a psychiatric disorder has undergone significant change from the DSM-I to the DSM-V. By the DSM-IV, it had become classified as an anxiety disorder, onset occurring and lasting at least one month following a stressful event (4) (see Figure 2).

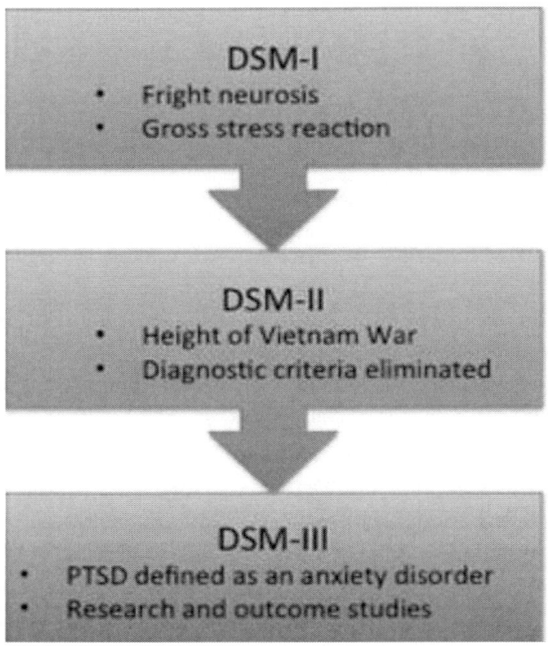

Figure 2. Historical framework of PTSD in the DSM. Adapted from Bush (2010).

Currently, the DSM-IV lists six criteria to warrant a formal diagnosis of post-traumatic stress disorder:

1. experiencing an event in which the life, physical safety or physical integrity of the client was threatened or actually harmed, resulting in feelings of intense fear, helplessness or horror
2. continuing to re-experience the traumatic event after it is over
3. seeking to avoid reminders of the event
4. exhibiting signs of persistent arousal
5. symptoms last more than one month
6. disturbance causes significant distress in important areas of functioning (23).

As previously reviewed, in cancer patients some of the most common symptoms of PTSD presentation include flashbacks or re-experiencing a traumatic moment, avoidance, helplessness/hopelessness and intrusive symptoms. While most cancer patients in general will not exhibit all six criteria, many patients will experience some or most of these aspects in their cancer journey, which the literature demonstrates may impact the course of their disease and treatment. DSM-V has been recently released, and provides an even narrower definition, requiring the medical incident to be "sudden" and "catastrophic" to be considered as a formal PTSD diagnosis (22). However, the cancer experience is fraught with potentially traumatic moments; patients know that without treatment, they will die, and they may also die as a result of their treatment. As the research with this unique population continues to build, the characteristics specific to cancer will continue to inform diagnosis.

Assessment

In the United States (US), a national study reported 65% of oncologists reported screening for distress in their patients, but only 14.3% used a standardized measure. Similarly only 10% in the United Kingdom (UK) used a standardized measure (24). Bultz (24) conducted a Canadian study on the use of the previously validated Edmonton Symptom Assessment System (ESAS) and a Canadian Problem Checklist (CPC) to screen for distress (Appendix A). These authors found both assessments relatively easy to administer in a busy clinic and an important first step to screening. He encourages each cancer clinic to identify their own barriers to implementation (24).

The Beck Depression Inventory (BDI) and the Hospital Anxiety and Depression Screening Inventory (HADS) are also common depression screening tools used in medical clinical and research settings (see appendix B). The BDI can be time-consuming in a busy clinic, and one Australian study (similar health system to Canada) found the modified HADS-Anxiety and HADS-Depression more useful in cancer patients than the HADS-Total (25). Our first and most widely used assessment tools for PTSD come from the military, and generally are specific to the experiences of military roles. The Post-traumatic Stress Disorders Checklist (PCL-C) has been developed for civilians, intended for everyone outside of the military, including patients with life-threatening illnesses (26). The PCL-C has demonstrated excellent reliability and validity, and studies have confirmed its use for screening for adult oncology patients (27).

Interventions

What are the most commonly prescribed interventions for cancer patients with emotional distress? Many patients are referred to the cancer centre's social workers or psychotherapists for counselling, some patients are prescribed an SSRI for depression, and even beta-blockers have been found to benefit cancer patients' psychological adjustment following diagnosis (28). While in general, CBT has the most evidenced based support for use in depression and anxiety; it is not always a home run for other mental illnesses. One study demonstrated that for cancer patients in the follow-up stage, Eye Movement Desensitization and Reprocessing

(EMDR) were associated with the absence of PTSD after the treatment rather than CBT (29). EMDR is a psychotherapy technique developed by Francine Shapiro, emphasizing disturbing memories as the cause of psychopathology, and it is used to alleviate the symptoms of PTSD. In a study examining the effects of EMDR versus CBT in cancer patients, EMDR was found to be significantly more effective than CBT in reducing scores on the Impact of Event Scale—Revised (IES-R) and Clinician-Administered PTSD Scale (CAPS) intrusive symptom sub-scale (29).

However, a randomized controlled trial of CBT versus non-directing supportive counselling (SC) found CBT to be superior in reducing PTSD and anxiety symptoms both in the short and longer term in head and neck cancer (HNC) patients. At the study conclusion, up to 67% of patients in the CBT program no longer met clinical or sub-clinical PTSD, anxiety and/or depression by 12 months post-treatment, compared with 25% of patients who received SC (30). The significance the authors of this trial emphasized was that both interventions were helpful, and it was perhaps the presence of an early intervention that alleviated these patients psychological distress, rather than no intervention at all.

Nenova (31) conducted a review of randomized controlled trials, looking to validate the use of CBT in cancer patients with PTSD or PTSS, looking particularly at symptoms of intrusion and avoidance. Most of the studies were not designed to target traumatic stress symptoms in highly distressed cancer patients and didn't include previously validated CBT components, such as cognitive restructuring or exposure. However, it was clear interventions with CBT components may have potential for the reduction of PTSD symptoms in highly distressed patients, and the authors conclude future research should be directed here (31).

As previously noted by Kangas (30), some intervention is better than no intervention, even if it is non-directive and simply supportive. A strong therapeutic alliance might be one of the best predictors of the strength of a healing relationship in psychotherapy, without which, the healing work cannot be done. A CBT telephone administered study with hematopoietic stem cell transplant survivors found the therapeutic alliance to be critical to maximizing psychotherapeutic benefits for cancer survivors (32). Therefore, this study recommends techniques for maximizing the therapeutic alliance be incorporated into early phases of creating the care plan for a cancer patient. While oncology clinicians in Canada might have some expertise in this area, this data demonstrates the significance of focusing on this as an important aspect of care.

Other psychotherapeutic interventions for PTSD have included trauma focused cognitive behavioral therapy (TF-CBT). Briefly, trauma focused-CBT involves repeated exposure to the trauma memory in imagination, or by writing a narrative, and "*in vivo* exposure to situations associated with the traumatic event that are objectively safe yet cause anxiety or are avoided, and/or challenging maladaptive trauma-related appraisals" (33). However, the literature has not yet examined cancer patients and the cancer experience. Most of its use has historically been in clients with childhood abuse, road accidents and military operations.

Finally, a psychotherapeutic approach that is thousands of years old, and recently gaining in popularity, is mindfulness, or more recently, mindfulness based stress reduction (MBSR). A 2015 Canadian study confirms is use and validity in 122 cancer patients (34). The authors noted, "In cancer settings, results from nine randomized controlled trials (RCTs) indicate a beneficial effect of MBIs (mindfulness based interventions) on symptoms of stress, mood disturbance, depression, anxiety, perceived stress, quality of life, physical functioning, sleep, fatigue, energy, spirituality, meaning, and positive states of mind" (34). It is important to note these were not patients who necessarily had PTSD, but reported emotional distress. However, the patients in the MBI groups reported a decrease in experiential avoidance, which is a key symptom in cancer patients who have PTSS. Another study investigated the effect of MBSR on the potential for PTG, and found that MBSR subjects (cancer patients) demonstrated increased spirituality, PTG, and mindfulness, relative to controls (35).

A technique more commonly associated with PTSD experienced by military personnel that could be potentially used with cancer patients, is grounding techniques, particularly those experiencing avoidance or flashbacks. Grounding techniques help people remain focused and in the present and are used by clinicians to prevent patient emotional arousal from getting too high during trauma reprocessing. The objective of a grounding exercise is to reconnect to the present moment, remind the patient of the here and now, connect her to her body and sense of personal control and connect her to the therapist and the safe context of the therapy room (23) (see Figure 3).

Grounding Techniques: Visual & Auditory cues:
Say to clients:
Use your visual senses by looking around the room. Name what you see. Auditory clues are helpful.
You can say to the client:
Listen to my voice. I am _____, your therapist. You are in my office. Can you hear my voice? Nod your head if you can hear my voice.

Grounding Techniques: Cognitive skills:
Reorient yourself in place and time by asking yourself some or all of these questions:
- Where am I?
- What is today?
- What is the date?
- How old am I?
- What season is it?

Adapted from *Working Toward Change: Therapeutic Techniques* (n.d.).

Figure 3.

CONCLUSION

PTSD is a serious anxiety disorder, widely recognized in military personnel, victims of childhood abuse, violence or accidental (vehicular) trauma. Increasingly, cancer patients are being included in the group of clients with chronic or terminal illness. Research supports the validity of this diagnosis in this patient group, and further warns that trauma unchecked can also adversely affect disease and treatment outcomes. PTS and PTSD should be distinguished with assessments validated for cancer patients from emotional distress. While many of the treatments used with other trauma victims, like CBT, EMDR or MBSR might prove useful with cancer patients with PTSD, the data is still forthcoming. Thorough assessments might help pinpoint specific areas of concern for a patient, such as avoidance coping, flashbacks or anxious preoccupation, which can inform treatment techniques and categories of intervention. An individualized approach should be adapted for each patient's unique journey. The data also supports the notion that some treatment is better than no treatment at all. Supporting patients "where they are at" will also allow clinicians to be mindful of opportunities for teachable moments and PTG. Clinicians are also encouraged to help patients navigate and source the best options for their psychological care, through both publically and privately funded options.

APPENDIX A. EDMONTON SYMPTOM ASSESSMENT SYSTEM (ESAS) AND A CANADIAN PROBLEM CHECKLIST (CPC) (24)

Completed by:
- ❒ Patient
- ❒ Family
- ❒ Health Professional
- ❒ Assisted by family or health

Date of Completion: ____________________ **Time:** ____________

1. Edmonton Symptom Assessment System (ESAS):

Please circle the number that best describes:

No pain	0	1	2	3	4	5	6	7	8	9	10	Worst possible pain
Not tired	0	1	2	3	4	5	6	7	8	9	10	Worst possible tiredness
Not nauseated	0	1	2	3	4	5	6	7	8	9	10	Worst possible nausea
Not depressed	0	1	2	3	4	5	6	7	8	9	10	Worst possible depression
Not anxious	0	1	2	3	4	5	6	7	8	9	10	Worst possible anxiety
Not drowsy	0	1	2	3	4	5	6	7	8	9	10	Worst possible drowsiness
Best appetite	0	1	2	3	4	5	6	7	8	9	10	Worst possible appetite
Best feeling of wellbeing	0	1	2	3	4	5	6	7	8	9	10	Worst possible feeling of wellbeing
No shortness of breath	0	1	2	3	4	5	6	7	8	9	10	Worst possible shortness of breath
Other problem	0	1	2	3	4	5	6	7	8	9	10	

2. Canadian Problem Checklist:

Please check all of the following items that have been a concern or problem for you in the past week including today:

Emotional:
- ❒ Fears/Worries
- ❒ Sadness
- ❒ Frustration/Anger
- ❒ Changes in appearance
- ❒ Intimacy/Sexuality

Practical:
- ❒ Work/School
- ❒ Finances
- ❒ Getting to and from appointments
- ❒ Accommodation

Informational:
- ❒ Understanding my illness and/or treatment
- ❒ Talking with the health care team
- ❒ Making treatment decisions
- ❒ Knowing about available resources

Spiritual:
- ❒ Meaning/Purpose of life
- ❒ Faith

Social/Family:
- ❒ Feeling a burden to others
- ❒ Worry about family/friends
- ❒ Feeling alone

Physical:
- ❒ Concentration/Memory
- ❒ Sleep
- ❒ Weight

**Questionnaire from the Cancer Journey Advisory Group, Canadian Partnership Against Cancer's Minimum Data Set*

APPENDIX B. THE HOSPITAL ANXIETY AND DEPRESSION SCREENING TOOL (36)

Hospital Anxiety and Depression Scale (HADS)

Tick the box beside the reply that is closest to how you have been feeling in the past week.
Don't take too long over you replies: your immediate is best.

D	A		D	A	
		I feel tense or 'wound up':			**I feel as if I am slowed down:**
	3	Most of the time	3		Nearly all the time
	2	A lot of the time	2		Very often
	1	From time to time, occasionally	1		Sometimes
	0	Not at all	0		Not at all
		I still enjoy the things I used to enjoy:			**I get a sort of frightened feeling like 'butterflies' in the stomach:**
0		Definitely as much		0	Not at all
1		Not quite so much		1	Occasionally
2		Only a little		2	Quite Often
3		Hardly at all		3	Very Often
		I get a sort of frightened feeling as if something awful is about to happen:			**I have lost interest in my appearance:**
	3	Very definitely and quite badly	3		Definitely
	2	Yes, but not too badly	2		I don't take as much care as I should
	1	A little, but it doesn't worry me	1		I may not take quite as much care
	0	Not at all	0		I take just as much care as ever
		I can laugh and see the funny side of things:			**I feel restless as I have to be on the move:**
0		As much as I always could		3	Very much indeed
1		Not quite so much now		2	Quite a lot
2		Definitely not so much now		1	Not very much
3		Not at all		0	Not at all
		Worrying thoughts go through my mind:			**I look forward with enjoyment to things:**
	3	A great deal of the time	0		As much as I ever did
	2	A lot of the time	1		Rather less than I used to
	1	From time to time, but not too often	2		Definitely less than I used to
	0	Only occasionally	3		Hardly at all
		I feel cheerful:			**I get sudden feelings of panic:**
3		Not at all		3	Very often indeed
2		Not often		2	Quite often
1		Sometimes		1	Not very often
0		Most of the time		0	Not at all
		I can sit at ease and feel relaxed:			**I can enjoy a good book or radio or TV program:**
	0	Definitely	0		Often
	1	Usually	1		Sometimes
	2	Not Often	2		Not often
	3	Not at all	3		Very seldom

Please check you have answered all the questions

Scoring:
Total score: Depression (D) ___________ Anxiety (A) _____________
0-7 = Normal
8-10 = Borderline abnormal (borderline case)
11-21 = Abnormal (case)

REFERENCES

[1] Mehnert AU. Prevalence of acute and post-traumatic stress disorder and comorbid mental disorders in breast cancer patients during primary cancer care: a prospective study. Psycho-Oncology 2007;16(3):181-8.

[2] Mystakidou K, Parpa E, Tsilika E, Panagiotou I, Roumeliotou A, Galanos A, et al. Traumatic experiences of patients with advanced cancer. J Loss Trauma 2012;17(2):125-136. Doi:10.1080/ 15325024 .2011.595296.

[3] Shand LA. Symptoms of post-traumatic stress in Australian women with ovarian cancer. Psycho-Oncology 2015;24(2):190-6.

[4] Bush NJ. Post-traumatic stress disorder related to cancer: Hope, healing, and recovery. Oncol Nurs Forum 2010;37(5):E331-E43. Doi:10.1188/10.ONF.E331-E343.

[5] Bell K. Remaking the self: Trauma, teachable moments, and the biopolitics of cancer survivorship. Cult Med Psychiatry 2012;36(4):584-600.

[6] Holland JC, Andersen B, Breitbart WS, Buchmann LO, Compas B, Deshields TL, et al. Distress management. J Natl Compr Canc Netw 2013;11(2):190-209.

[7] Hirai K, Shiozaki M, Motooka H, Arai H, Koyama A, Inui H, et al. Discrimination between worry and anxiety among cancer patients: development of a brief cancer-related worry inventory. Psycho-Oncology 2008;17(12): 1172-9. Doi:10.1002/pon.1348.

[8] Vin-Raviv N, Hillyer GC, Hershman DL, Galea S, Leoce N, Bovbjerg DH, et al. Racial Disparities in Post-traumatic Stress after Diagnosis of Localized Breast Cancer: The BQUAL Study. J Natl Cancer Inst 2013;105(8):563-72. Doi:10.1093/jnci/djt024.

[9] Butler LD, Koopman C, Classen C, Spiegel D. Traumatic stress, life events, and emotional support in women with metastatic breast cancer: Cancer-related traumatic stress symptoms associated with past and current stressors. Health Psychol 1999;18(6):555-60.

[10] Bulotienė G, Matuizienė J. Post-traumatic stress in breast cancer patients. Acta Med Litu 2014;21(2):43-9.

[11] The Adverse Childhood Experiences Study. (n.d.). URL: http://www.acestudy.org/home.

[12] Brown DW, Anda RF, Felitti VJ, Edwards VJ, Malarcher AM, Croft JB, et al. Adverse childhood experiences are associated with the risk of lung cancer: a prospective cohort study. BMC Public Health 2010;101-12. Doi:10.1186/1471-2458-10-20.

[13] Goldsmith RE, Jandorf L, Valdimarsdottir H, Amend KL, Stoudt BG, Rini C, et al. Traumatic stress symptoms and breast cancer: The role of childhood abuse. Child Abuse Negl 2010;34(6):465-70. Doi:10.1016/j.chiabu.2009.10.007.

[14] Lanche M. Higher risk of PTSD in patients with history of mood and anxiety disorders. Prim Psychiatry 2008;15(6):20-1.

[15] Nordin K, Rissanen R, Ahlgren J, Burell G, Fjïllskog M, Bïrjesson S, et al. Design of the study: How can health care help female breast cancer patients reduce their stress symptoms? A randomized intervention study with stepped-care. BMC Cancer 2012;12(1):167-72. Doi:10.1186/1471-2407-12-167.

[16] Type C Personality. (n.d.) Segen's medical dictionary, 2011. URL: http://medicaldictionary.thefree dictionary.com/Type+C+Personality

[17] Pérez SE. Post-traumatic stress symptoms in breast cancer patients: Temporal evolution, predictors, and mediation. J Trauma Stress 2014;27(2):224-31.

[18] Gold JI, Douglas MK, Thomas ML, Elliott JE, Rao SM, Miaskowski C. The relationship between post-traumatic stress disorder, mood states, functional status, and quality of life in oncology outpatients. J Pain Symptom Manage 2012;44(4):520-31. Doi:10.1016/j.jpainsymman.2011.10.014.

[19] Morath J, Moreno-Villanueva M, Hamuni G, Kolassa S, Ruf-Leuschner M, Schauer M, et al. Effects of Psychotherapy on DNA Strand Break Accumulation Originating from Traumatic Stress. Psychother Psychosom 2014;83(5):289-97. Doi:10.1159/000362739.

[20] Cordova MJ, Giese-Davis J, Golant M, Kronenwetter C, Chang V, Spiegel D. Breast Cancer as Trauma: Post-traumatic Stress and Post-traumatic Growth. J Clin Psychol Med Settings 2007;14(4):308-19. Doi:10.1007/s10880-007-9083-6.

[21] Ubogy S, Olson K. The trauma symptom checklist for children and misdiagnosis of PTSD in a youth with acute lymphocytic leukemia: A brief report. J Child Adolesc Trauma 2014;7(1):13-5. Doi:10.1007/s40653-014-0004-1.

[22] Vuotto SC, Perez KM, Krull KR, Brinkman TM. A narrative review of the occurrence of post-traumatic stress responses in adolescent and young adult cancer survivors. Clin Oncol Adolesc Young Adults 2015;519-33. Doi:10.2147/COAYA.S49175.

[23] Working toward change: Therapeutic techniques. (n.d.). Centre for Mental Health and Addiction. URL: http://knowledgex.camh.net/amhspecialists/specialized_treatment/trauma_treatment/Documents/first_stage_trauma_143_147.pdf

[24] Bultz BC. Implementing screening for distress, the 6th vital sign: a Canadian strategy for changing practice. Psycho-Oncology 2011;20(5):463-9.

[25] Lambert SD, Pallant JF, Boyes AW, King MT, Britton B, Girgis, A. A Rasch analysis of the Hospital Anxiety and Depression Scale (HADS) among cancer survivors. Psychol Assess 2013;25(2):379-90. Doi:10.1037 /a0031154.

[26] Post-traumatic stress disorders self-assessment (n.d.). PTSD Association (Canada). URL: http://www.ptsdassociation.com/ptsd-self-assessment.php.

[27] Meyer R, Amariglio N, Gold J. Psychometric Properties of the PTSD Checklist Civilian Version in a Sample of Patients With Cancer. American Psychological Association meeting 2014.

[28] Lindgren MK. Beta-blockers may reduce intrusive thoughts in newly diagnosed cancer patients. Psycho-Oncology 2013;22(8):1889-94.

[29] Capezzani L, Ostacoli L, Cavallo M, Carletto S, Fernandez I, Solomon R, et al. EMDR and CBT for cancer patients: Comparative study of effects on PTSD, anxiety, and depression. J EMDR Pract Res 2013;7(3):134-43. Doi:10.1891/1933-3196.7.3.134.

[30] Kangas MA. A pilot randomized controlled trial of a brief early intervention for reducing post-traumatic stress disorder, anxiety and depressive symptoms in newly diagnosed head and neck cancer patients. Psycho-Oncology 2013;22(7):1665-73.

[31] Nenova MK. Psychosocial interventions with cognitive-behavioral components for the treatment of cancer-related traumatic stress symptoms: A review of randomized controlled trials. J Cogn Psychother 2013;27(3):258-84.

[32] Applebaum AJ, DuHamel KN, Winkel G, Rini C, Greene PB, Mosher CE, et al. Therapeutic alliance in telephone-administered cognitive–behavioral therapy for hematopoietic stem cell transplant survivors. J Consul Clin Psychol 2012;80(5):811-6. Doi:10.1037/a0027956.

[33] Ponniah K, Hollon SD. Empirically supported psychological treatments for adult acute stress disorder and post-traumatic stress disorder: a review. Depress Anxiety 2009;26(12):1086-1109. Doi:10.1002/da.20635.

[34] Labelle LE, Campbell TS, Faris P, Carlson LE. Mediators of Mindfulness-Based Stress Reduction (MBSR): Assessing the Timing and Sequence of Change in Cancer Patients. J Clin Psychol 2015;71(1):21-40. doi:10.1002/jclp.22117.

[35] Labelle LE, Lawlor-Savage L, Campbell TS, Faris P, Carlson LE. Does self-report mindfulness mediate the effect of Mindfulness-Based Stress Reduction (MBSR) on spirituality and post-traumatic growth in cancer patients? J Posit Psychol 2015;10(2):153-66. Doi:10.1080/17439760.2014.927902.

[36] Hospital Anxiety and Depression Scale. (n.d.). URL: http://opencourses.emu.edu.tr/pluginfile.php/8619/mod_resource/content/1/HADS.pdf.

Submitted: March 05, 2015. *Revised:* April 02, 2015. *Accepted:* April 06, 2015.

In: Pain Management Yearbook 2015
Editor: Joav Merrick

ISBN: 978-1-63484-515-1

Chapter 21

BURNOUT AND SELF-CARE CONSIDERATIONS FOR ONCOLOGY PROFESSIONALS

Christina Crowe*[*], *HBSc, MA, Counselling Psych
Faculty of Behavioral Sciences, Yorkville University,
Fredericton, New Brunswick, Canada

The focus of a health care professional's career is to care for other people. Over a lifetime, this often occurs at the expense of his/her own physical and mental health. An increased public awareness about mental health in general leads us to the question, who is taking care of those who take care of us? In the specialty of oncology, physicians and nurses are at increased risk for burnout or burnout syndrome. This review provides a brief look at literature supporting the view that oncology physicians and nurses are at increased risk for burnout, and discusses protective measures.

Keywords: cancer, oncology, oncologists, oncology nurses, burnout, burnout syndrome, self-care, Ontario, Canada

INTRODUCTION

Health care providers take on an enormous task embarking on a career built on providing medical care for the general public's physical and emotional lives. A question worth asking is who is taking care of them? Patient after patient, day after day, often with no time to eat, let alone time to take ten minutes to reflect on how tough cases are affecting them, doctors and nurses have to get through the day. In particular, oncology health care professionals have been shown to be at a greater risk for burnout, in part due to the complex and challenging nature of the clinical work, and also in part due to the high rates of patient death. One thing new and current oncology physicians have to figure out is how to do their jobs efficiently,

[*] Correspondence: Christina Crowe, HBSc, MA Counselling Psychology, Faculty of Behavioral Sciences, Yorkville University, Yorkville Landing Suite 102, 100 Woodside Lane, Fredericton, New Brunswick E3C 2R9, Canada. E-mail: Christina@christinacrowe.ca.

accurately and with as much compassion as possible and also cope with their feelings each time they lose a patient to cancer.

Studies have shown caregivers supporting cancer patients feel they can't show negative emotions as frequently as they normally would, yet at the same time they are expected to show understanding and express sympathy to the patient (1). If the caregivers are at home with the patient, they often do not have an opportunity for a break. If the caregivers are the clinicians at the hospital, they too do not get a break: there are always more patients to be seen. There is no doubt, being a doctor is emotionally challenging, and oncology physicians have some unique challenges.

WHAT IS 'BURNOUT'?

Specifically, burnout is a stress-related syndrome, and is characterized by some of the following symptoms: high emotional exhaustion, high depersonalization, and reduced personal accomplishment. In medical school students, burnout similarly presents as high emotional exhaustion, high cynicism, and also low academic efficacy. Medical school students with emotional exhaustion report feeling totally drained of all emotional resources, have a detached attitude toward their learning, and start to feel incompetent (2). Burnout is typically a slow developing condition. Many health care professionals fail to recognize the signs of burnout in themselves, potentially because they are simply too busy and primarily focused on caring for others. Some common questions a health care provider can ask himself or herself include:

- Do you care less about work, or dreading going to work?
- Are you anxious, irritable or snapping at your colleagues?
- Do you feel disengaged, or have a loss of passion for what you were once passionate about?

Some of the issues oncology professionals face include serious work overload (large patient volumes, insufficient resources, or poorly managed centres) and a lack of control over their work environment. Women physicians have a tougher time, and working alone in a solo practice and being young are also risk factors. Studies have shown some of the things that help to buffer against burnout include being married and having children, which suggests the importance of having healthy, supportive relationships (3). Strategies to support these factors will be addressed further on.

Traditionally, medical and popular culture views a patient's death as the physician failure, and it's no different in oncology. In addition to the intensity of the clinical challenges oncology professionals encounter, as well as facing a higher frequency of patient death, there are other complex issues that must be dealt with on a regular basis. End-of-life concerns often require confronting one's own belief system, facing resistance from patients and their families, colleagues, and also their own institutional culture. This is referred to as moral distress. Physicians find themselves with the inability to act in a manner consistent with their personal and professional values due to institutional or other constraints, and compassion fatigue, marked by diminished emotional energy needed to care for patients (4).

How do oncology professionals cope?

In Ontario, 20 oncologists were interviewed at three hospitals exploring what coping strategies they used to deal with burnout and grief. The results showed they engaged in various rituals, including meeting with families, participating in bereavement rituals in their centre, making a phone call or sending a condolence card to the family. Specific coping strategies that they reported using included social support, activity-oriented coping (such as exercise), turning to faith, compartmentalization, and also withdrawing from patients and families. There is no question that these oncologists grieved for their patients, however, the ability to demonstrate that grief or find good coping strategies may still be needed (3). More often than not, a busy day might get in the way, and at least a third of medical, radiation and surgical oncologists surveyed in Canada never participate in these practices (5).

Oncology nurses also suffer from burnout, high levels of job dissatisfaction and distress from their clinical work. Oncology nurses deal with multiple deaths, providing close care for patients, as well as families/caregivers. After a patient death, a nurse is also expected to continue working. However, being able to talk about one's feelings really does help: one study found many benefits when nurses got together though a support group, including,

- a reduction in end-of-life care stress,
- an increase in self-care, and
- improved patient and team care (6)

Another study confirmed the validity and benefits of bereavement programs for oncology health care professionals (7). Some of the types of activities health care professionals can engage in include: attending funerals, holding alternative rituals, calling families, posting photographs and/or sending cards. Staff can take turns each month leading the signing of the sympathy cards, enabling all to personally sign their names and express condolences. These programs tend to garner positive feedback from participants as well as from patients families.

Reflecting on burnout

As previously reviewed, validated in studies with oncology professionals, burnout syndrome was described by three main dimensions (also called Maslach's dimensions): emotional exhaustion (EE), depersonalization (DP) and low personal accomplishment (PS) (2, 8). Maslach describes components of these further as:

- Exhaustion: Feeling over-extended, both emotionally and physically.
- Cynicism: Taking a cold, cynical attitude toward responsibilities.
- Ineffectiveness: When people feel ineffective, they feel a growing sense of inadequacy.

Oncologists have self-reported rates of emotional exhaustion as high as 69% (4). This warrants our attention because physicians with burnout are also at risk for making more clinical errors and showing poorer clinical judgment. A study from the Netherlands, surveying over 2,000 medical residents and physicians found burnout does in fact impact patient care. Residents and physicians used the Maslach Burnout Inventory-Health and Social Services scale, and the Utrecht Work Engagement Scale and self-assessed patient care practices. The results of this survey showed:

- 94% of the residents reported making one or more mistake without negative consequences for the patient during their training.
- 71% reported performing procedures for which they did not feel properly trained.
- More than half (56%) of the residents stated they had made a mistake with a negative consequence.
- 76% felt they had fallen short in the quality of care they provided on at least one occasion.
- Men reported more errors in action/judgment than women. Significant effects of specialty and clinical setting were found on both types of errors.
- Residents with burnout reported significantly more errors ($p < 0.001$) (9).

It's also important to note if a clinician has burnout, it might not be that the individual clinician's poor coping skills are necessarily the problem, but because of the social work environment they are in. Further, residents in general feel they often make errors over the course of their training (10). They potentially could engage in more productive self-care strategies, but they might not be in an environment that is supportive.

Self-care: Beyond 'coping'

A Canadian study looking at physician's current coping strategies for stress was consistent with previous data discussed showing strategies like working through stress, talking with co-workers, taking a time out, using humor, exercise, quiet time and spending time with family were all used, but to different degrees. However, analysis of the data from the questionnaire used in the study showed that the three most often used strategies were positively correlated with feeling emotionally exhausted (specifically, keeping stress to oneself ($r = .23$), concentrating on what to do next ($r = .16$), and going on as if nothing happened ($r = .07$)). The authors conclude that not all strategies are equally effective, and physician stress reduction interventions are needed (10). Similarly, a study revealed oncology nurses in Japan are distressed about their own mental health, feel they need more training to support their patients' mental health and that they would like more stress management education (11).

How do we move from coping to self-care for health care providers?

> "Self-care is a spectrum of knowledge, skills, and attitudes including self-reflection and self-awareness, identification and prevention of burnout, appropriate professional boundaries, and grief and bereavement." (12)

Unfortunately, there are not any mandatory courses on self-care or wellness management in Canadian medical schools. Where there have been wellness courses, they are student-led, and elective. However, there are validated strategies that can be used and sometimes stating the obvious is important. There are many ways to live a healthy, well-balanced life, including recognizing our inner lives, families, work, community and spirituality. A widely available tool called The Wellness Wheel, developed by Vanderbilt University, refers to six types of wellness – physical, intellectual, emotional, spiritual, social and occupational – and allows individuals to reflect on current life balance and self-care (13).

Health care providers can also use the Wellness Wheel to improve job satisfaction and overall well-being, reducing the likelihood of stress and burnout. Some of these strategies for personal self-care include:

- prioritizing close relationships such as those with family,
- ensuring adequate sleep,
- regular exercise,
- time for vacations,
- fostering recreational activities and hobbies,
- practicing mindfulness and meditation, and
- pursuing spiritual development.

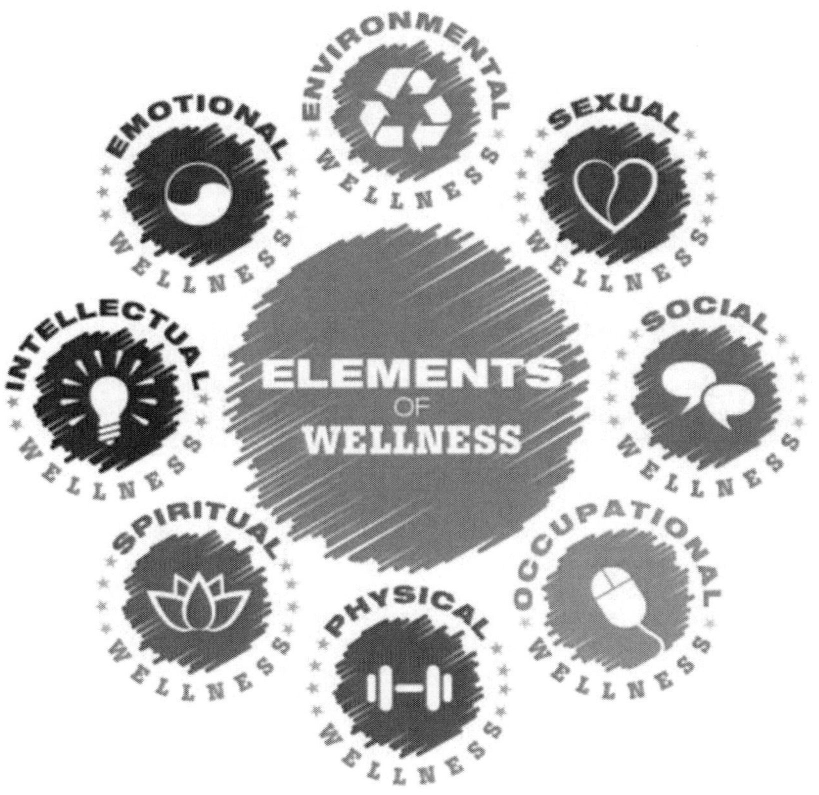

Figure 1. The wellness wheel (13).

Many health care providers do not automatically include self-care activities in their lives, however they can reach out for psychoeducation from a qualified therapist or seek support from their colleagues, and investigate what kinds of programs they might be able to set up in their institution. Self-care skills are strategies everyone can learn, and have proven benefits, including decreasing the impairment from burnout, compassion fatigue, and moral distress. It also encourages personal and professional well-being, job engagement, compassion satisfaction and resilience (4). In fact, many physicians and nurses may be practicing some of these skills and not specially identifying it as 'self-care.'

The bottom line is, oncology care professionals are people too. Doctors and nurses, pharmacists, social workers and care navigators are all also deeply affected by the nature of the work in cancer care. The system is perpetually stressed, and that isn't changing anytime soon. Supporting all medical professionals to do the job they have been trained to do is a worthwhile pursuit. Support can be found in many places, whether it's within one's own cancer centre, religious/faith community, social community or with a professional therapist, and ultimately might improve patient care.

References

[1] Kovács M. Is emotional dissonance more prevalent in oncology care? Emotion work, burnout and coping. Psychooncology 2010;19(8):855-62.

[2] Pagnin D, De Queiroz V, Oliveira Filho M, Gonzalez N, Salgado A, Melo R, et al. Burnout and career choice motivation in medical students. Med Teacher 2013; 35(5):388-94.

[3] Granek L. Oncologists' protocol and coping strategies in dealing with patient loss. Death Stud 2013;37(10):937-52.

[4] Sanchez-Reilly S, Morrison LJ, Carey E, Bernacki R, O'Neill L, Kapo J, et al. Caring for oneself to care for others: physicians and their self-care. J Support Oncol 2013;11(2):75-81.

[5] Chau NG, Zimmermann C, Ma C, Taback N, Krzyzanowska MK. Bereavement practices of physicians in oncology and palliative care. Arch Intern Med 2009; 169(10):963-71.

[6] Wittenberg-Lyles E, Goldsmith J, Reno J. Perceived benefits and challenges of an oncology nurse support group. Clin J Oncol Nurs 2014;18:E71-6. Doi:10.1188/14.CJON.E71-E76.

[7] Marshall G. Bringing a bereavement program back to life. Oncol Nurs Forum 2007; 34(2):506.

[8] Trufelli D, Bensi C, Garcia J, Narahara J, Abrao M, Diniz R, et al. Burnout in cancer professionals: a systematic review and meta-analysis. Eur J Cancer Care 2008;17(6):524-31.Doi:10.1111/j.1365-2354.2008.00927.x.

[9] Prins JT, van der Heijden FMA, Hoekstra-Weebers JEHM, Bakker AB, van de Wiel HBM, Jacobs B, et al. Burnout, engagement and resident physicians' self-reported errors. Psychol Health Med 2009;14(6):654-66.

[10] Lemaire JB, Wallace JE. Not all coping strategies are created equal: A mixed methods study exploring physicians self-reported coping strategies. BMC Health Serv Res 2010;10:208-17.

[11] Kaneko MR, Mariko R, Shuhei N, Hiroshi T, Kumi S, Yuiko N, et al. Nurses' recognition of the mental state of cancer patients and their own stress management: A study of Japanese cancer-care nurses. Psychooncology 2013;22(7):1624-9.

[12] Richards KC, Campenni CE, Muse-Burke JL. Self-care and well-being in mental health professionals: The mediating effects of self-awareness and mindfulness. J Ment Health Couns 2010;32(3):247-64.

[13] Vanderbilt.edu. Wellness wheel. Wellness Center, Vanderbilt University, 2015 URL: http://www.vanderbilt.edu/recreationandwellnesscenter/wellness/wellness-wheel

Submitted: June 01, 2015. *Revised:* July 02, 2015. *Accepted:* July 09, 2015.

In: Pain Management Yearbook 2015
Editor: Joav Merrick

ISBN: 978-1-63484-515-1

Chapter 22

IMPAIRED MENTAL CAPACITY UNDERMINES AUTONOMY AND SELF-DETERMINATION AMONG PATIENTS WITH BONE AND BRAIN METASTASES PARTICIPATING IN PALLIATIVE RADIATION THERAPY CLINICAL TRIALS IN CANADA: ETHICAL AND METHODOLOGICAL IMPLICATIONS FOR THE CLINICIAN INVESTIGATOR

Kristopher Dennis[1,*], MD, FRCPC, Kelly Linden[2], MRT(T), C Shun Wong[3], MD, FRCPC, and Edward Chow[3], MBBS, FRCPC, MSc, PhD

[1]Division of Radiation Oncology, University of Ottawa, Ottawa Hospital Research Institute, Ottawa, Ontario, Canada
[2]Radiation Medicine Program, The Ottawa Hospital, Ottawa, Ontario, Canada
[3]Department of Radiation Oncology, Odette Cancer Centre, Sunnybrook Health Sciences Centre, University of Toronto, Toronto, Ontario, Canada

There are many threats to mental capacity among patients with bone and brain metastases who participate in palliative radiation therapy clinical trials in Canada. Lapses in capacity compromise autonomy and self-determination, and erode trial result validity. Unfortunately, changes in capacity can easily go undetected. We discuss the ethical and methodological consequences of overlooking impaired capacity, and we explore the systemic factors that contribute to the problem: the subtle modulating effects of bone and brain metastases or their therapies on cognition, the urgency for palliation among

* Correspondence: Kristopher Dennis, MD, FRCPC, Division of Radiation Oncology, University of Ottawa; Ottawa Hospital Research Institute, The Ottawa Hospital, 501 Smyth Road, Ottawa, Ontario, K1H8L6, Canada. E-mail: krdennis@toh.on.ca.

symptomatic patients, the academic pressures within Canadian radiation oncology departments and potential conflicts of interest among clinician investigators, deficiencies in the process of informed consent, the lack of capacity assessments within clinical trial designs, and psychosocial dynamics unique to the palliative radiation therapy setting. We reference specific oncology literature and cooperative research groups, and examples of palliative radiation oncology research in Canada to illustrate issues that are applicable to other countries. Our aim is to be provocative and to promote discussion.

Keywords: autonomy, bone metastases, brain metastases, capacity, consent, ethics, palliative care, radiation therapy, radiotherapy

INTRODUCTION

The Canadian Cancer Society estimates that 196,900 Canadians will be diagnosed with a new cancer in 2015 (1). More than half of them will require radiation therapy at some time during their disease course (2, 3). Palliative radiation treatments in particular make up a considerable proportion of the total treatments delivered in modern cancer centres. In most cases these treatments aim to relieve symptoms and improve quality of life, rather than prolong survival. Patients whose cancers have metastasised to the bones or brain commonly receive palliative radiation therapy, and the majority of palliative radiation therapy trials focus on these populations. The demand for treatment will rise in the future because the general population is aging and access to radiation therapy is improving. Patients also now survive longer after they are diagnosed with bone or brain metastases than they did years ago. The unintended consequence of this progress has been a longer duration of time during which they can develop symptoms from their disease.

RADIATION ONCOLOGY IS A SMALL ACADEMIC SPECIALTY

In Canada radiation therapy is usually administered in tertiary centres. The entire Canadian population of over 30 million residents is serviced by only 42 centres and just over 400 radiation oncologists (4). Most Canadian radiation oncology departments train medical students, residents and fellows, and radiation oncologists typically have university appointments. As such the specialty has a rich academic culture, and many treatment centres serve jointly as research institutions. Research activity is an expectation for most radiation oncologists, which places them daily in the role of the clinician investigator.

With respect to palliative radiation therapy, many centres operate specialised rapid-access clinics that expedite palliative treatments for patients with symptomatic metastases. Depending on the specific model employed, compared to other clinics they can be generously staffed and their patients prioritised. Their efficiencies and predictable patient populations also make them ideal settings for research. These clinics have become useful sources of academic productivity.

THE PALLIATIVE ONCOLOGY RESEARCH IMPERATIVE

Palliative radiation therapy clinical trial designs attempt to balance the need for rigorous methodology with the feasibility of enrolling patients. Exclusion criteria can be made strict to minimise bias and strengthen validity, but this can cause many patients to be deemed ineligible. For example, patients receiving these treatments are usually old and have reduced functional independence. Some are admitted to hospital or long-term care facilities which can be logistically challenging. They typically have multiple comorbidities and take numerous medications. The symptoms from their metastases can be overwhelming and exhausting. Depending on how rigorously a trial is designed, any one of these factors can deem patients ineligible for participation.

Consequently, when a patient functions reasonably well and meets the selection criteria for a clinical trial, the interested clinician investigator can feel a sense of urgency to 'get the patient on study.' Reasons for this urgency can range from the narrow and personal (e.g., the researcher is intellectually committed to the trial or desires academic productivity), to the broad and general (e.g., there is public interest in conducting research within the setting at hand). Indeed, there is international recognition that research among elderly patients with advanced malignancy must be promoted and increased (5). The special task force of palliative care experts convened by the influential American Society of Clinical Oncology (ASCO) asserted in 2009 that the case for increasing research among patients with advanced oncologic disease is "now more compelling than ever, as the overall burden of suffering increases" (6). Cooperative research groups now have committees dedicated to advancing palliative and symptom control research agendas (7). Investigators have proposed more pragmatic trial designs that are less burdensome by keeping trial durations short, limiting the number of necessary encounters, and omitting overly strict exclusion criteria. Clearly at present there is enthusiasm for advancing palliative radiation therapy research.

THE MODULATING EFFECTS OF BONE AND BRAIN METASTASES ON MENTAL CAPACITY, AUTONOMY, AND SELF-DETERMINATION

Autonomy is a precondition for a patient's consent to participate in a clinical trial to be morally valid. Patients must understand information provided and be competent about possible courses of action (8). They must appreciate the nature of the trial procedures, the risks and potential benefits, and the alternatives (9). Emanuel states that the purpose of informed consent is "... to ensure that individuals control whether or not they enrol in clinical research and participate only when the research is consistent with their values, interests, and preferences" (10). In this setting autonomy affords patients the right to self-determination (11); the freedom to make decisions for themselves. However, if patients have diminished mental capacity, the assumption of autonomy can be violated, self-determination precluded, and the informed consent process invalidated.

The Canadian Institutes of Health Research (CIHR), the Natural Sciences and Engineering Research Council of Canada (NSERC) and the Social Sciences and Humanities Research Council of Canada (SSHRC) are Canada's three federal research agencies. Their *Tri-Council Policy Statement: Ethical Conduct for Research Involving Humans*, defines 'capacity' as "the ability of prospective or actual participants to understand relevant information presented about a research project, and to appreciate the potential consequences of their decision to participate or not participate" (12). The *Statement* further recognises that capacity is not a static determination; it may vary according to the choice being made, the circumstances surrounding the decision, and the point in time at which consent is sought. The National Commission for the Protection of Human Subjects of Biomedical and Behavioural Research also published their *Belmont Report: Ethical Principles and Guidelines for the Protection of Human Subjects of Research* which similarly recognises that some individuals may lose their capacity "wholly or in part because of illness" and that a "judgement that any individual lacks autonomy should be periodically re-evaluated...." It is implied in this statement that the loss of autonomy is due to a preceding loss of capacity (13).

These issues are important when patients with bone and brain metastases consider participating in clinical trials. Their cancers and the treatments they receive can easily modulate their mental capacity at the time of radiation therapy, as shown in the following examples:

Pain is the most common manifestation of bone metastases, and it distresses and interferes with concentration. Opioid-, corticosteroid-, anticonvulsant - and antidepressant medications given to relieve pain can themselves sedate, impair cognition and cause emotional labiality. This is especially true among the elderly and frail, the very populations most likely to be approached regarding palliative radiation therapy trials. Bone metastases also give rise to subclinical hypercalcemia that can cause transient bouts of confusion and delirium. During radiation therapy, depending on the targeted anatomic region patients may develop fatigue, nausea, vomiting, cramping, coughing, pain or other sequelae that can easily disrupt their delicate equilibriums and threaten competency.

Brain metastases can interfere with cognition and capacity by physically damaging specialised executive centres or by increasing global intracranial pressure which depresses central nervous system activity. The default reactive treatment in this setting is a corticosteroid, as without this type of medication it is uncommon for symptoms to resolve during radiation therapy. Unfortunately, corticosteroids themselves can adversely affect mood, personality, motivation and sleep. Patients can be impacted by these symptoms and have impaired mental capacity as a result for weeks or even months following treatment completion.

However, despite these well-known complications of bone and brain metastases it is easy for mental incapacity to go undetected during radiation therapy, during the enrolment process for clinical trials, and throughout the duration of the therapy and trial periods. This should concern clinician investigators because overlooking capacity among potential or established trial participants can have serious consequences.

Most palliative radiotherapy treatments aim to deliver the highest possible radiation dose to a tumor target while sparing the surrounding normal tissues. Recent advances in radiotherapy technologies have ushered in a host of new clinical trials where extremely high doses of radiation are being delivered to tumor targets intimately related to radio-sensitive vital structures such as the brain, brainstem, spinal cord and bowel. The risks that newer treatments pose to these structures are incompletely understood. Indeed the goals of many new trials are to establish safe and tolerable radiotherapy doses to deliver with these new technologies. Only patients capable of making informed decisions should be allowed to subject themselves to these risks, some of which can be life-threatening.

Given the emphasis placed on informed consent in North American bioethics, the betrayal of this process is likely the most serious consequence. Patients with bone and brain metastases are vulnerable, and when they lack the capacity for self-determination they can be subjected to unjustifiable risk on trial. Another consequence that should be obvious to the researcher is that impaired capacity can compromise a trial's findings and validity. Most palliative radiation therapy trials use patient-reported signs and symptoms as clinical endpoints, and impaired cognition can result in misleading patient reports that will bias results. Beyond the immediate methodological problems this can pose to a trial, there is also a risk to future patients as their care takers may look to the results of such compromised trials to guide their practice patterns.

FACTORS CONTRIBUTING TO INADEQUATE ASSESSMENT OF MENTAL CAPACITY

How is mental capacity overlooked among patients who are clearly at risk of losing it? A few specific factors may contribute to the problem. The first is an inconsistent approach to the informed consent process in Canadian radiation therapy centres. Even for patients receiving treatment off-study, many do so without any formal consent process; a surprising fact given the potential toxicities associated with radiation therapy. In a provocative article, Freeman et al. from the Department of Radiation Oncology at McGill University in Montreal surveyed the heads of all 38 radiation oncology departments in Canada in April 2008 (14). The heads were asked if their departments used a written consent form for external beam radiotherapy, and to send a copy if they did. Twenty-nine departments responded (76%). Twelve of 29 used no consent forms. Nine used only a generic hospital or centre form that contained no information specific to radiation. Five used a form specific to radiotherapy in general that mentioned the need for multiple visits, the need for photographs in the treatment position, the use of tattoos to aide with treatment set-up and other general radiotherapy factors. Only 2 departments used forms with information specific to the type of cancer being irradiated. By comparison all research studies now obviously employ consent forms, but some of the underlying issues from this paper inform our discussion about informed consent in research as well. Freeman suggested that for centres without any informed consent process, consent is understood to take place in the context of the consultation, when discussion revolves around the risks and proposed benefits of treatment. This discussion is then summarised in a dictated note by the attending radiation oncologist. However, these notes are not typically seen by patients, they do not necessarily summarise the entirety of the discussion, and they do not answer the question of whether or not the patients understood what was discussed. The assumption that appropriate informed consent takes place in such an unstructured manner is a pervasive underlying threat to the autonomy of patients enrolling to palliative radiation therapy trials.

The second factor is the lack mental capacity assessments within entry procedures for many oncology trials. For example, the last two completed palliative radiation therapy trials for bone metastases from the National Cancer Institute of Canada Clinical Trials Group (NCIC CTG SC20 and SC23 did not incorporate assessments of mental capacity in their entry procedures (15). It is likely assumed that assessments are done informally by trial staff at the time of informed consent.

The most common metric for assessing overall fitness for trial (including mental capacity) is performance status. Various scales purport to measure this index of general functionality. Depending on the threshold eligibility value chosen, as long as a patient is not in bed more than 50% of the time (16) or can care for most of their personal needs (with assistance) (17), they may be deemed 'fit' and eligible. These scales only indirectly measure mental capacity, they are completed by care providers and not patients themselves, and they are notorious for their lack of inter-rater reliability. These deficiencies stand in the face of a growing consensus that standards for assessing capacity are necessary in research studies. Such standards guide the American Psychiatric Association (APA)'s recommended process for reviewing and assessing potential trial participants (18). If the APA recognises the potential harms of reduced capacity among its vulnerable patients, should not the oncology research community with its similarly vulnerable patients?

The third factor is that many outcomes in palliative radiation therapy trials are measured during the acute or 'on therapy' period. Logistically this usually occurs during standard once-weekly patient review appointments. These assessments typically last only a few minutes and focus on specific symptoms related to the anatomic regions being irradiated. They can be carried out by nurses, trainees, therapists or radiation oncologists. Patients will sometimes be assessed by a different team member at each appointment. Subtle changes in mental status over time can go undetected in the absence of a dedicated longitudinal care provider, or protocol-specified on-trial assessments by study staff. The problem is worsened when one considers that due to lapses in patient education, many of them feel compelled to minimise and under-report their symptoms for fear that treatment will be discontinued and their metastases will go untreated.

A final factor results from the unfortunate reality that despite improvements in recent years, palliative radiation therapy can still be difficult and costly for many Canadian patients to access (19). Once they do they are usually motivated to proceed as recommended, especially those who are acutely symptomatic. Second opinions are rarely sought. Patients feel grateful to their physicians and treating institutions and can feel as though they should reciprocate the 'favour' by enrolling in trials. Indeed, a forthcoming senior clinical researcher interviewed by President Clinton's Advisory Committee on Human Radiation Experiments (20) admitted that: "Most patients, we were told, readily agree to almost anything presented by their physicians. The nicer the patient, the poorer the prognosis, the more dependent and eager to please the patient generally becomes." The *Tri-Council Statement* also characterises these situations as potential threats to autonomy, because patients have fears of alienating "those in positions of authority, such as professional or personal caregivers, researchers, leaders, larger groups, or a community to which one belongs" (12). Therapeutic misconception can also easily occur; the risk only increases when clinician investigators are also primary care givers. The *Tri-Council Statement* states that clinicians in this situation may "...be overly optimistic about the prospects of an experimental intervention and overstate potential benefits or understate foreseeable risks to prospective participants" (12).

These problems are worsened by other dynamics that play out in clinic. Patients can defer decision making to their family and take a passive role in decision making. This often happens when the prognosis is dire (9, 21) and radiation oncologists must adapt to and accommodate their preferences. Although the goal of palliative therapy is to decrease symptoms, radiation usually induces an acute transient phase of side effects. Some radiation oncologists advocate not troubling patients with this information as it will lead to unnecessary anxiety. They contend that independent of acute side effects, anxiety levels can increase in the first stages of treatment due solely to extensive pre-treatment discussions and deliberations regarding the risks of treatment. They argue that it is unethical to raise these concerns as dose prescriptions are typically designed to subject patients to a 5% maximum theoretical risk of serious toxicity. In fact for many common palliative treatments the true incidence of acute side effects is unclear. Others go further and argue that for patients who are ill and require palliative therapy, autonomy can be a burden and cause of 'overstrain' (22). With these considerations in mind, one can understand how a well-meaning radiation oncologist might selectively filter information and how full disclosure of potential side effects might not occur. This 'protective' approach could by extension be taken when carrying out the informed consent conversation for a clinical trial. Although ethics review boards can modify the composition of research protocols and consent forms, they cannot monitor the physical encounters between patients and clinician investigators when the informed consent process plays out. It is here where a patient's autonomy can be easily compromised.

COUNTERARGUMENTS

One could argue that assessing mental capacity is unnecessary, as there is no ethical quandary with enrolling compromised patients. The *Tri-Council Statement* actually states that "While autonomy may be considered a necessary condition for participation in research, involving those who *lack* capacity to make their own decisions to participate can be valuable, just and even necessary" (12). However, due to the significant number of suitable potential participants for palliative radiation therapy trials, there should not be a need to exercise this kind of strategy. The strategy also does not in and of itself address the fact that radiation can cause serious and irreversible complications that are unjustifiable for unknowing patients.

Proxy decision making could be another 'way around the problem' of patients with reduced capacity, but currently there is great controversy regarding the discretion that proxies should exercise over these patients due to uncertainties associated with trial risks and potential benefits. The National Bioethics Advisory Commission has urged that proxies exercise "great caution" in making judgments about a patient's best interests regarding research (23). Similarly the *Tri-Council Statement* sets out a number of conditions that need to be met for authorised third parties to give consent on behalf of patients without the capacity for self-determination (12). For this type of consent to be admissible for a palliative radiation therapy trial, the trial therapy would presumably need to be the only means to reverse the process that has led to the loss of capacity in the first place. In practice this is exceedingly unlikely to ever be the case.

Another admissible scenario could be that overwhelming symptoms could only be effectively treated on trial. Again this is unlikely as new radiation treatments under investigation would have less evidence supporting their ability to do so compared with established standard techniques.

What Needs to Be Done

Formal assessments of mental capacity must be built into entry requirements for clinical trials in palliative radiation therapy. A number of short assessment tools have been investigated for patients with metastatic disease such as the Mini Mental State Examination and the Montréal Cognitive Assessment, but their ability to detect mild yet clinically important changes in cognition has been questioned, and their validity among different groups of patients with metastatic disease requires further investigation (24). Mental capacity must be assessed at numerous times as trials proceed. Weekly review appointments need to be lengthened to accommodate this. Just as informed consent should be an ongoing and revisited process, so too should assessments of capacity. Advance research directives should also be made as specific as possible in the case of patients enrolling to trials who are deemed at risk for losing capacity later on. However, it is important to note that an advance directive is not consent, but rather guidance to the proxy regarding what to consent to if capacity is later lost. Finally, trial stopping rules should also incorporate changes in mental capacity along with the typical lists of other standardised adverse events.

Conclusion

Patients with bone and brain metastases have specific threats to their mental capacity resulting from their cancers and the treatments they receive. Palliative radiation therapy trials have inherent risks that should only be accepted by those with the capacity for self-determination throughout the entire trial period. Unfortunately changes in mental capacity can easily go undetected for these patients. We have explored the methodological and ethical consequences of this problem and the systemic patient-, physician-, treatment- and environmental factors that may explain why it occurs. Changes should be made to the designs of palliative radiation therapy trials, and to the culture of informed consent within Canadian radiation oncology departments. If they are not, vulnerable patients may be unjustifiably subjected to the risks of clinical trials.

References

[1] Canadian Cancer Society's Advisory Committee on Cancer Statistics. Canadian Cancer Statistics 2015. Toronto, ON: Canadian Cancer Society, 2015.

[2] Halperin EC, Perez CA, Brady LW. Preface. In: Halperin EC, Perez CA, Brady LW, eds. Principles and practice of radiation oncology, 5th ed. Philadelphia PA: Lippincott Williams Wilkins, 2008:xix.

[3] National Cancer Insitute. Radiation Therapy for Cancer. URL: http://www.cancer.gov/cancertopics/factsheet/Therapy/radiation.

[4] Canadian Association of Radiation Oncology. Accessed Jul 6th 2015. URL: http://www.caro-acro.ca/Links/Canadian_Radiation_Oncology_Centres.htm.

[5] Aapro MS, Kohne CH, Cohen HJ, Extermann M. Never too old? Age should not be a barrier to enrollment in cancer clinical trials. Oncologist 2005;10(3):198-204.

[6] Ferris FD, Bruera E, Cherny N, Cummings C, Currow D, Dudgeon D, et al. Palliative cancer care a decade later: Accomplishments, the need, next steps -- from the American Society of Clinical Oncology. J Clin Oncol 2009;27(18):3052-8.

[7] Profile of the Canadian Palliative Radiation Oncology Group (CPROG). Multinational Association of Supportive Care in Cancer NEWS. URL: http://www.mascc.org/assets/documents/Newsletters/masccnews_dec2014.pdf.

[8] Brown RF, Butow PN, Butt DG, Moore AR, Tattersall MHN. Developing ethical strategies to assist oncologists in seeking informed consent to cancer clinical trials. Soc Sci Med 2004;58(2):379-90.

[9] Schafer C, Herbst M. Ethical aspects of patient information in radiation oncology. An introduction and a review of the literature. Strahlenther Onkol 2003;179(7):431-40.

[10] Emanuel EJ, Wendler D, Grady C. What makes clinical research ethical? JAMA 2000;283(20):2701-11.

[11] Appelbaum PS, Grisso T. Assessing patients' capacities to consent to treatment. N Engl J Med 1988;319(25):1635-8.

[12] Canadian Institutes of Health Research Natural Sciences and Engineering Research Council of Canada, and Social Sciences and Humanities Research Council of Canada. Tri Council Policy Statement: Ethical Conduct for Research Involving Humans. Ottawa: Interagency Secretariat on Research Ethics, 2010.

[13] The National Commission for the Protection of Human Subjects of Biomedical and Behavioural Research. Belmont Report - Ethical Principles and Guidelines for the Protection of Human Subjects of Research. Washington, DC: Superintendent Government Documents, 1979.

[14] Freeman C, Lamed H, Gingras C, Shenouda G. Consent to external-beam radiotherapy. Curr Oncol 2010;17(6):9-11.

[15] National Cancer Institute of Canada Clinical Trials Group. URL: http://www.ctg.queensu.ca/.

[16] Oken MM, Creech RH, Tormey DC, Horton J, Davis TE, McFadden ET, et al. Toxicity and response criteria of the Eastern Cooperative Oncology Group. Am J Clin Oncol 1982;5(6):649-55.

[17] Karnofsky DA, Burchenal JH. The clinical evaluation of chemotherapeutic agents in cancer. In: MacLeod CM, ed. Evaluation of chemotherapeutic agents. New York: Columbia University Press, 1949:196.

[18] Guidelines for assessing the decision-making capacities of potential research subjects with cognitive impairment. American Psychiatric Association. Am J Psychiatry 1998;155(11):1649-50.

[19] Sutton DS, Kong W, Ding K, Mackillop WJ. The use of palliative radiotherapy for bone metastasis. Radiother Oncol 2010;97(3):548-53.

[20] United States Advisory Committee on Human Radiation Experiments. Final report of the Advisory Committee on Human Radiation Experiments. New York: Oxford University Press, 1996.

[21] Mackillop WJ. The principles of palliative radiotherapy: a radiation oncologist's perspective. Can J Oncol 1996;6(1 Suppl):5-11.

[22] Gattellari M, Voigt KJ, Butow PN, et al. When the treatment goal is not cure: Are cancer patients equipped to make informed decisions? J Clin Oncol 2002;20(2):503-13.

[23] Saks ER. Competency to decide on treatment and research: The MacArthur Capacity Instruments. Rockville, MD: National Bioethics Advisory Commission, 1998.

[24] Olson R, Tyldesley S, Carolan H, Parkinson M, Chhanabhai T, McKenzie M. Prospective comparison of the prognostic utility of the Mini Mental State Examination and the Montreal Cognitive Assessment in patients with brain metastases. Support Care Cancer 2011;19(11):1849-55.

Submitted: June 2, 2015. *Revised:* July 5, 2015. *Accepted:* July 11, 2015.

In: Pain Management Yearbook 2015
Editor: Joav Merrick

ISBN: 978-1-63484-515-1

Chapter 23

REVIEW OF THE MANAGEMENT OF MUCOSITIS IN THE RADIATION TREATMENT OF HEAD AND NECK CANCER

Tony Yiu Sang Yuen**, MBChB, FRCR,
Kam Hung Wong, MBChB, FRCR, FHKCR, FHKAM
and Roger Kai Cheong Ngan, MBBS, FRCR, FHKCR, FHKAM
Department of Clinical Oncology, Queen Elizabeth Hospital,
Hong Kong, China

Mucositis secondary to radiation in head and neck cancer is common. It has a negative impact on patient's quality of life as well as various disease outcomes. A basic understanding of mechanism of its development and its proper assessment is essential in order to provide timely management.

Keywords: mucositis, head and neck, cancer, radiotherapy, oncology

INTRODUCTION

Mucositis is defined as inflammatory and/or ulcerative lesions of the oral and/or gastrointestinal tract. Onset of oral mucositis usually occurs approximately two weeks after the initiation of radiotherapy. Clinical features include erythema, edema, tenderness, pain, difficulty in swallowing and hoarseness. Symptoms generally peak at about weeks 5 to 6 and typically resolve during weeks 8 to 12 of follow-up (1).

Oral mucositis has significant consequences. Apart from reducing quality of life and patient's compliance to treatment, odynophagia limits appetite and causes weight loss. Mucositis impairs swallowing function and increases risk of aspiration pneumonia. Weakened mucosal barrier also serves as a portal for invasive infection. In terms of radiotherapy

* Correspondence: Tony Yiu Sang Yuen, MBChB, FRCR, Queen Elizabeth Hospital, Hong Kong, China, Email: yuentys@yahoo.com.hk.

treatment, shrinkage of subcutaneous fat from anorexia undermines immobilization, so greater error from patient setup can lead to suboptimal dose delivery to target volumes while put sensitive structures at risk of overdose. In severe cases, radiotherapy has to be suspended, and treatment interruption is known to jeopardize disease control rate.

INCIDENCE

Radiotherapy frequently causes mucositis. Incidence over 90% has been reported on patients receiving radiotherapy for head and neck cancer (2). Severe mouth or throat pain has also been reported in 76% of subjects (3). Use of concurrent chemotherapy is a well-known risk factor. Ulcerative mucositis can develop in 61% of patients treated with chemoradiation for head and neck cancer (4).

BURDEN

On top of the cancer itself, treatment complications like mucositis also burden the healthcare system. The incremental costs of mild to moderate mucositis were noted to be around US$2,000, and rose to around US$4,000 when severe grades were considered (5, 6). For head and neck cancer specifically, the reported costs were even more dramatic (around US$20,000). One study showed that, 30% of the subjects were hospitalized directly as a consequence of mucositis, 51% received feeding tubes and 78% received opioid prescriptions for mouth and throat pain (3). Another study found that 40% of those with mucositis visited emergency department while only <6% of those without did (2). Mucositis patients spent US$100 more on medications than the unaffected (4).

PATHOPHYSIOLOGY

A detailed description of mucositis mechanism is beyond the scope of this book. The 5-phase model developed by Sonis is illustrated here (7, 8):

- Initiation: generation of reactive oxygen species by radiation.
- Up-regulation with generation of messengers: cellular injury leads to activation of nuclear factor-κB (NK-κB) as well as other enzymatic pathways, which in turn promote the release of pro-inflammatory cytokines like TNF-α, IL-1β, and IL-6. NK-κB has also been shown to up-regulate cyclooxygenase-2 (COX-2), which enhances the release prostaglandin (9).
- Signaling and amplification: pro-inflammatory cytokines provide positive feedback signals to augment aforementioned pathways, promoting their further production.
- Ulceration with inflammation: bacterial colonization and their cell wall products exacerbate the release of pro-inflammatory cytokines.
- Healing: renewal of epithelial proliferation and differentiation, and reestablishment of the local microbial flora.

Assessment

A number of assessment tools are available to gauge mucositis in clinical as well as research settings. One example is National Cancer Institute – Common Terminology Criteria for Adverse Events (CTCAE) version 4 (2009):

Adverse Event	Grade				
	1	2	3	4	5
Oral mucositis	Asymptomatic or mild symptoms; intervention not indicated	Moderate pain; not interfering with oral intake; modified diet indicated	Severe pain; interfering with oral intake	Life-threatening consequences; urgent intervention indicated	Death
Dysphagia	Symptomatic, able to eat regular diet	Symptomatic and altered eating/swallowing	Severely altered eating/swallowing; tube feeding or TPN or hospitalization indicated	Life-threatening consequences; urgent intervention indicated	Death

Regardless of the tools used, training and standardization are vital to improve accuracy and consistency of assessment. The importance of adequate illumination during examination cannot be over-emphasized.

Management

Multinational Association of Supportive Care in Cancer and International Society of Oral Oncology (MASCC/ISOO) provide updated joint guidelines for the management of mucositis secondary to cancer therapy. "Recommendation" was reserved for guidelines based on level I or II evidence, "suggestion" was used for guidelines based on level III, IV and V evidence. The latest version was published in 2014 (10), and a brief summary focusing on oral mucositis secondary to head and neck radiation is summarized below:

Recommendation in favor of an intervention

1. Recommend benzydamine mouthwash for *prevention* for moderate-dose radiotherapy (up to 50 Gy) in patients not receiving concomitant chemotherapy

Suggestion in favor of an intervention

1. Suggest oral care protocol (tooth-brushing, dental flossing, mouth rinse) to maintain oral hygiene for *prevention*
2. Suggest low-level laser therapy (wavelength around 632.8 nm) for *prevention* (without concomitant chemotherapy)
3. Suggest zinc supplement for *prevention* in patients with *oral cancer* undergoing (chemo-)radiation

4. Suggest 2% morphine mouthwash may be effective to *treat pain* due to oral mucositis from chemoradiation
5. Suggest 0.5% doxepin (tricyclic antidepressant) mouthwash may be effective to *treat pain* due to oral mucositis

Recommendation against an intervention

1. Recommend against polymyxin, tobramycin and amphotericin B (PTA)/ Bacitracin, clotrimazole and gentamicin (BCoG) lozenges, and PTA paste for *prevention*
2. Recommend against iseganan (broad-spectrum antimicrobial) mouthwash for *prevention*
3. Recommend against sucralfate mouthwash for *prevention* or *treatment*

Suggestion against an intervention

1. Suggest against chlorhexidine mouthwash for *prevention*
2. Suggest against misoprostol mouthwash for *prevention*
3. Suggest against systemic (oral) pilocarpine for *prevention*

Despite the fact that normal saline and bicarbonate mouthwashes are widely used to promote oral hygiene and patient comfort, there is insufficient or conflicting evidence supporting their use for prevention or treatment of oral mucositis. Chlorhexidine mouthwash, though being suggested against for prevention, may still be indicated in treatment of gingivitis and in patients with limited access for plaque control.

No guideline is possible on amifostine (an organic thiophosphate thought be a free radical scavenger), aspirin, corticosteroid or diphenhydramine mouthwash and oral indomethacin for the prevention of oral mucositis due to insufficient or conflicting evidence.

Analgesics play a central role in treatment of mucositis. Apart from oral analgesics, 2% morphine or 0.5% doxepin mouthwash can be prescribed, after proper patient education. Effort should be made to prevent patients from mixing up morphine of two different concentrations (e.g., 2% for mouthwash and 0.2% for oral use) and from swallowing doxepin, which can potentiate drowsiness if analgesic with sedative effect is concurrently prescribed.

Nutritional status should be evaluated at baseline, during and after radiotherapy. Dietitian input is crucial to prevent weight loss and malnutrition. Swallowing function needs to be monitored. In case of poor oral intake or choking, tube feeding should actively be considered.

CONCLUSION

A number of agents have been used for the prevention of oral mucositis during head and neck radiotherapy. Nevertheless, many of them are not supported by robust evidence. Simple mouthwashes (normal saline and sodium bicarbonate), albeit not evidence-based, can still be advised to patients as they are harmless and help to promote oral hygiene and patient comfort. Oral care protocol is suggested for mucositis prevention. Mouthwash or lozenge with antimicrobial component should be reserved for treatment of mucositis in appropriate setting.

Management of patients undergoing head and neck radiotherapy requires a multidisciplinary approach, involving radiation oncologist, dosimetrist, nurse, dietitian and speech therapist. Patients should be closely reviewed and severity of mucositis be clearly documented. Infection intensifies mucositis and can result in invasive complications, and should therefore be treated with appropriate antibiotics and antifungal agents. Pain needs to be assessed and addressed with adequate analgesics.

REFERENCES

[1] Blanco AI, Chao C. Management of radiation-induced head and neck injury. In: Small W, Woloschak GE, eds. Radiation toxicity: A practical guide. New York: Springer, 2006:23-42.

[2] Elting LS, Cooksley CD, Chambers MS, Garden AS. Risk, outcomes, and costs of radiation-induced oral mucositis among patients with head-and-neck malignancies. Int J Radiat Oncol Biol Phys 2007;68(4):1110–20.

[3] Murphy BA, Beaumont JL, Isitt J, Garden AS, Gwede CK, Trotti AM, et al. Mucositis-related morbidity and resource utilization in head and neck cancer patients receiving radiation therapy with or without chemotherapy. J Pain Symptom Manage 2009;38(4):522–32.

[4] Nonzee NJ, Dandade NA, Patel U, Markossian T, Agulnik M, Argiris A, et al. Evaluating the supportive care costs of severe radiochemotherapy-induced mucositis and pharyngitis. Cancer 2008;113(6):1446–52.

[5] Elting LS, Cooksley C, Chambers M, Cantor SB, Manzullo E, Rubenstein EB. The burdens of cancer therapy: clinical and economic outcomes of chemotherapy induced mucositis. Cancer 2003;98(7):1531–9.

[6] Elting L, Shih Y. The economic burden of supportive care of cancer patients. Support Care Cancer 2004;12(4):219–26.

[7] Sonis ST, Elting LS, Keefe D, Peterson DE, Schubert M, Hauer-Jensen M, et al. Perspectives on cancer therapy-induced mucosal injury. Pathogenesis, measurement, epidemiology, and consequences for patients. Cancer 2004;100:1995-2025.

[8] Al-Dasooqi N, Sonis ST, Bowen JM, Bateman E, Blijlevens N, Gibson RJ, et al. Emerging evidence on the pathobiology of mucositis. Support Care Cancer 2013;21:3233-41.

[9] Sonis ST, O'Donnell KE, Popat R, Bragdon C, Phelan S, Cocks D, et al. The relationship between mucosal cyclooxygenase-2 (COX-2) expression and experimental radiation-induced mucositis. Oral Oncol 2004;40:170-6.

[10] Lalla RV, Bowen J, Barasch A, Elting L, Epstein J, Keefe DM. et al., and The Mucositis Guidelines Leadership Group of the Multinational Association of Supportive Care in Cancer and International Society of Oral Oncology (MASCC/ISOO). MASCC/ISOO clinical practice guidelines for the management of mucositis secondary to cancer therapy. Cancer 2014;120:1453–61.

Submitted: June 2, 2015. *Revised:* July 5, 2015. *Accepted:* July 11, 2015.

In: Pain Management Yearbook 2015
Editor: Joav Merrick

ISBN: 978-1-63484-515-1

Chapter 24

TARGETED THERAPIES AND RADIOTHERAPY IN TREATMENT OF BRAIN METASTASES

Derek S Tsang, MD and May N Tsao*, MD
Department of Radiation Oncology, Odette Cancer Centre,
Sunnybrook Health Sciences Centre,
University of Toronto, Toronto, Ontario, Canada

Brain metastases are commonly found in patients with advanced cancer. The incidence of brain metastasis is highest from lung, melanoma, renal, and breast carcinomas. Although primary treatment for brain metastases is surgery and radiation therapy, many targeted therapies (including tyrosine kinase inhibitors and monoclonal antibodies) that are effective in controlling systemic disease are also effective in controlling brain metastases. These agents can be used alone, sequentially with radiation, or concurrently with radiation. In this chapter, efficacy of targeted therapies for brain metastases and potential associated toxicities with sequential or concurrent radiotherapy are discussed.

Keywords: brain metastases, tyrosine kinase inhibitors, immunotherapy, radiation therapy, radiotherapy

INTRODUCTION

Brain metastases are the most common intracranial tumour in adults (1, 2). Carcinomas and melanomas are the most common neoplasms causing brain metastases; among carcinomas, lung, kidney, and breast have the highest propensity to metastasize to brain parenchyma (2, 3). In a population-based study from Detroit (3), the incidence of brain metastasis was 9.6% for all primary cancers, and was highest for lung (19.9%), melanoma (6.9%), renal (6.5%), and breast (5.1%). Thus, many efforts to find targeted therapies against brain metastases have focused on these histologies.

* Correspondence: Dr. May Tsao, Odette Cancer Centre, Sunnybrook Health Sciences Centre, 2075 Bayview Ave, Toronto ON M4N 3M5, Canada. E-mail: may.tsao@sunnybrook.ca.

The mainstay of treatment for brain metastases is surgery and radiation therapy (radiotherapy) (1). Treatment with chemotherapy for brain metastases has not traditionally been emphasized due to the reduced blood-brain barrier penetration of many cytotoxic agents (4). Recently, newer drugs have been adopted into clinical use that may have better blood-brain barrier penetration (1). Availability of these agents has renewed interest in their use for treatment of brain metastases. Targeted therapies can be classified into several categories; examples are listed in Table 1.

Targeted therapies have particular importance for the top histologies causing brain metastases. For metastatic non-small cell lung cancer (NSCLC), tumours harbouring an epidermal growth factor receptor (EGFR) mutation or anaplastic lymphoma kinase (ALK) fusion oncogene may respond to tyrosine kinase inhibitors (TKIs) (5, 6). Metastatic melanoma treatment is tailored to specific tumour mutations; patients with a BRAF mutation may receive vemurafenib, a BRAF inhibitor; those without a BRAF mutation may receive immune therapies (7). Renal cell carcinomas (RCC) typically harbour mutations that inactivate the Von Hippel-Lindau gene (*VHL*), leading to upregulation of hypoxia-inducible factor (HIF) and stimulation of vascular endothelial growth factor (VEGF). TKIs that target the VEGF receptor are effective in treatment of patients with metastatic RCC (8). Finally, many breast cancers overexpress human epidermal growth factor receptor 2 (HER2), which may be targeted by monoclonal antibodies or TKIs (9).

Table 1. Categories of targeted therapies

Category	Sub-category	Suffix	Examples	Histology
Tyrosine kinase inhibitors		-nib		
	ALK inhibitor		crizotinib	Lung
	B-Raf inhibitor		dabrafenib, vemurafenib	Melanoma
	EGFR inhibitor		erlotinib, gefitinib	Lung
	HER2 inhibitor		lapatinib	Breast
	VEGFR inhibitor		sorafenib, sunitinib	Renal
Monoclonal antibodies		-mab		
	CTLA-4 inhibitor		ipilimumab	Melanoma
	HER2 inhibitor		trastuzumab, trastuzumab emtansine	Breast
	PD-1 inhibitor		nivolumab	Melanoma

ALK = anaplastic lymphoma kinase; CTLA-4 = cytotoxic T-lymphocyte-associated protein 4; EGFR = epidermal growth factor receptor; HER2 = human epidermal growth factor receptor 2; PD-1 = programmed cell death 1; VEGFR = vascular endothelial growth factor receptor.

This review will discuss the role of targeted therapies for each of these histologies in turn, with a focus on combining targeted therapies with radiation therapy for brain metastases. It should be noted that use of targeted agents for brain metastases remains experimental, and patients should be offered enrollment in clinical trials when possible.

LUNG (NON-SMALL CELL LUNG CANCER)

Therapies targeted against EGFR

The two best-studied agents for brain metastases in NSCLC carrying an EGFR mutation are erlotinib and gefitinib. Erlotinib is particularly promising, due to its increased blood-brain barrier penetration (1). In this section, representative studies of targeted therapies in the context of radiotherapy will be discussed.

Porta et al. (10) retrospectively studied the outcomes of patients with brain metastases from NSCLC treated with erlotinib. In their study, just over half of patients had received whole brain radiotherapy (WBRT) and erlotinib sequentially. 8 of 9 patients had an intracranial response to treatment with erlotinib and WBRT, while 6 of 8 patients had intracranial response to erlotinb alone. The median time between WBRT and erlotinib was 42 days. Although limited by a small sample size, this study demonstrated two things: first, brain metastases can respond to erlotinib; second, treatment toxicity with sequential radiation followed by erlotinib was manageable.

Wu et al. (11) performed a prospective phase II single-arm study using erlotinib as second-line treatment for asymptomatic brain metastases after first-line platinum doublet cytotoxic therapy. 48 patients with stable extracranial disease were included (regardless of EGFR mutation status); individuals with tumour EGFR mutations had longer median progression-free survival than those with wild-type EGFR (15.2 months vs 4.4 months, $p = 0.02$). WBRT was given to 35% of patients for progression while on-study.

In an attempt to improve outcomes, concurrent WBRT and erlotinib has been studied. Concurrent therapy permits ongoing systemic disease control while potentially improving intracranial disease response, at a risk of increased neurotoxicity (12). Hendriks et al. published a systematic review of concurrent brain radiotherapy with TKIs (12); two important studies in this area are discussed here (12).

Welsh et al. (13) performed a prospective, two-institution, phase II, single-arm study using erlotinib concurrent with WBRT followed by maintenance erlotinib. The initial protocol-specified WBRT dose was initially 30 Gy in 10 fractions; however, after ten patients were enrolled, the WBRT schedule was changed to 35 Gy in 14 fractions to reduce the dose-per-fraction in an attempt to ameliorate the risk of neurotoxicity. Any EGFR status was permitted. 40 patients were enrolled, but only 17 had known EGFR status. Overall response rate was 86%. Survival results broken down by EGFR status are challenging to interpret due to a small sample size; overall survival was 9.3 months for EGFR wild-type and 19.1 months for patients with EGFR mutations ($p = 0.534$). Toxicities were manageable; acneiform rash was the most common. Two patients had possible neurotoxicity related to treatment, with one case of dementia and one case of radiation necrosis after subsequent SRS for progression.

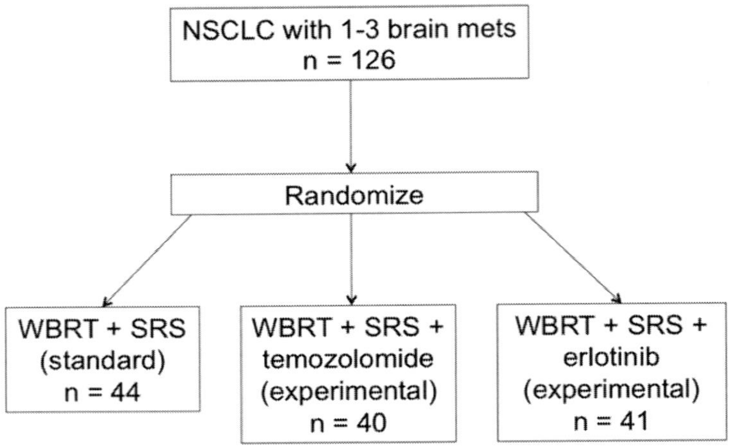

Figure 1. Schema for RTOG 0320 (14); target study accrual was 381. One patient was not randomized (not eligible) (NSCLC = non-small cell lung cancer; SRS = stereotactic radiosurgery; WBRT = whole brain radiotherapy).

The above phase II study paved the way for a multi-institutional phase III randomized controlled trial by the Radiation Therapy Oncology Group (RTOG 0320) (14). The treatment arms were designed based on the known blood-brain barrier penetration of temozolomide (TMZ), an oral alkylating agent, and erlotinib. Furthermore, the radiation treatment in RTOG 0320 was selected based on the results of RTOG 9508, demonstrating a survival benefit for the addition of SRS to WBRT for a subgroup of patients with NSCLC and 1-3 brain metastases (15, 16). As such, RTOG 0320 randomized 126 NSCLC patients with 1-3 brain metastases to three treatment arms (Figure 1).

Any EGFR status was permitted. Unfortunately, the study was stopped after enrollment of 126 patients due to poor accrual; the target sample size was 381. Again, a small sample size made interpretation challenging; patients receiving standard therapy (WBRT + SRS alone) had a median survival of 13.4 months; patients who also received TMZ had a median survival of 6.3 months ($p = 0.93$) and those who received erlotinib had a median survival of 6.1 months ($p = 0.95$). There was a statistically significant increase in proportion of patients experiencing deterioration in performance status among those receiving experimental therapy (TMZ or erlotinib, 85.7% vs standard therapy, 52.5%). 11% of those receiving standard therapy had grade 3 toxicity and none had grade 4 or 5 (no deaths), whereas 33% in the temozolomide arm had grade 3 toxicity and 8% had grade 4-5 toxicity (1 death). 42% in the erlotinib arm experienced grade 3 toxicity and 7% had grade 4-5 toxicity (1 death). Limitations of this study included incomplete accrual and lack of enrichment of the patient population for EGFR mutation, which could have improved the therapeutic ratio.

These studies in NSCLC demonstrate that brain metastases can respond to erlotinib alone. Treatment toxicity with sequential radiation and erlotinib appears to be manageable. Treatment toxicity with concurrent radiation and erlotinib or temozolomide is increased, without an apparent clinical benefit; concurrent therapy may be detrimental to survival. Further studies of brain metastases in NSCLC should take into account EGFR mutation status, as individuals with an EGFR mutation appear to have better response to targeted therapies such as erlotinib.

Targeted therapies against ALK

Between 2-7% of NSCLC patients with wild-type EGFR carry a different genetic alteration involving inversion on chromosome arm 2p, resulting in formation of a fusion oncogene *EML4-ALK* (5, 6). Crizotinib is an ALK inhibitor that targets such tumours. Studies of crizotinib in brain metastases are limited. A sub-group analysis of patients with ALK-rearrangement positive patients and asymptomatic brain metastases within two large randomized trials identified 275 patients (17). 60.3% of these patients had received prior WBRT and/or SRS. Among those who had prior received brain radiotherapy, the 12-week intracranial disease control rate was 62% and median time to intracranial progression was 13.2 months. For those who had not received brain radiation, intracranial disease control at 12 weeks was 56% with median time to intracranial progression at 7 months. This study demonstrated that crizotinib provides transient control of asymptomatic brain metastases, but acquired resistance to ALK inhibition may result in disease progression. As such, radiotherapy continues to play an important role in control of brain metastases in this population. No studies are available about concurrent ALK inhibitors and radiotherapy (12) except for a case report (18).

MELANOMA

Treatment for brain metastases caused by melanoma is tailored to the patient's clinical condition and number of metastatic deposits. Surgery and post-operative radiation play an important role in control of solitary or large lesions. In particular, melanoma metastases may be prone to hemorrhage, requiring upfront craniotomy and resection (19). Multiple lesions may be successfully treated with WBRT and/or SRS (20), though melanoma is believed to be somewhat more radioresistant than other histologies, such as carcinomas (21). On the other hand, targeted therapies and immune therapies have changed treatment for extracranial metastatic melanoma and have been shown to improve overall survival over cytotoxic chemotherapy (7). Furthermore, many case reports have emerged demonstrating an abscopal effect after radiotherapy (22, 23). This section will discuss examples of use of both targeted and immune therapies in brain metastases from melanoma.

Targeted therapies against melanoma

Dabrafenib is an inhibitor of BRAF kinase that targets a constitutively activated signalling pathway in BRAF-mutated melanoma (7). This agent has been found to have activity against brain metastases in a multi-institution, phase II non-randomized trial by Long et al. (24). In this study, patients were divided into two groups: no prior intracranial local treatment (cohort A), or progressive brain metastases after local treatment (cohort B). Eligibility was restricted to patients with V600E or V600K mutations. Cohort A had a 39.2% intracranial response rate, whereas cohort B had a 30.8% intracranial response rate. 22% developed grade 3 or worse toxicity. This study demonstrated modest activity of dabrafenib in BRAF-mutated melanoma brain metastases, even for patients who received prior intracranial local therapy.

Vemurafenib, another BRAF kinase inhibitor, has been studied in a two-institution, prospective, non-randomized trial by Dummer et al. (25). In their study of 24 patients, more than half of all patients had received prior intracranial local therapy (WBRT, SRS, and/or surgery). At study enrollment, 19 of 24 patients had measurable brain metastases. 37% achieved intracranial disease response. 17% experienced grade 3 toxicity. Results were corroborated in a retrospective study by Harding et al., which included patients with BRAF-mutant melanoma and brain metastases treated with vemurafenib (26). 44% had prior intracranial local therapy. A 50% response rate was observed intracranially in 22 patients assessable for response; among the 10 patients with prior WBRT, 3 experienced radiation dermatitis or a radiation recall reaction.

Data from the above studies are consistent and indicate that sequential treatment with brain radiotherapy and a BRAF inhibitor appears to be tolerable, though radiation recall reactions may occur. Prior intracranial local therapy may reduce response to a BRAF inhibitor. Outcomes are summarized in Table 2.

Table 2. Studies of BRAF inhibitors for brain metastases in melanoma

Study	n	BRAF inhibitor	Prior intracranial local therapy*	Intracranial response	Any grade 3 toxicity
Dummer et al. (25)	24	vemurafenib	>79%	37%	17%
Harding et al. (26)	22	vemurafenib	44%	50%	>22%
Long et al. (24)	172	dabrafenib	0% (Cohort A) 100% (Cohort B)	39.2% (Cohort A) 30.8% (Cohort B)	22% (similar between both groups)

* Includes whole brain radiotherapy, stereotactic radiosurgery, and/or surgery.

Concurrent therapy with vemurafenib or dabrafenib should be approached with caution due to radiosensitization. In a multi-institution analysis from Hecht et al., 32 patients receiving concurrent WBRT and BRAF inhibitors were compared with patients receiving WBRT alone; grade 2 dermatitis was observed among 44% receiving concurrent therapy versus 8% receiving WBRT alone ($p < 0.001$) (27). No toxicities were reported among 19 patients receiving stereotactic radiotherapy (which included all body sites). Vemurafenib appeared to be a more potent radiosensitizer than dabrafenib (27). Merten et al. reported a case of radiation dermatitis and severe mucositis requiring hospitalization and parental nutrition when radiation was given to a truncal bone metastasis concurrent with vemurafenib (28). The same patient received radiation before vemurafenib therapy for a separate bone metastasis without any noted toxicity. Finally, two cases of grade 2 and two cases of grade 3 radiation dermatitis were reported by Satzger et al. in patients receiving concurrent dabrafenib or vemurafenib and radiation (29).

Even short-interval sequential therapy may result in toxicity. In the previously-mentioned study by Harding et al., radiation recall was noted with vemurafenib that was commenced 6 weeks after WBRT (26). Boussemart et al. published two case reports of severe cutaneous toxicity with sequential therapy (30); the first patient started vemurafenib one day after completion of radiation to two truncal sites; the second patient developed recall dermatitis with vemurafenib that commenced 23 days after the last radiotherapy fraction.

Given the toxicity associated with concurrent and sequential BRAF inhibitors and radiotherapy, it would be prudent to temporally separate the two therapies if possible. As always, clinical judgement and an informed discussion with the patient are required, particularly for cases that require urgent or emergent commencement of therapy.

Immune therapies against melanoma

Traditional immune treatment for metastatic melanoma used interleukin-2 (IL-2), which resulted in low response rates and high toxicity (31). Ipilimumab is a monoclonal antibody that blocks cytotoxic T-lymphocyte-associated protein 4 (CTLA-4). CTLA-4 inhibits T-cell activation pathways; thus, ipilimumab is believed to up-regulate innate immune responses against tumour cells (7, 32). Finally, the role of programmed death 1 (PD-1) blockade will be briefly discussed.

Chu et al. reported on the results of 8 patients with brain metastases from melanoma treated with high-dose IL-2 therapy (31). One out of 7 patients with active intracranial disease at the time of IL-2 therapy achieved a partial response; median survival was 8.7 months for all patients.

Sequential ipilimumab and SRS for brain metastases has been prior studied and shown to have effect (see Table 3). A retrospective study by Kniesley et al. (33) reviewed 77 patients who received SRS for melanoma brain metastases; 35% received ipilimumab. Among these, 11 received ipilimumab before SRS and 16 received ipilimumab after SRS. Median survival was 21.3 months in patients receiving ipilimumab and 4.9 months without ipilimumab (statistically significant). Intracranial disease control was not reported. A similar study by Silk et al. reviewed 70 patients who received WBRT or SRS for melanoma brain metastases; 47% received ipilimumab (34). Median survival was 18.3 months for patients who received ipilimumab versus 5.3 months without ipilimumab ($p = 0.009$). 42 patients were evaluable for intracranial response. 40% of patients who received ipilimumab prior to radiation had intracranial response; 17% of patients who received ipilimumab after radiation had intracranial response; 9% of patients who received radiation alone (WBRT) had intracranial response. Finally, Mathew et al. retrospectively reviewed 58 patients who received SRS with or without ipilimumab (35). In contrast to the study by Kniesley, there was no statistically significant difference in toxicity, local control, distant brain control, or overall survival between the two groups.

Effect of sequential ipilimumab and radiation has also been studied prospectively by Margolin et al. in a prospective, multi-institution, phase II non-randomized clinical trial of 72 patients (36). In this study, patients must have completed any radiation at least 14 days prior to commencement of ipilimumab. Study subjects with asymptomatic (cohort A, no corticosteroids) and symptomatic (cohort B, receiving corticosteroids) brain metastases were analyzed separately. 31% had prior intracranial brain radiotherapy; only 6% received SRS. Intracranial disease response, taking into account the effect of ipilimumab only, was observed in 16% of cohort A patients and 5% of cohort B patients. Median survival was 7 months in cohort A and 3.7 months in cohort B. Grade 4 toxicities were uncommon (2 patients, confusion); the most common grade 3 toxicities were fatigue (7 patients), diarrhea (6 patients), hyperglycemia (4 patients) and dehydration (4 patients). This prospective study concluded that ipilimumab had modest activity in asymptomatic patients with brain metastases.

Table 3. Survival for patients treated with SRS with or without sequential ipilimumab for metastatic melanoma

Study	Survival		Statistical significance
	Without ipilimumab	*With ipilimumab*	
Kniesley et al. (33)	4.9 months (MS), 95% CI 6.4-26.7	21.3 months (MS), 95% CI 24.8-66.8	Significant (p-value not reported)
Mathew et al. (35)	45% (6 month OS)	56% (6 month OS)	p = 0.18
Silk et al. (34)	4.0 months (MS), 95% 3.2-14.6	19.9 months (MS), 95% 15.9-NR	p = 0.009

CI = confidence interval; MS = median survival; NR = not reached; OS = overall survival.

Finally, concurrent SRS and ipilimumab has been studied retrospectively (37). 15 patients received concurrent therapy, 19 received SRS before ipilimumab, and 12 received SRS after ipilimumab. The median SRS dose was 21 Gy. Individuals who received SRS before or during ipilimumab had longer overall survival and distant brain control than patients receiving ipilimumab after SRS (see table 4). There was also a trend towards improved local control in patients receiving SRS during ipilimumab. 20% of patients experienced any grade 3 or 4 toxicity (including hemorrhage from metastasis and seizures). Interestingly, 50% of patients had an increase in size of tumours on follow-up MRI if they received SRS during or before ipilimumab, compared with 13% who received SRS after ipilimumab, possibly due to immune-mediated tumour inflammation.

Further studies of ipilimumab in brain metastases are needed due to small patient numbers (32). Ipilimumab appears to have modest effect in controlling brain metastases, but radiation treatment remains a mainstay of intracranial disease control. Retrospective data support the safety of concurrent ipilimumab and radiation. Provocative suggestions of improved disease control when radiation is given during ipilimumab require confirmation in well-designed prospective clinical trials (32).

Table 4. Results of ipilimumab timing with SRS by Kiess et al. (37)

Patient group	SRS before ipilimumab (n = 19)	SRS during ipilimumab (n = 15)	SRS after ipilimumab (n = 12)	p-value
1 year overall survival	56%	65%	40%	0.008
Local recurrence	13%	0%	11%	0.21
Distant brain recurrence	64%	69%	92%	0.003

SRS = stereotactic radiosurgery.

To conclude discussion of immune therapies, nivolumab is a programmed death 1 (PD-1) immune checkpoint inhibitor antibody (38). Nivolumab has been shown to improve overall survival in patients with metastatic melanoma as compared with dacarbazine, but the phase 3 clinical trial studying nivolumab excluded patients with active brain metastases (38). There is no known information about the effect of nivolumab on brain metastases or its interaction with radiotherapy in melanoma, though pre-clinical studies are promising (39).

Abscopal effect

An abscopal effect is observed when local treatment to a single site (e.g., WBRT) induces regression in distant sites without local treatment; this effect may be potentiated by immune therapies (22, 23). Radiation is hypothesized to act as a local form of immune therapy that can provoke a systemic abscopal response (40). Here, abscopal responses triggered by intracranial radiotherapy are briefly discussed.

Teulings et al. described a case of persistent abscopal response after WBRT (20 Gy in 5 fractions) and dacarbazine, without further immune therapy (40). WBRT can also trigger abscopal response during interleukin-2 therapy (41); disease control was lost with time but subsequent treatment with ipilimumab then vemurafenib maintained disease control. Finally, Grimaldi et al. reported 11 cases prior treated with ipilimumab with abscopal response after radiotherapy; 4 had received WBRT and 3 received stereotactic radiotherapy (23). Authors hypothesized that local response to radiotherapy may predict for abscopal response.

Vemurafenib and radiotherapy have been associated with an abscopal response. Sullivan et al. reported a case of metastatic melanoma treated with vemurafenib on a clinical trial (42). After 9 months of treatment, a mixed response with new brain metastases were seen. After vemurafenib was discontinued, the patient received SRS to three intracranial metastatic sites. 11 months after SRS, fluorodeoxygluose-position emission tomography (FDG-PET) revealed no residual metastatic lesions and brain magnetic response imaging (MRI) showed near complete resolution of the brain metastasis.

Although exciting, it should be noted that abscopal responses remain rare and challenging to predict. Further studies with immunologic correlates are required to determine predictors of abscopal response and to better study this oncologic phenomenon.

Renal

Renal cell carcinomas (RCC) often harbour mutations that inactivate the Von Hippel-Lindau gene (*VHL*), leading to stimulation of vascular endothelial growth factor (VEGF). TKIs (such as sunitinib, sorafenib, pazopanib, or axitinib) that target the VEGF receptor have been shown to be effective in treatment of patients with metastatic RCC (43, 44). However, there is limited information about treatment of metastatic RCC lesions in the brain. Relevant studies are discussed here.

The TARGET trial was a multi-institution, phase III, prospective, placebo-controlled randomized controlled trial evaluating sorafenib in unresectable or metastatic RCC (45). A sub-group analysis of trial participants enrolled at two institutions in France and Poland (n =

139) found a reduced incidence of brain metastasis among patients receiving sorafenib (3%) as compared with those receiving placebo (12%, $p < 0.05$) (46). Crossover was permitted in the TARGET trial, which may have reduced the observed benefit of sorafenib. No information was provided about use of radiation.

Patients with brain metastases receiving sunitinib under an expanded access program were evaluated by Gore et al. (47). Out of 321 patients with brain metastases included in the study, 213 were evaluable for tumour response. Responses were not categorized by site (e.g., intracranial or elsewhere). Among those with brain metastases, 12% had disease response and 52% had stable disease ≥3 months, as compared with 18% and 59%, respectively, for those without brain metastases. Patients with brain metastases had decreased median survival (9.2 months versus 19.1 months, statistically significant). The most common toxicities were diarrhea, fatigue, nausea, and mucositis. One patient had grade 1 or 2 brain hemorrhage. The incidence of grade 3 or 4 toxicities was similar between patients with and without brain metastases. No information was available about use of radiation.

Cases have been reported regarding a possible increased risk of brain hemorrhage from TKI therapy, prompting suggestions of waiting 6 weeks between intracranial radiotherapy and commencement of a targeted agent (48). The risk of bleeding is not unique to RCC, but has also been observed in other histologies for which anti-VEGFR therapy is used. In a meta-analysis, Je et al. report a 16.7% incidence of bleeding from any site with sunitinib or sorafenib therapy (49).

Caution should be used when combining radiotherapy and TKIs for RCC due to possible radiosensitization. Inoue et al. reported two cases of gastrointestinal perforation after abdominal radiotherapy (50). In the first case, the patient had left femur and acetabulum bone metastases treated with 30 Gy in 10 fractions. The patient commenced on sorafenib 7 days after radiation; 4 weeks after starting sorafenib, she developed sigmoid colon perforation and died of sepsis one month after. The second patient had three brain metastases treated with SRS concurrent with sorafenib; no undue toxicity was reported with this course of radiation. Subsequent to the intracranial treatment, this patient developed lytic bone metastases in the lumbar spine. 30 Gy in 10 fractions were delivered concurrent with sorafenib. 2 months after competing radiation, sigmoid perforation was observed requiring surgery.

Discontinuation of TKIs before and after radiation is often done; despite this, there is a reported case of bowel perforation after lumbar spine radiotherapy (8 Gy in 1 fraction) even though sorafenib was stopped 2 days before radiation and resumed 3 days after radiation (51). Toxicity is not limited to the abdomen; a case of bronchial fistula after mediastinal radiotherapy to a subcarinal deposit of RCC (30 Gy in 10 fractions) was reported (52). One week after completing cranial and mediastinal radiotherapy, sunitinib was commenced. Two months later, dramatic tumour regression was noted and a bronchial fistula formed. Although the authors noted the association with sequential radiotherapy and sunitinib therapy, it is also possible that tumour response to sunitinib resulted in the bronchial fistula.

In summary, TKIs used for RCC may help prevent development of brain metastases. These agents may have some activity against active brain metastases, but more data are required. Treating clinicians should be aware of the unique toxicities associated with sorafenib and sunitinib (Table 5) (53). Unusual and severe adverse effects may be seen when radiotherapy is used concurrently or in close temporal association with sorafenib or sunitinib.

As with any radiosensitizing agent, clinical judgement and an informed discussion are required before starting radiotherapy or a VEGF inhibitor.

Table 5. Common toxicities observed with VEGFR inhibitors for RCC, by frequency (adapted from Bhojani et al.) (53)

Sorafenib				Sunitinib			
All grades	%	Grade 3 or 4	%	All grades	%	Grade 3 or 4	%
Hypophospha-temia	45	Hypophosphatemia, lymphopenia	13	Hypothyroidism	71	High lipase	16
Anemia	44	High lipase	12	High creatinine	66	Neutropenia, lymphopenia	12
High lipase	41	Hand-foot syndrome	6	Thrombocytopenia	65	Hypertension, thrombocy-topenia	8
Diarrhea	43	Mucositis	6	Lymphopenia	60	Fatigue	7
Rash	40	Fatigue, neutropenia	5	Fatigue	58	Diarrhea, hand-foot syndrome, hypopho-sphatemia	5
Fatigue	37			Diarrhea	53		
Hand-foot syndrome	30			High lipase	52		
Alopecia	27			Mucositis	45		
Nausea, lymphopenia	23			Nausea, dysgeusia	44		
Mucositis	21			Dyspepsia, anorexia	28		

BREAST

Targeted therapies against HER2

A proportion of breast carcinomas have overexpression of the human epidermal growth factor receptor 2 (HER2) gene (54). These tumours are responsive to targeted therapies directed against the HER2 pathway, including monoclonal antibodies (trastuzumab), TKIs (lapatinib), or trastuzumab emtansine (T-DM1) (9, 55).

Trastuzumab has poor blood-brain barrier penetration; although it may delay the development of brain metastases (56), its effect on established brain metastases is unclear (57). Furthermore, most patients with HER2-positive breast cancer who develop brain metastases have typically already received trastuzumab (57). Use of other HER2-targeted agents to treat brain metastases is discussed here.

The LANDSCAPE trial was a prospective, multi-institution, phase II, single-arm trial that enrolled 45 patients with HER2-positive breast cancer and brain metastases without prior WBRT (58). Patients were treated with lapatinib and capecitabine. 65.9% of patients had objective intracranial response (all partial responses). 49% had grade 3 or 4 toxicity; the most common grade 3-4 toxicities were diarrhea (20%) and hand-foot syndrome (20%). No grade 5 toxicities were observed. This trial indicated activity of lapatinib and capecitabine in previously unirradiated brain metastases from breast cancer.

A number of studies have evaluated lapatinib as salvage treatment after prior intracranial therapy (see table 6). Lin et al. evaluated lapatinib alone in 242 patients with HER2-positive breast cancer and progressive brain metastases after prior trastuzumab and cranial radiotherapy (WBRT or SRS) (59). Among these heavily pre-treated patients, 6% experienced an objective response (defined as ≥ 50% volumetric reduction in CNS lesions). 21% experienced ≥ 20% volume reduction. 13% experienced grade 3 diarrhea. In a sub-trial of 50 patients evaluating lapatinib and capecitabine, 20% had objective CNS response. In this sub-trial, the most common grade 3 toxicities were hand-foot syndrome (8%) and nausea (8%). These and other studies (Table 6) suggest effect of targeted therapy on brain metastases, even in patients who had previously received cranial radiotherapy.

Table 6. Treatment and response of brain metastases in HER2-positive breast cancer with targeted therapy

Study	Design	Patients	Prior cranial RT	Therapy	Objective response*	Partial** or complete response
LANDSCAPE (58)	Prospective	45	No	lapatinib and capecitabine	66%	
Lin et al. main trial (59)	Prospective	242	Yes	lapatinib	6%	
Lin et al. sub-trial (59)	Prospective	50	Yes	lapatinib and capecitabine	20%	
Ro et al. (60)	Retrospective	58 (47 evaluable)	Yes (most)	lapatinib and capecitabine		17%

* Objective response defined as ≥ 50% volumetric reduction in brain lesion. ** Partial response defined as ≥ 30% reduction in longest diameter of brain lesion. RT = radiotherapy.

Safety of targeted breast cancer therapies with radiation

The safety of trastuzumab has been established when given concurrently with breast radiotherapy (61, 62). However, trastuzumab is associated with congestive heart failure and decline in left ventricle ejection fraction (LVEF) (63). Given that radiotherapy to the left breast is also associated with cardiotoxicity (64), many investigators have looked at whether concurrent trastuzumab and radiation could increase cardiac events. The two largest studies did not show a difference in cardiac toxicity between left-sided or right-sided breast radiotherapy with trastuzumab (61, 62). Nonetheless, longer-term follow-up is required to definitively exclude late cardiac morbidity (65).

Radiotherapy to the brain concurrent with trastuzumab is less well-studied. Chargari et al. retrospectively reviewed 31 patients who received concurrent WBRT (30 Gy in 10 fractions) with trastuzumab; 19% had complete radiologic response and 55% had partial response (overall response of 74%) (66). Nonetheless, brain progression was the sole cause of death in 83% of patients, likely due to lack of use of SRS. Within the limitations of small sample size and retrospective collection of toxicity data, adverse effects were uncommon. 26% had headache (grade 1), 13% experienced nausea/vomiting, and 3 patients had a decrease in LVEF (two grade 1, one grade 2). The authors concluded that concurrent therapy was feasible, and further study of trastuzumab as a radiosensitizer for brain metastases was warranted.

Lapatinib and concurrent radiotherapy has been evaluated in some small phase I studies. Kimple et al. prospectively enrolled 19 patients who received concurrent lapatinib and breast radiotherapy (35-70 Gy in 1.8-2.0 Gy daily fractions) (67). The only grade 3 toxicities observed were radiation dermatitis (7 patients) and pain (2 patients). Complete response was seen in 4 patients, and partial response in 6 patients. Lin et al. evaluated concurrent lapatinib and WBRT, 37.5 Gy in 15 fractions (68). The maximum tolerated dose of lapatinib was 1 250 mg daily; at this dose level, 7 of 27 participants experienced dose-limiting toxicity. Intracranial objective response rate was 79%. Ongoing study of concurrent lapatinib and WBRT is underway in an international, multi-institution phase II study by the RTOG (RTOG 1119, NCT01622868).

Trastuzumab emtansine is an emerging therapy for metastatic breast cancer (69), although its activity in brain metastases is not well studied. The drug is an antibody-cytotoxic drug conjugate that links trastuzumab with the microtubule inhibitor DM1 (69). Carlson et al. reported radiation necrosis in four patients who received T-DM1 a median of 8.5 days (range, 3-449 days) after SRS for brain metastases (70). SRS doses ranged from 16-24 Gy. Two patients experienced symptoms of radiation necrosis immediately after the first T-DM1 infusion.

In summary, targeted therapy for brain metastases from HER2-positive breast cancer appears to have clinical efficacy in both previously-irradiated or unirradiated patients. Currently available data suggest that lapatinib and capecitabine may be the most promising regimen for future study. Limited data are available about safety of intracranial radiotherapy and trastuzumab, but this combination appears to be feasible. Cases of radionecrosis have been reported among patients treated with sequential SRS and T-DM1.

Role of hormone therapy for brain breast metastases

Anti-hormone therapy (commonly called "hormone therapy") is used as adjuvant treatment and treatment for metastatic breast carcinomas that express estrogen receptor (ER) and/or progesterone receptor (PR) (71). Commonly used agents include tamoxifen and aromatase inhibitors (letrozole or anastrazole) (71). Cases have been reported of brain metastases responding to systemic hormone therapy, demonstrating effect of tamoxifen (72), letrozole (73), or megesterol acetate (74). Although hormone therapy may have some effect, high-quality data are lacking. The mainstay of treatment for breast brain metastasis remains radiotherapy (WBRT and/or SRS), as breast cancer patients developing brain metastases may be resistant to further hormone manipulation (55, 75).

Table 7. Summary of possible interactions between targeted therapies and radiation therapy

Probably tolerable with radiation	Associated with increased toxicity	No information available
Concurrent therapy		
ipilimumab	dabrafenib	crizotinib
trastuzumab	erlotinib*	nivolumab
lapatinib	sorafenib	trastuzumab emtansine
	sunitinib	
	vemurafenib	
Sequential therapy		
erlotinib	dabrafenib	crizotinib
ipilimumab	sorafenib	nivolumab
trastuzumab	sunitinib	
lapatinib	trastuzumab emtansine	
	vemurafenib	

* Increased toxicity with concurrent erlotinib and radiotherapy is probably tolerable but further study is required to establish safety (12).

CONCLUSION

Targeted therapies are available to treat cancers commonly associated with brain metastases. In lung cancer, erlotinib appears to have activity against EGFR-mutated carcinomas. Sequential erlotinib and radiation to the brain appears to be safe, but concurrent therapy may be associated with toxicity. In melanoma, vemurafenib has effect on brain metastases; sequential treatment with a BRAF inhibitor and radiation may modestly increase toxicity whereas concurrent therapy is associated with severe radiosensitization and an increased risk of severe toxicity. On the other hand, concurrent ipilimumab and radiation appears to be safe and may increase treatment efficacy. In renal cell carcinoma, VEGFR-targeted tyrosine kinase inhibitors have been shown to delay development of brain metastases and may produce intracranial disease response but data are poor. Both sorafenib and sunitinib are potent radiosensitizers and concurrent therapy with radiation increases the risk of severe adverse effects. Lastly, lapatinib and capecitabine have modest activity for brain metastases in HER2-positive breast cancer. Use of targeted agents for brain metastases remains experimental, and patients should be offered enrollment in a clinical trial when possible. When considering a targeted therapy, potential interaction with other treatment modalities, especially radiotherapy (Table 7), should be carefully evaluated in the context of the site to be treated, histology, drug involved, and patient prognosis.

REFERENCES

[1] Owonikoko TK, Arbiser J, Zelnak A, Shu HK, Shim H, Robin AM, et al. Current approaches to the treatment of metastatic brain tumours. Nat Rev Clin Oncol 2014;11(4):203-22.

[2] Johnson JD, Young B. Demographics of brain metastasis. Neurosurg Clin North Am 1996;7(3):337-44.

[3] Barnholtz-Sloan JS, Sloan AE, Davis FG, Vigneau FD, Lai P, Sawaya RE. Incidence proportions of brain metastases in patients diagnosed (1973 to 2001) in the Metropolitan Detroit Cancer Surveillance System. J Clin Oncol 2004;22(14):2865-72.

[4] Deeken JF, Loscher W. The blood-brain barrier and cancer: transporters, treatment, and Trojan horses. Clin Cancer Res 2007;13(6):1663-74.

[5] Lindeman NI, Cagle PT, Beasley MB, Chitale DA, Dacic S, Giaccone G, et al. Molecular testing guideline for selection of lung cancer patients for EGFR and ALK tyrosine kinase inhibitors: guideline from the College of American Pathologists, International Association for the Study of Lung Cancer, and Association for Molecular Pathology. J Mol Diagn 2013;15(4):415-53.

[6] Leighl NB, Rekhtman N, Biermann WA, Huang J, Mino-Kenudson M, Ramalingam SS, et al. Molecular testing for selection of patients with lung cancer for epidermal growth factor receptor and anaplastic lymphoma kinase tyrosine kinase inhibitors: American Society of Clinical Oncology endorsement of the College of American Pathologists/International Association for the study of lung cancer/association for molecular pathology guideline. J Clin Oncol 2014;32(32):3673-9.

[7] Gedye C, Hogg D, Butler M, Joshua AM. New treatments for metastatic melanoma. CMAJ 2014;186(10):754-60.

[8] Atkins MB. Management of advanced renal cancer. Kidney Int 2005;67(5):2069-82.

[9] Yu Q, Zhu Z, Liu Y, Zhang J, Li K. Efficacy and Safety of HER2-Targeted Agents for Breast Cancer with HER2-Overexpression: A Network Meta-Analysis. PLoS One 2015;10(5):e0127404.

[10] Porta R, Sanchez-Torres JM, Paz-Ares L, Massuti B, Reguart N, Mayo C, et al. Brain metastases from lung cancer responding to erlotinib: the importance of EGFR mutation. Eur Respir J 2011;37(3):624-31.

[11] Wu YL, Zhou C, Cheng Y, Lu S, Chen GY, Huang C, et al. Erlotinib as second-line treatment in patients with advanced non-small-cell lung cancer and asymptomatic brain metastases: a phase II study (CTONG-0803). Ann Oncol 2013;24(4):993-9.

[12] Hendriks LE, Schoenmaekers J, Zindler JD, Eekers DB, Hoeben A, De Ruysscher DK, et al. Safety of cranial radiotherapy concurrent with tyrosine kinase inhibitors in non-small cell lung cancer patients: A systematic review. Cancer Treat Rev 2015 May 13.

[13] Welsh JW, Komaki R, Amini A, Munsell MF, Unger W, Allen PK, et al. Phase II trial of erlotinib plus concurrent whole-brain radiation therapy for patients with brain metastases from non-small-cell lung cancer. J Clin Oncol 2013;31(7):895-902.

[14] Sperduto PW, Wang M, Robins HI, Schell MC, Werner-Wasik M, Komaki R, et al. A phase 3 trial of whole brain radiation therapy and stereotactic radiosurgery alone versus WBRT and SRS with temozolomide or erlotinib for non-small cell lung cancer and 1 to 3 brain metastases: Radiation Therapy Oncology Group 0320. Int J Radiat Oncol Biol Phys 2013;85(5):1312-8.

[15] Andrews DW, Scott CB, Sperduto PW, Flanders AE, Gaspar LE, Schell MC, et al. Whole brain radiation therapy with or without stereotactic radiosurgery boost for patients with one to three brain metastases: phase III results of the RTOG 9508 randomised trial. Lancet 2004;363(9422):1665-72.

[16] Sperduto PW, Shanley R, Luo X, Andrews D, Werner-Wasik M, Valicenti R, et al. Secondary analysis of RTOG 9508, a phase 3 randomized trial of whole-brain radiation therapy versus WBRT plus stereotactic radiosurgery in patients with 1-3 brain metastases; poststratified by the graded prognostic assessment (GPA). Int J Radiat Oncol Biol Phys 2014;90(3):526-31.

[17] Costa DB, Shaw AT, Ou SH, Solomon BJ, Riely GJ, Ahn MJ, et al. Clinical experience with crizotinib in patients with advanced ALK-reearranged non-small-cell lung cancer and brain metastases. J Clin Oncol 2015 Jan 26.

[18] Pinto IG, Lee M, Graziano S, Lacombe M, Gajra A. Concurrent crizotinib and whole-brain radiation for brain metastases in ALK-positive lung adenocarcinoma. Lung Cancer Management 2014;3(5):369-71.

[19] Kondziolka D, Bernstein M, Resch L, Tator CH, Fleming JF, Vanderlinden RG, et al. Significance of hemorrhage into brain tumors: clinicopathological study. J Neurosurg 1987;67(6):852-7.

[20] Bernard ME, Wegner RE, Reineman K, Heron DE, Kirkwood J, Burton SA, et al. Linear accelerator based stereotactic radiosurgery for melanoma brain metastases. J Cancer Res Ther 2012;8(2):215-21.

[21] Khan MK, Khan N, Almasan A, Macklis R. Future of radiation therapy for malignant melanoma in an era of newer, more effective biological agents. OncoTargets and therapy 2011;4:137-48.

[22] Postow MA, Callahan MK, Barker CA, Yamada Y, Yuan J, Kitano S, et al. Immunologic correlates of the abscopal effect in a patient with melanoma. N Engl J Med 2012;366(10):925-31.

[23] Grimaldi AM, Simeone E, Giannarelli D, Muto P, Falivene S, Borzillo V, et al. Abscopal effects of radiotherapy on advanced melanoma patients who progressed after ipilimumab immunotherapy. Oncoimmunology 2014;3:e28780.

[24] Long GV, Trefzer U, Davies MA, Kefford RF, Ascierto PA, Chapman PB, et al. Dabrafenib in patients with Val600Glu or Val600Lys BRAF-mutant melanoma metastatic to the brain (BREAK-MB): a multicentre, open-label, phase 2 trial. Lancet Oncol 2012;13(11):1087-95.

[25] Dummer R, Goldinger SM, Turtschi CP, Eggmann NB, Michielin O, Mitchell L, et al. Vemurafenib in patients with BRAFV600 mutation-positive melanoma with symptomatic brain metastases: Final results of an open-label pilot study. Eur J Cancer 2014;50(3):611-621.

[26] Harding JJ, Catalanotti F, Munhoz RR, Cheng DT, Yaqubie A, Kelly N, et al. A retrospective evaluation of vemurafenib as treatment for BRAF-mutant melanoma brain metastases. Oncologist 2015 May 8.

[27] Hecht M, Zimmer L, Loquai C, Weishaupt C, Gutzmer R, Schuster B, et al. Radiosensitization by BRAF inhibitor therapy-mechanism and frequency of toxicity in melanoma patients. Ann Oncol 2015;26(6):1238-44.

[28] Merten R, Hecht M, Haderlein M, Distel L, Fietkau R, Heinzerling L, et al. Increased skin and mucosal toxicity in the combination of vemurafenib with radiation therapy. Strahlenther Onkol 2014;190(12):1169-72.

[29] Satzger I, Degen A, Asper H, Kapp A, Hauschild A, Gutzmer R. Serious skin toxicity with the combination of BRAF inhibitors and radiotherapy. J Clin Oncol 2013;31(13):e220-2.

[30] Boussemart L, Boivin C, Claveau J, Tao YG, Tomasic G, Routier E, et al. Vemurafenib and radiosensitization. JAMA Dermatol 2013;149(7):855-7.

[31] Chu MB, Fesler MJ, Armbrecht ES, Fosko SW, Hsueh E, Richart JM. High-dose interleukin-2 (HD IL-2) therapy should be considered for treatment of patients with melanoma brain metastases. Chemother Res Pract 2013;2013:726925.

[32] Patel KR, Lawson DH, Kudchadkar RR, Carthon BC, Oliver DE, Okwan-Duodu D, et al. Two heads better than one? Ipilimumab immunotherapy and radiation therapy for melanoma brain metastases. Neuro-oncology 2015 May 25.

[33] Knisely JP, Yu JB, Flanigan J, Sznol M, Kluger HM, Chiang VL. Radiosurgery for melanoma brain metastases in the ipilimumab era and the possibility of longer survival. J Neurosurg 2012;117(2):227-33.

[34] Silk AW, Bassetti MF, West BT, Tsien CI, Lao CD. Ipilimumab and radiation therapy for melanoma brain metastases. Cancer Med 2013;2(6):899-906.

[35] Mathew M, Tam M, Ott PA, Pavlick AC, Rush SC, Donahue BR, et al. Ipilimumab in melanoma with limited brain metastases treated with stereotactic radiosurgery. Melanoma Res 2013;23(3):191-5.

[36] Margolin K, Ernstoff MS, Hamid O, Lawrence D, McDermott D, Puzanov I, et al. Ipilimumab in patients with melanoma and brain metastases: an open-label, phase 2 trial. Lancet Oncol 2012;13(5):459-65.

[37] Kiess AP, Wolchok JD, Barker CA, Postow MA, Tabar V, Huse JT, et al. Stereotactic radiosurgery for melanoma brain metastases in patients receiving ipilimumab: safety profile and efficacy of combined treatment. Int J Radiat Oncol Biol Phys 2015;92(2):368-75.

[38] Robert C, Long GV, Brady B, Dutriaux C, Maio M, Mortier L, et al. Nivolumab in previously untreated melanoma without BRAF mutation. N Engl J Med 2015;372(4):320-30.

[39] Barker CA, Postow MA. Combinations of radiation therapy and immunotherapy for melanoma: a review of clinical outcomes. Int J Radiat Oncol Biol Phys 2014;88(5):986-97.

[40] Teulings HE, Tjin EP, Willemsen KJ, Krebbers G, van Noesel CJ, Kemp EH, et al. Radiation-induced melanoma-associated leucoderma, systemic antimelanoma immunity and disease-free survival in a patient with advanced-stage melanoma: a case report and immunological analysis. Br J Dermatol 2013;168(4):733-8.

[41] Okwan-Duodu D, Pollack BP, Lawson D, Khan MK. Role of radiation therapy as immune activator in the era of modern immunotherapy for metastatic malignant melanoma. Am J Clin Oncol 2015;38(1):119-25.

[42] Sullivan RJ, Lawrence DP, Wargo JA, Oh KS, Gonzalez RG, Piris A. Case records of the Massachusetts General Hospital. Case 21-2013. A 68-year-old man with metastatic melanoma. N Engl J Med 2013;369(2):173-83.

[43] Atkins E, Zamora S, Candia BJ, Baca A, Orlando RA. Development of a Mammalian suspension culture for expression of active recombinant human urokinase-type plasminogen activator. Cytotechnology 2005;49(1):25-37.

[44] Funakoshi T, Lee C, Hsieh JJ. A systematic review of predictive and prognostic biomarkers for VEGF-targeted therapy in renal cell carcinoma. Cancer Treat Rev 2014;40(4):533-47.

[45] Escudier B, Eisen T, Stadler WM, Szczylik C, Oudard S, Staehler M, et al. Sorafenib for treatment of renal cell carcinoma: Final efficacy and safety results of the phase III treatment approaches in renal cancer global evaluation trial. J Clin Oncol 2009;27(20):3312-8.

[46] Massard C, Zonierek J, Gross-Goupil M, Fizazi K, Szczylik C, Escudier B. Incidence of brain metastases in renal cell carcinoma treated with sorafenib. Ann Oncol 2010;21(5):1027-31.

[47] Gore ME, Hariharan S, Porta C, Bracarda S, Hawkins R, Bjarnason GA, et al. Sunitinib in metastatic renal cell carcinoma patients with brain metastases. Cancer 2011;117(3):501-9.

[48] Pouessel D, Culine S. High frequency of intracerebral hemorrhage in metastatic renal carcinoma patients with brain metastases treated with tyrosine kinase inhibitors targeting the vascular endothelial growth factor receptor. Eur Urol 2008;53(2):376-81.

[49] Je Y, Schutz FA, Choueiri TK. Risk of bleeding with vascular endothelial growth factor receptor tyrosine-kinase inhibitors sunitinib and sorafenib: a systematic review and meta-analysis of clinical trials. Lancet Oncol 2009;10(10):967-74.

[50] Inoue T, Kinoshita H, Komai Y, Kawabata T, Kawa G, Uemura Y, et al. Two cases of gastrointestinal perforation after radiotherapy in patients receiving tyrosine kinase inhibitor for advanced renal cell carcinoma. World J Surg Oncol 2012;10:167.

[51] Peters NA, Richel DJ, Verhoeff JJ, Stalpers LJ. Bowel perforation after radiotherapy in a patient receiving sorafenib. J Clin Oncol 2008;26(14):2405-6.

[52] Basille D, Andrejak M, Bentayeb H, Kanaan M, Fournier C, Lecuyer E, et al. Bronchial fistula associated with sunitinib in a patient previously treated with radiation therapy. Ann Pharmacother 2010;44(2):383-6.

[53] Bhojani N, Jeldres C, Patard JJ, Perrotte P, Suardi N, Hutterer G, et al. Toxicities associated with the administration of sorafenib, sunitinib, and temsirolimus and their management in patients with metastatic renal cell carcinoma. Eur Urol 2008;53(5):917-30.

[54] Zhang H, Berezov A, Wang Q, Zhang G, Drebin J, Murali R, et al. ErbB receptors: from oncogenes to targeted cancer therapies. J Clin Invest 2007;117(8):2051-8.

[55] Lin NU. Breast cancer brain metastases: new directions in systemic therapy. Ecancermedicalscience 2013;7:307.

[56] Yap YS, Cornelio GH, Devi BC, Khorprasert C, Kim SB, Kim TY, et al. Brain metastases in Asian HER2-positive breast cancer patients: anti-HER2 treatments and their impact on survival. Br J Cancer 2012;107(7):1075-82.

[57] Larsen PB, Kumler I, Nielsen DL. A systematic review of trastuzumab and lapatinib in the treatment of women with brain metastases from HER2-positive breast cancer. Cancer Treat Rev 2013;39(7):720-7.

[58] Bachelot T, Romieu G, Campone M, Dieras V, Cropet C, Dalenc F, et al. Lapatinib plus capecitabine in patients with previously untreated brain metastases from HER2-positive metastatic breast cancer (LANDSCAPE): a single-group phase 2 study. Lancet Oncol 2013;14(1):64-71.
[59] Lin NU, Dieras V, Paul D, Lossignol D, Christodoulou C, Stemmler HJ, et al. Multicenter phase II study of lapatinib in patients with brain metastases from HER2-positive breast cancer. Clin Cancer Res 2009;15(4) :1452-9.
[60] Ro J, Park S, Kim S, Kim TY, Im YH, Rha SY, et al. Clinical outcomes of HER2-positive metastatic breast cancer patients with brain metastasis treated with lapatinib and capecitabine: an open-label expanded access study in Korea. BMC Cancer 2012;12:322.
[61] Halyard MY, Pisansky TM, Dueck AC, Suman V, Pierce L, Solin L, et al. Radiotherapy and adjuvant trastuzumab in operable breast cancer: tolerability and adverse event data from the NCCTG Phase III Trial N9831. J Clin Oncol 2009;27(16):2638-44.
[62] Tan-Chiu E, Yothers G, Romond E, Geyer CE, Jr, Ewer M, Keefe D, et al. Assessment of cardiac dysfunction in a randomized trial comparing doxorubicin and cyclophosphamide followed by paclitaxel, with or without trastuzumab as adjuvant therapy in node-positive, human epidermal growth factor receptor 2-overexpressing breast cancer: NSABP B-31. J Clin Oncol 2005;23(31):7811-9.
[63] Moja L, Tagliabue L, Balduzzi S, Parmelli E, Pistotti V, Guarneri V, et al. Trastuzumab containing regimens for early breast cancer. Cochrane Database Syst Rev 2012;4:CD006243.
[64] Darby SC, Ewertz M, McGale P, Bennet AM, Blom-Goldman U, Bronnum D, et al. Risk of ischemic heart disease in women after radiotherapy for breast cancer. N Engl J Med 2013;368(11):987-98.
[65] Marinko T, Dolenc J, Bilban-Jakopin C. Cardiotoxicity of concomitant radiotherapy and trastuzumab for early breast cancer. Radiol Oncol 2014;48(2):105-12.
[66] Chargari C, Idrissi HR, Pierga JY, Bollet MA, Dieras V, Campana F, et al. Preliminary results of whole brain radiotherapy with concurrent trastuzumab for treatment of brain metastases in breast cancer patients. Int J Radiat Oncol Biol Phys 2011;81(3):631-6.
[67] Kimple RJ, Horton JK, Livasy CA, Shields JM, Lawrence JA, Chiu WM, et al. Phase I study and biomarker analysis of lapatinib and concurrent radiation for locally advanced breast cancer. Oncologist 2012;17(12):1496-1503.
[68] Lin NU, Freedman RA, Ramakrishna N, Younger J, Storniolo AM, Bellon JR, et al. A phase I study of lapatinib with whole brain radiotherapy in patients with Human Epidermal Growth Factor Receptor 2 (HER2)-positive breast cancer brain metastases. Breast Cancer Res Treat 2013;142(2):405-14.
[69] Verma S, Miles D, Gianni L, Krop IE, Welslau M, Baselga J, et al. Trastuzumab emtansine for HER2-positive advanced breast cancer. N Engl J Med 2012;367(19):1783-91.
[70] Carlson JA, Nooruddin Z, Rusthoven C, Elias A, Borges VF, Diamond JR, et al. Trastuzumab emtansine and stereotactic radiosurgery: an unexpected increase in clinically significant brain edema. Neuro Oncol 2014;16(7):1006-9.
[71] Rugo HS. The breast cancer continuum in hormone-receptor-positive breast cancer in postmenopausal women: evolving management options focusing on aromatase inhibitors. Ann Oncol 2008;19(1):16-27.
[72] Salvati M, Cervoni L, Innocenzi G, Bardella L. Prolonged stabilization of multiple and single brain metastases from breast cancer with tamoxifen. Report of three cases. Tumori 1993;79(5):359-62.
[73] Madhup R, Kirti S, Bhatt ML, Srivastava PK, Srivastava M, Kumar S. Letrozole for brain and scalp metastases from breast cancer--a case report. Breast 2006;15(3):440-2.
[74] Stewart DJ, Dahrouge S. Response of brain metastases from breast cancer to megestrol acetate: a case report. J Neurooncol 1995;24(3):299-301.
[75] Lee SS, Ahn JH, Kim MK, Sym SJ, Gong G, Ahn SD, et al. Brain metastases in breast cancer: prognostic factors and management. Breast Cancer Res Treat 2008;111(3):523-30.

Submitted: June 5, 2015. *Revised:* July 6, 2015. *Accepted:* July 13, 2015.

In: Pain Management Yearbook 2015
Editor: Joav Merrick
ISBN: 978-1-63484-515-1

Chapter 25

Palliative radiotherapy for locally advanced non-small cell lung cancer (NSCLC): The Rapid Response Radiotherapy Program (RRRP) Experience

Cyril Danjoux*[1,*]*, MD, Breanne Lechner*[1]*, MD(C), Natalie Pulenzas*[1]*, MD(C), May Tsao*[1]*, MD, Elizabeth Barnes*[1]*, MD, Alysa Fairchild*[2]*, MD and Edward Chow*[1]*, MBBS

[1]Rapid Response Radiotherapy Program,
Department of Radiation Oncology, Odette Cancer Centre,
Sunnybrook Health Sciences Centre,
University of Toronto, Toronto, Ontario, Canada
[2]Cross Cancer Institute, Edmonton, Alberta, Canada

The majority of lung cancer patients have locally advanced or metastatic disease at diagnosis. Many of patients with locally advanced or metastatic lung cancer are treated with palliative intent to help relieve symptoms and improve quality of life. This article summarizes some of our experience with palliative thoracic RT for NSCLC at the Rapid Response Radiotherapy Program (RRRP).

Keywords: lung cancer, palliative, thoracic radiotherapy

Introduction

The cure rate of non-small cell lung cancer (NSCLC) by irradiation is disappointingly low, with a 5 year survival of about 10% (1). Only 15% of patients with NSCLC remain

* Correspondence: Cyril Danjoux MD, FRCPC, Odette Cancer Centre, Sunnybrook Health Sciences Centre, 2075 Bayview Ave, Toronto, Ontario M4N 3M5, Canada. E-mail: Cyril.danjoux@sunnybrook.ca.

asymptomatic through the course of their disease (2). The majority of patients with locally advanced or metastatic lung cancer are treated with palliative intent to help relieve symptoms and improve quality of life (3). Nearly one third of all palliative radiotherapy (RT) courses are administered to patients with lung cancer (4, 5). Those with intra-thoracic symptoms respond to palliative thoracic radiotherapy in over two thirds of cases (6).

The majority of lung cancer patients have locally advanced or metastatic disease at diagnosis. These patients may have minimal or no symptoms, or more commonly, complain of loco-regional symptoms. Symptoms caused by disease within the thorax can be addressed by palliative-intent external beam radiotherapy (EBRT) or endo-bronchial brachytherapy alone, or in combination. Selected patients with limited 3-5 oligo-metastases to bone, brain or liver may be considered for stereotactic body radiotherapy (SBRT). Following palliative thoracic EBRT over two thirds have improvement of their symptoms (6). The current article summarizes some of our experience with palliative external beam thoracic radiotherapy for lung cancer at the RRRP.

METHODS

A review of the literature regarding palliative radiotherapy for NSCLC was conducted. The relevant studies were summarized and included in this review. The data for the RRRP was collected from an existing database with record of each patient referred to the RRRP, the patient demographics, and the reason for referral.

NSCLC patients seen in the RRRP

The RRRP was initiated in 1996 to meet the demands for timely palliative RT for patients in the terminal phase of their illness (7-9). We see approximately 600 new patients in the RRRP annually. Demographics of patients seen at the RRRP between 2009 and 2014 are reported in Table 1.

NSCLC accounted for 29.6% of all cases referred. In comparison, between 1999 and2006, approximately 10% were referred to the RRRP for RT for a symptomatic lesion in the thorax (7), consistent with the 7% reported by the practice pattern in the United States (4). Table 2 lists symptoms for which patients were referred for treatment.

Fairchild (6) in 2008 reviewed if the pattern of practice in the prescription of RT for the palliation of thoracic symptoms had changed between 1999 and 2006 at the RRRP and concluded that:

1. There was a great deal of variability in RT prescribed, with 13 different dose-fractionation schedules. The most common schedules were 20Gy/5 (64%) and 30Gy/10 (13%).
2. Such variability was likely due to a combination of case mix, patient and disease factors, resource consideration, and a lack of consensus on standard practice (4) which existed at the time.

3. RT for palliation of intra-thoracic symptoms did not mirror the results of sequential, conflicting published randomized controlled trials (RCT).

Table 1. Demographics of all RRRP patients (January 2009 - December 2014, N=3,675)

Age (years)	
Mean	68.3
Median	69.0
Range	(20-97)
Sex, n (%)	
Male	1974 (53.7%)
Female	1701 (46.3%)
Karnofsky Performance Status (KPS)	
Median	60.0
Range	(10-100)
Primary Cancer Site, n (%)	
Lung	1089 (29.6%)
Breast	775 (21.1%)
Genitourinary (GU) – Prostate	704 (19.2%)
Genitourinary (GU) – Bladder, Renal	317 (8.6%)
Gastrointestinal (GI)	286 (7.8%)
Gynecological (GYN)	36 (0.9%)
Unknown	278 (7.6%)
Other	190 (5.2%)

Table 2. Site of symptoms for NSCLC patients referred to RRRP (January 2009 – December 2014; N=1,089)

Intra-Thoracic	**Number (%)**
Lung mass	30 (2.8%)
SVCO symptoms	20 (1.8%)
Shortness of breath	17 (1.6%)
Hemoptysis/Bleeding in the lung	16 (1.5%)
Chest pain	4 (0.4%)
Pleural effusion	3 (0.3%)
Difficulty swallowing	1 (0.09%)
Cough	1 (0.09%)
Extra-Thoracic	**Number (%)**
Skeletal (bone pain, post-surgery)	495 (45.5%)
Central Nervous System (CNS), Brain	447 (41.0%)
CNS, Spinal cord compression/Cauda Equina	24 (2.2%)

Each patient may have more than one site of symptom recorded.

Should patients with minimal or no symptoms receive immediate palliative RT?

In a prospective study of patients referred to the palliative care unit at diagnosis with advanced NSCLC, only 50% had cancer related symptoms (10).

One multicentre RCT addressing the timing of RT for patients with minimal or no symptoms randomised 230 patients to receive immediate treatment (10 Gy/1 or 17Gy/2) versus the same RT delayed until symptom progression. No difference in survival, QOL, or symptom control was found between the study arms. In addition, 56% of patients untreated at baseline never needed any thoracic RT (11). These findings were confirmed in two RCT which also reported no benefit in survival, symptom control or QOL in the use of immediate radiotherapy when compared to delayed radiotherapy (11, 12). There is therefore no good evidence for immediate thoracic radiotherapy in patients with minimal or no symptoms secondary to incurable disease.

How effective is RT in relieving intra-thoracic symptoms?

Thoracic symptoms which may respond to radiotherapy are hemoptysis, cough, chest pain, dyspnoea, obstructive pneumonia, dysphagia due to esophageal compression, or superior vena cava syndrome (SVCS). Symptoms of malignant pleural effusion, lymphangitic carcinomatosis and multilobar parenchymal disease are not suitable for palliative EBRT (15).

Two reviews, one in 2008 (6) and the other in 2010 (16), concluded there was no strong evidence favouring one schedule over another; 2) acute toxicity was greater with higher dose regimens; 3) patients with better performance status (PS) might have a survival benefit with a higher dose regimen (5% at 1 year and 3% at 2 years); and 4) RT myelopathy may be associated with some regimens (17Gy in 2 fractions) (17).

Response rates in RCT of palliative RT for hemoptysis are 70-90%, chest pain 50-80%, dyspnoea 37-57% and cough 20-80% (16). The lower rate of response for cough may be due to radiation side effects, which can result in a non-productive cough.

Fairchild et al. published a systematic review of 13 RCT of palliative thoracic radiotherapy involving 3473 patients, comparing the response of high dose (30 Gy/10 fractions equivalent or higher [HD]) and low dose (LD) RT on symptom control (Table 3). Higher dose schedules resulted in higher survival (Table 4) and side effects (Table 5).

In 2010, the ASTRO clinical practice guideline (15) included 3708 patients enrolled in 14 RCT. All studies showed a beneficial effect of palliative RT, without any specific schedule being favoured. Quality of life (QOL) when reported also showed no major differences (18-20). Higher dose regimens were associated with increased toxicity particularly esophagitis (15).

Based on those results it is recommended that:

1. Palliative thoracic RT be considered for symptom control as it offers a high probability of response with minimal toxicity.
2. For patients with good PS, higher dose schedules, such as 30 Gy/10 equivalent or greater, may be considered because of the observed modest survival benefit. Patients

should be informed of the trade-off of survival benefit and against a higher complication rate.

Table 3. Response to palliative RT by dose schedules (Modified from Fairchild et al.)

Symptom	Complete Response (%)	All Response (%)
	High Dose vs Low Dose	High Dose vs Low Dose
Hemoptysis	73.7 vs 68.9 (p=0.19)	80.2 vs 81.2 (p=0.91)
Cough	27.9 vs 32.1 (p=0.04)	53.5 vs 48.2 (p=0.04)
Chest Pain	57.5 vs 51.9 (p=0.03)	63.8 vs 64.8 (p=0.94)
Overall Symptom burden	16.2 vs 10 (p=0.15)	60.9 vs 55.5 (p=0.03)

Table 4. Survival by dose schedules

	Survival (%)
	High Dose vs Low Dose
1 year	26.5 vs 21.7 (p=0.02)
2 year	8.1 vs 6.7 (p=0.84)

Table 5. Toxicity rate (%)

	Toxicity (%)
	High Dose vs Low Dose
Dysphagia (assessed by physician)	20.5 vs 14.9 (p=0.01)
Pneumonitis	3.6 vs 1.8 (p=0.68)
Myelopathy	0.5 vs 0.08

RT RE-TREATMENT

Re-irradiation for relapse or progression within a previously irradiated field is limited by normal tissue tolerance. There are no prospective studies indicating the value of thoracic re-irradiation. Published small retrospective series with variable dose schedules for a variety of symptoms, suggest a high (70%) response rate and acceptable complication rates (16). Median survival post re-irradiation ranged from 3 to 14 months (21-30).

Combined RT and Chemotherapy

Palliative chemotherapy alone is often used in advanced NSCLC based on a 1995 meta-analysis showing a survival benefit with platinum-based regimens (13, 14). One RCT of 234 patients treated by 4 cycles of chemotherapy (Cisplatin/Etoposide) or RT (42Gy in 15 fractions) reported that the palliative response rate of radiotherapy is double that of chemotherapy (42% for RT compared to 21%) (p=0.009). There was no difference in median survival between the two arms, however, as patients received crossover treatment at progression (31).

There is no good RCT comparing concurrent versus sequential chemo-radiotherapy for palliation of symptoms in NSCLC. The standard of care at present is a sequential approach of chemotherapy with thoracic radiotherapy when and if required (15).

Conclusion

Current treatment guidelines are based on studies which span a period from 1985 and does not take into account newer technologies such as intensity-modulated RT (IMRT), volumetric modulated arc therapy (VMAT), Stereotactic Body radiotherapy (SBRT), image guided radiotherapy (IGRT) or the integration of CT, MRI and PET scanning based treatment planning. Future prospective trials may explore those with different fractionation schedules with different treatment planning and delivery options to optimize palliative thoracic radiotherapy.

References

[1] Jassem J. The role of radiotherapy in lung cancer: where is the evidence? Radiother Oncol 2007;83(2):203-13.

[2] Hawson G, Zimmerman PV, Ford CA, Johnston NG, Firouz-Abadi A. Primary lung cancer: characterization and survival of 1024 patients treated in a single institution. Med J Aust 1990;152(5): 230-4.

[3] Sirzen F, Kjellen E, Sorenson S, Cavallin-Ståhl E. A systematic overview of radiation therapy effects in non-small cell lung cancer. Acta Oncol 2003;42:493–515.

[4] Coia LR, Hanks GE, Martz K, Steinfeld A, Diamond JJ, Kramer S. Practice patterns of palliative care for the United States 1984–1985. Int J Radiat Oncol Biol Phys 1988;14:1261–9.

[5] Hoegler D. Radiotherapy for palliation of symptoms in incurable cancer. Curr Probl Cancer 1997;21:129–83.

[6] Fairchild A, Harris K, Barnes E, Wong R, Lutz S, Bezjak A, et al. Palliative thoracic radiotherapy for lung cancer: a systematic review. J. Clin. Oncol. 2008;26(24): 4001-11.

[7] Danjoux C, Chow E, Drossos A, Holden L, Hayter C, Tsao M, et al. An innovative Rapid Response Radiotherapy Program to reduce waiting time for palliative radiotherapy. Support Care Cancer 2006;14:38-43.

[8] Danjoux C, Szumacher E, Andersson L, Franssen E, Wong R, Chow E, et al. Palliative radiotherapy at Toronto-Sunnybrook Regional Cancer Centre: the Rapid Response Radiotherapy Program. Curr Oncol 2000;7(1):52-6.

[9] Fairchild A, Goh P, Sinclair E, Barnes E, Ghosh S, Danjoux C, et al. Has the pattern of practice in the prescription of radiotherapy for the palliation of thoracic symptoms changed between 1999 and 2006 at the Rapid Response Radiotherapy Program? Int J Radiat Oncol Biol Phys 2008;70(3):693-700.

[10] Temel JS, Jackson VA, Billings JA, Dahlin C, Block SD, Buss MK, et al. Phase II study: integrated palliative care in newly diagnosed advanced non-small cell lung cancer patients. J Clin Oncol 2007; 25(17): 2377-82.

[11] Falk S, Girling DJ, White RJ, Hopwood P, Harvey A, Qian W, et al. Immediate versus delayed palliative thoracic radiotherapy in patients with unresectable locally advanced non-small cell lung cancer and minimal thoracic symptoms: randomised controlled trial. BMJ 2002;325(7362): 465-72.

[12] Sundstrøm S, Bremnes R, Brunsvig P, Aasebø U, Olbjørn K, Fayers PM, et al. Immediate or delayed radiotherapy in advanced non-small cell lung cancer (NSCLC)? Data from a prospective randomised study. Radiother Oncol 2005;75(2):141-8.

[13] NSCLC Meta-Analyses Collaborative Group. Chemotherapy in addition to supportive care improves survival in advanced non-small-cell lung cancer: a systematic review and meta-analysis of individual patient data from 16 randomized controlled trials. J Clin Oncol 2008;26(28): 4617-25.

[14] Higgins MJ, Ettinger DS. Chemotherapy for lung cancer: the state of the art in 2009. Expert Rev. Anticancer Ther 2009; 9(10): 1365-78.

[15] Rodrigues G, Videtic G, Sur R, Bezjak A, Bradley J, Hahn CA, et al. Palliative thoracic radiotherapy in lung cancer: an American Society for Radiation Oncology evidence-based clinical practice guideline. Practical Radiat Oncol 2011;1(2):60-71.

[16] Kepka, L, Olszyna-Serementa, M. Palliative thoracic radiotherapy for lung cancer. Expert Rev Anticancer Ther 2010;10:559–69

[17] Lester JF, Macbeth FR, Toy E, Coles B. Palliative radiotherapy regimens for non-small cell lung cancer. Cochrane Database Syst Rev 2006;18(4): CD002143.

[18] Bezjak A, Dixon P, Brundage M, Tu D, Palmer MJ, Blood P, et al. Randomized Phase III trial of single versus fractionated thoracic radiation in the palliation of patients with lung cancer. Int J Radiat Oncol Biol Phys 2002;54(3):719-29.

[19] Sundstrøm S, Bremnes R, Aasebø U, Aamdal S, Hatlevoll R, Brunsvig P, et al. Hypofractionated palliative radiotherapy (17Gy per 2 fractions) in advanced non-small cell lung carcinoma is comparable to standard fractionation for symptom control and survival: a national phase III trial. J Clin Oncol 2004; 22: 801–10.

[20] Erridge SC, Gaze MN, Price A, Kelly CG, Kerr GR, Cull A, et al. Symptom control and quality of life in people with lung cancer: a randomised trial of two palliative radiotherapy fractionation schedules. Clin Oncol. 2005;17:61–7.

[21] Green N, Melbye RW. Lung cancer: retreatment of local recurrence after definitive irradiation. Cancer 1982;49(5): 865-8.

[22] Jackson MA, Ball DL. Palliative retreatment of locally-recurrent lung cancer after radical radiotherapy. Med J Aust 1987;147(8):391-4.

[23] Montebello JF, Aron BS, Manatunga AK, Horvath JL, Peyton FW. The reirradiation of recurrent bronchogenic carcinoma with external beam irradiation. Am J Clin Oncol 1993; 16(6): 482-8.

[24] Gressen EL, Werner-Wasik M, Cohn J, Topham A, Curran WJ Jr. Thoracic reirradiation for symptomatic relief after prior radiotherapeutic management for lung cancer. Am J Clin Oncol 2000; 23(2):160-3.

[25] Okamoto Y, Murakami M, Yoden E, Sasaki R, Okuno Y, Nakajima T, et al. Reirradiation for locally recurrent lung cancer previously treated with radiation therapy. Int J Radiat Oncol Biol Phys 2002;52(2):390-6.

[26] Wu KL, Jiang GL, Qian H, Wang LJ, Yang HJ, Fu XL, et al. Three-dimensional conformal radiotherapy for locoregionally recurrent lung carcinoma after external beam irradiation: a prospective Phase I-II clinical trial. Int J Radiat Oncol Biol Phys 2003;57(5):1345-50.

[27] Kramer GW, Gans S, Ullmann E, van Meerbeeck JP, Legrand CC, Leer JW. Hypofractionated external beam radiotherapy as retreatment for symptomatic non-small-cell lung carcinoma: an effective treatment? Int J Radiat Oncol Biol Phys 2004;58(5): 1388-93.

[28] Tada T, Fukuda H, Matsui K, Hirashima T, Hosono M, Takada Y, et al. Non-small-cell lung cancer: reirradiation for loco-regional relapse previously treated with radiation therapy. Int J Clin Oncol 2005;10(4): 247-50.

[29] Ebara T, Tanio N, Etoh T, Shichi I, Honda A, Nakajima N. Palliative re-irradiation for in-field recurrence after definitive radiotherapy in patients with primary lung cancer. Anticancer Res 2007;27(1B): 531-4.

[30] Cetingoz R, Arican-Alicikus Z, Nur-Demiral A, Durmak-Isman B, Bakis-Altas B, Kinay M. Is re-irradiation effective in symptomatic local recurrence of non-small cell lung cancer patients? A single institution experience and review of the literature. J Buon 2009; 14(1):33-40.

[31] Kaasa S, Thorud E, Host H, Lien HH, Lund E, Sjolie I. A randomized study evaluating radiotherapy versus chemotherapy in patients with inoperable non-small cell lung cancer. Radiother Oncol 1988;11(1):7-13.

Submitted: June 7, 2015. *Revised:* July 6, 2015. *Accepted:* July 14, 2015.

In: Pain Management Yearbook 2015
Editor: Joav Merrick
ISBN: 978-1-63484-515-1

Chapter 26

A RANDOMIZED PILOT STUDY COMPARING OLANZAPINE (ZYPREXA) TO APREPITANT (EMEND) FOR TREATMENT OF CHEMOTHERAPY-INDUCED NAUSEA AND VOMITING

***Nathan M Shumway*[1,*]*, Sandra E Terrazzino*[1] *and Christopher B Jones*[2]**

[1]Department of Medicine, San Antonio Military Medical Center (SAMMC), San Antonio, TX, US

[2]NorthEast Oncology Associates, Concord, NC, US

Chemotherapy-induced nausea and vomiting in patients receiving highly emetogenic chemotherapy is prevalent. The NK_1 antagonist, aprepitant (Emend) is currently used in the setting of highly emetogenic chemotherapy, and with increased use, the cost of supportive care is rising. Olanzapine (Zyprexa) has been shown to be safe and effective for preventing chemotherapy-induced nausea and vomiting and is less expensive than aprepitant at our institution. Objectives: Perform a pilot study to determine the efficacy of olanzapine containing anti-emetic regimens when compared to standard of care aprepitant containing regimens. Methods: We conducted a randomized, double-blind, placebo controlled pilot study to evaluate the efficacy of olanzapine compared to aprepitant for prevention of chemotherapy-induced nausea and vomiting. Twenty patients consented to the protocol and 19/20 were evaluable (1 lost daily diary). Episodes of emesis and use of rescue medicines were recorded using a daily diary and nausea was measured using the MD Anderson Symptom Inventory (MDASI) for the first 2 cycles of chemotherapy. Results: Complete response (CR) rates for both cycles during the acute period were 62.5% for olanzapine versus 33.3% for aprepitant, and CR rates for the delayed period were 66.7% for olanzapine versus 55.6% for aprepitant. Conclusion: Olanzapine containing regimens were well tolerated and offered similar efficacy as aprepitant containing regimens.

* Correspondence: Lieutenant Colonel Nathan M Shumway DO, MC, USA, FACP, Program Director, Hematology/Oncology Fellowship, SAMMC, 3551 Roger Brooke Drive, Fort Sam Houston, TX 78234, United States. E-mail: nathanshumway@mac.com.

Keywords: cancer, chemotherapy, nausea, vomiting, olanzapine

Introduction

Chemotherapy-induced nausea and vomiting (CINV) can severely affect quality of life in cancer patients. (1) This in turn can adversely affect treatment outcomes due to non-compliance or untoward side effects from vomiting (electrolyte disturbances, poor nutrition, injury to healing wound sites, or injury to the gastrointestinal tract) which can delay or prevent further therapy (2). Estimates of the prevalence of CINV have been as high as 70-80% (3).

Newer agents have been introduced which have led to improvement in the incidence of CINV. These include serotonin 5-HT_3 receptor antagonists, dopamine receptor antagonists, dopamine-serotonin receptor antagonists, cannabinoids, and neurokinin-1 receptor antagonists. Despite providers' best efforts and the use of these newer anti-emetics, the frequency of CINV is still high. In 2004, Grunberg et al. performed a prospective observational study looking at the incidence of CINV after the use of modern anti-emetics (4). In those patients receiving moderately emetogenic chemotherapy (MEC) or highly emetogenic chemotherapy (HEC), 35% of patients experienced acute nausea and 13% experienced acute emesis. For delayed CINV, 60% of patients receiving HEC experienced nausea and 50% experienced emesis. Another conclusion by the authors was that nurses and physicians overestimated the control of CINV by 30%.

Newer targeted agents have been investigated to help improve CINV rates. In 2003, the FDA approved aprepitant (Emend) for prevention of CINV in HEC. Two phase III trials looked at complete response (CR) rates (no emesis + no use of rescue meds) in patients receiving cisplatin-based chemotherapy regimens with the addition of aprepitant to standard anti-emetic regimens (5, 6). The CR rates for the two studies during the acute period were 83% and 89% respectively and the CR rates for the delayed period were 68% and 75% respectively in the groups receiving the aprepitant containing anti-emetic regimen. Despite these newer targeted therapies, CINV remains a challenge for both patients and providers. Further investigation is warranted to help maximize efficacy, decrease toxicity, and maintain cost-effective care. One approach has been the investigation of dopamine antagonists to help prevent CINV. Metoclopramide (Reglan) has been used in the past, but is limited by extrapyramidal adverse reactions (7). The dopamine antagonist metopimazine (Vogalene), when added to the serotonin antagonist ondansetron (Zofran), was found to significantly reduce nausea and vomiting in patients receiving MEC (8). These early findings suggest that dopamine blockade could have additive contributions in preventing CINV. In fact, recent evidence has emerged using olanzapine (Zyprexa), a potent dopamine antagonist, for prevention of acute and delayed CINV.

Olanzapine is FDA approved for the treatment of schizophrenia and manic episodes in bipolar disorders. It blocks multiple neurotransmitters including: dopamine at D_1, D_2, D_3, and D_4, serotonin at 5-HT_{2a}, 5-HT_{2c}, 5-HT_3, and 5-HT_6, catecholamine receptors, α1-adrenergic receptors, and histaminic receptors (9). The most common side effects are agitation, change in personality, constipation, dizziness, dry mouth, increased appetite, indigestion, low blood pressure upon standing, sedation, tremor, weakness, and weight gain. Initial trials with olanzapine for use in preventing CINV are described below.

Passik et al. (10) performed a retrospective chart review for the use of olanzapine for prevention of CINV. They found that 28 patients had received olanzapine for the prevention of delayed emesis and therapy was well tolerated. The results of this retrospective review along with a previous pilot study using olanzapine for prevention of CINV (11), led to the development of phase I testing of olanzapine for prevention of CINV. In this phase I study, the investigators used olanzapine for the prevention of delayed CINV (12). 15 patients completed the study and there were no grade IV toxicities. 4/6 patients that received HEC and 9/9 patients receiving MEC had CR (no emesis + no use of rescue meds). This same study group published 2 phase II trials looking at olanzapine for prevention of CINV. In the first study, 30 patients getting MEC or HEC received standard 5-HT_3 antagonists with steroids plus olanzapine (5mg orally D-2, D-1, then 10mg orally D1-4) (13). CR rates were 100% for the acute period and 80% for the delayed period. In 2007, a second phase II study was published. In this study, 40 patients getting MEC and HEC received palonosetron (Aloxi) and steroids plus olanazapine (14) For cycle one, the CR rates for the acute period were 97% (MEC) and 100% (HEC). The delayed CR rates were 75% in both the MEC and HEC groups. There were no grade III/IV toxicities noted.

Based on these phase II trials, we decided to test our hypothesis that olanzapine containing regimens are just as efficacious in preventing CINV as aprepitant containing regimens in patients receiving HEC. To date, there have been no published data assessing the efficacy of olanzapine containing anti-emetic regimens to standard of care aprepitant containing regimens.

METHODS

We conducted a prospective, randomized, double-blind pilot study using olanzapine versus aprepitant containing anti-emetic regimens for the prevention of acute and delayed CINV. 20 consecutive patients who were chemotherapy naïve receiving HEC as defined by the National Comprehensive Cancer Network (NCCN) were enrolled. HEC is defined as chemotherapy that is associated with >90% frequency of emesis per the Hesketh model (15). Per NCCN guidelines, this included patients receiving doxorubin (Adriamycin) or epirubicin (Ellence) in combination with cyclophoshamide (Cytoxan).

Randomization was computer generated and performed by the central oncology pharmacy. Patients were randomized into either the standard (aprepitant) containing arm or the experimental (olanzapine) containing arm. Both groups were treated according to randomization for the first 2 cycles of chemotherapy and data was collected. For all subsequent cycles of chemotherapy, the patients were treated per their primary oncologist's discretion.

The standard (aprepitant) arm received placebo for D-2 and D-1 prior to each cycle of chemotherapy given as a black gel capsule prepared by the central oncology pharmacy. On D1, patients received standard pretreatment with dexamethasone (Decadron) at a dose of 12mg given intravenously. In addition, all patients received palonosetron (Aloxi) given at the dose of 0.25mg intravenously. Aprepitant was given at a dose of 125mg orally on D1 and was placed in a black gel capsule to ensure blinding. On D2-3, patients in the standard (aprepitant) arm received dexamethasone at a dose of 4mg orally twice daily and aprepitant at a dose of 80mg orally given daily (placed in black gel capsules). On D4, patients received dexamethasone at a dose of 4mg orally twice daily along with a placebo, black gel capsule. Breakthrough or rescue medicines were prescribed by the treating physician per their discretion (see Figure 1).

The experimental (olanzapine) arm received olanzapine 5mg orally for D-2 and D-1 given in black gel capsules. On D1, patients received standard pretreatment with dexamethasone at a dose of 12mg given intravenously. In addition, all patients received palonosetron given at the dose of 0.25mg intravenously. Olanzapine was given at a dose of 10mg orally and was placed in a black gel capsule to ensure blinding. On D2-4, patients in the experimental (olanzapine) arm received dexamethasone at a dose of 4mg orally twice daily and olanzapine given at a dose of 10mg orally once daily (placed in black gel capsules). Breakthrough or rescue medicines were prescribed by the treating physician per their discretion (see Figure 1).

	D-2	D-1	D1	D2	D3	D4
STANDARD ARM	Placebo	Placebo	Aprepitant 125mg po Decadron 12mg IV Palonosetron 0.25mg IV	Aprepitant 80 mg po Decadron 4mg po bid	Aprepitant 80 mg po Decadron 4mg po bid	Placebo Decadron 4mg po bid
EXPERIMENTAL ARM	Olanzapine 5mg po	Olanzapine 5mg po	Olanzapine 10mg po Decadron 12mg IV Palonosetron 0.25mg IV	Olanzapine 10mg po Decadron 4mg po bid	Olanzapine 10mg po Decadron 4mg po bid	Olanzapine 10mg po Decadron 4mg po bid

Treatment medications were blinded from patients and providers using black gel capsules

Figure 1. Treatment Arms.

Patient demographic and pertinent medical history were collected at the start of enrollment and included age, gender, smoking status, alcohol use, height, weight, and Eastern Cooperative Oncology Group (ECOG) performance status. Medical and demographic history were collected from the outpatient electronic medical record system. Patients were given a daily diary to record episodes of emesis/retching and use of rescue medicines. In addition, patients were asked to fill out the MD Anderson Symptom Inventory (MDASI) (16). The MDASI measures symptoms experienced by patients with cancer. It consists of 13 core symptoms rated on their presence and severity along with six questions rating how much symptoms interfered with different aspects of a patient's life. Nausea was recorded as present if patients answered ≥ 1 for question number three on the MDASI ("Your nausea at its WORST?"). Significant nausea was recorded as present if patients answered ≥ 3. Daily queries from the investigators were performed to remind patients to fill out forms and ask about toxicities. Data was recorded for 6 days each cycle during treatment (D-1, D-2, D1, D2, D3, D4).

Inclusion criteria required patients ≥18 years of age with histologically or cytologically confirmed malignant disease who were chemotherapy naïve and scheduled to receive HEC as defined by the NCCN guidelines.

Patients were excluded if they had documented nausea or vomiting in the 24 hours prior to beginning anti-emetic therapy (D-2). Other exclusion criteria included serum creatinine ≥2mg/dL; serum bilirubin ≥2 mg/dL; SGOT or SGPT ≥ 3 times the upper limit of normal, and absolute neutrophil count ≤1500 mm^3. Patients of childbearing age (male and female) must have consented to use of adequate contraception throughout protocol therapy; women of childbearing age must have had a negative serum pregnancy test; no severe cognitive compromise; no history of CNS disease (e.g., uncontrolled brain mets, seizure disorder); no treatment with another antipsychotic agent such as risperidone (Risperdal), quetiapine (Seroquel), clozapine(Clozaril), phenothiazine, or butyrophenone for 30 days prior to or during protocol therapy. No chronic phenothiazine administration as an antipsychotic agent was allowed, but patients may have been receiving prochlorperazine (Compazine) and other phenothiazines as rescue antiemetic therapy. No concurrent use of amifostine (Ethyol); no concurrent abdominal radiotherapy; no concurrent use of quinolone antibiotic therapy; no chronic alcoholism (as determined by the investigator); no known hypersensitivity to olanzapine; no known cardiac arrhythmia, uncontrolled congestive heart failure, or acute myocardial infarction within the previous 6 months and no history of uncontrolled diabetes, no history of stroke, and no dementia related psychoses.

ETHICS

All patients gave written informed consent, and the study was approved by the institutional review committee.

Statistics

A pilot study was performed with 10 subjects per group. The primary endpoint for the efficacy analysis was the proportion of patients with complete response, defined as no emesis and no use of rescue medicines. This endpoint was recorded for the acute period (D1), the delayed period (D2-4), and the total period (D1-4). Additional endpoints included complete response rates for the anticipatory period (D-2, D-1 for the second cycle of chemotherapy only). Nausea was recorded as present if patients answered ≥1 for question number three on the MDASI ("Your nausea at its WORST?"). Significant nausea was recorded as present if patients answered ≥3. Toxicity rates using the Common Terminology Criteria for Adverse Events (CTCAE) version 3.0 were recorded by investigators via telephone consult for both cycles (D-2, D-1, D1, D2, D3, D4) Response rates were compared between groups using Fisher's exact test (two-tailed). Data was analyzed using SPSS for Windows (v. 17, SPSS Inc., Chicago, IL).

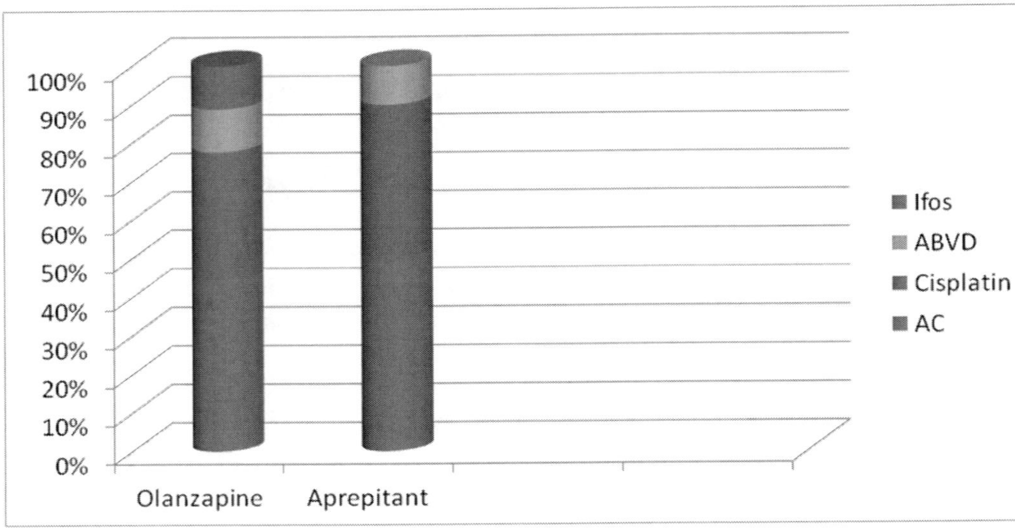

Abbreviations: Ifos, ifosfamide (Ifex); ABVD, doxorubicin (Adriamycin), bleomycin, vinblastine, dacarbazine (DTIC); AC, doxorubicin (Adriamycin), cyclophosphamide (Cytoxan)

Figure 2. Types of chemotherapy per treatment arm.

Results

20 patients were enrolled and randomized to either the olanzapine (OLN) or aprepitant (APR) containing regimen. 19 patients were evaluable (1 patient lost daily diary in the olanzapine group). 63% of the patients were women. In the OLN group 56% were women compared to 70% in the APR group. Median age was 54 in the OLN group compared to 60 in the APR group. ECOG PS, height, weight, smoking, alcohol use, and cancer type for both groups are presented on Table 1. Types of chemotherapy are presented on Figure 2 (see Figure 2).

During the acute period (D1) for both cycles combined the CR was 62.5% for OLN compared to 33.3% in the APR group ($p = 0.35$). For the delayed period (D2-4) for both cycles combined the CR was 66.7% for OLN compared to 55.6% in the APR group ($p = 0.99$). For the overall period (D1-4) for both cycles combined, the CR was 44.4% for OLN compared to 22.2% in the APR group ($p = 0.62$). CR rates for each cycle and both cycles combined are shown in Figure 2.

Anticipatory CR rates (cycle 2 only) were 88.9% in the OLN group compared to 100% in the APR group ($p = 0.99$). Rates of nausea for the overall period (D1-4) were 77.8% for OLN compared to 70% in the APR group ($p = 0.99$). Rates of significant nausea for the overall period were 33.3% in the OLN group compared to 40% in the APR arm ($p = 0.99$) (see Table 2)

Both treatment arms were well tolerated with only one grade III toxicity in the APR group (grade III heartburn requiring ER visit). Grade I fatigue was noted in 44.4% of OLN group compared to 20% in the APR group ($p = 0.35$). Grade I insomnia occurred in one patient in the OLN group.

Table 1. Patient baseline characteristics by treatment group

	Olanzapine **n = 9**	**Aprepitant** **n = 10**
Sex, female	55.6	70
Age, years Median	54	60.5
ECOG PS		
0	77.8	50
1	22.2	40
2	0	10
Height		
inches	67	65.5
Weight pounds	178	173
Smoking		
Never	55.6	40
Current	22.2	30
Past	22.2	30
Alcohol		
Never	33.3	30
Current or past	66.7	70
Cancer type		
Breast	44.4	50
Lung	22.2	40
Hodgkins	11.1	10
Head and neck	11.1	0
Sarcoma	11.1	0

NOTE. All data are given as percent of patients, unless otherwise noted.
Abbreviations: ECOG PS, Eastern Cooperative Oncology Group performance status.

Table 2. Percentages of patients reaching defined endpoints by study phase and treatment group

	Acute D1 **OLN**	Acute D1 **APR**	Delayed D2-4 **OLN**	Delayed D2-4 **APR**	Overall D1-4 **OLN**	Overall D1-4 **APR**
Complete response (Cycle 1)	87.5	70	100	70	87.5	60
Complete response (Cycle 2)	77.8	66.7	66.7	77.8	55.6	55.6
Complete response (both cycles)	62.5	33.3	66.7	55.6	44.4	22.2
Rates of nausea -both cycles	66.7	50	55.6	70	77.8	70
Rates of significant nausea -both cycles	22	20	11.1	30	33.3	40

NOTE: Complete response indicates no emesis or use of rescue medicine. Presence of nausea was defined as answering question 3 on the MDASI with a score of ≥ 1 and significant nausea defined as a score ≥ 3.

Grade I constipation occurred in 2 patients in the APR arm ($p = 0.47$). Grade I diarrhea occurred in 1 patient in the APR arm. Grade I xerostomia occurred in 2 patients in the OLN arm compared to 1 patient in the APR arm ($p = 0.58$).

Grade I hiccups occurred in 1 patient in the APR group. Grade I heartburn occurred in 1 patient the APR arm. Grade I sensory neuropathy occurred in one patient in the OLN arm with tingling of the tip of the tongue. Grade II fatigue was noted in 1 patient in the APR arm. Grade I dyspnea was recorded in 1 patient in the APR arm. Grade I dizziness was reported in 2 patients in the OLN arm and none in the APR arm ($p = 0.21$).

DISCUSSION

Despite recent advances in the treatment of CINV for HEC with the use of aprepitant, approximately 32% of patients will fail to achieve complete responses from antiemetics during both the acute and delayed periods (17). In addition to emesis and use of rescue medicines, this same pooled analysis showed that rates of nausea in the overall period were 52% in the aprepitant containing arm versus 58% in the control group ($p < 0.05$).

One reason for the difficulty in treating CINV may be its complex pathophysiology. In a recent review, key mechanisms of action for the etiology of CINV were discussed (18). The primary component deals with the generation of oxygen radicals produced after administration of systemic chemotherapy. These radicals cause release of 5-HT from the enterochromaffin cells in the gut, which in turn interact with 5-HT_3 receptors of vagal afferents leading to stimulation of the nucleus tractus solitarius (NTS) in the brain which can lead to emesis. Another mechanism involves the direct toxic effect of chemotherapy on the area postrema (AP), part of the dorsal vagal complex in the brain where the blood-brain barrier is more permeable. Both the NTS and AP have multiple receptors for several neurotransmitters. The most important include neurokinin-1, 5-HT_3, and D_2. Both newer and older agents that target these receptors may help our control of CINV.

Recently, data has been published showing the efficacy of a new, novel neurokinin-1 antagonist, casopitant mesylate (19, 20). Interestingly, casopitant was found to have similar efficacy as a single day dose when compared to 3-day dosing. Fosaprepitant (Emend for injection), a water soluble prodrug of aprepitant is currently approved by the FDA and the European union at a dose of 115mg given intravenously as an alternative to the 125mg oral dose of aprepitant on D1 of therapy. Currently, patients still require the 80mg oral dose of aprepitant for D2 and D3 of therapy (21). Future studies assessing the safety and efficacy of single dose fosaprepitant are ongoing.

Even with these new, active agents for better control of CINV, many patients fail to receive delayed CINV prophylaxis. Grunberg discussed some of the problems associated with implementation of antiemetic guidelines (22). Examples of improving guideline adherence were discussed including measures to cut costs such as improving in-house guidelines and use of standard antiemetic order sets. Another interesting program was described that encouraged providers to review patient symptom diaries which seemed to improve the providers adherence to antiemetic recommendations. With increased access to newer therapies and improvement in guideline adherence, the use of these agents for prevention of CINV will likely increase along with costs of supportive care.

At our military institution, the cost for aprepitant therapy is $180 per cycle. The cost of olanzapine as given in this study is $9.42 per cycle of chemotherapy. As new data emerges showing efficacy of aprepitant in MEC (23-25), we anticipate our use of aprepitant to increase along with our costs. In this setting, we sought to evaluate olanzapine for the treatment of CINV in patients receiving HEC. Our hypothesis was that olanzapine containing antiemetic regimens were just as efficacious as aprepitant containing regimens and much less expensive. Despite recent studies suggesting cost-effectiveness with use of aprepitant-containing regimens (26-28), further cost savings may be possible in our tertiary care military medical center with the use of older agents such as olanzapine.

In our randomized, double blind pilot study comparing olanzapine to aprepitant for prevention of CINV in HEC, it appears that both arms were efficacious and well tolerated. It is important to note that the majority of our patients were breast cancer patients receiving anthracycline-based therapy and therefore our results may not be applicable to patients receiving cisplatin-containing regimens. Our very small sample size also limits the applicability of our results. Sample size was too small to ensure balance between treatment arms or to enable statistically significant differences to be noted. In addition, adequate evaluation of toxicity with olanzapine, a medicine often described as having a low therapeutic index, is difficult to ascertain in a small pilot study. Despite these shortcomings, this pilot study represents the first time olanzapine-containing regimens have been compared to standard of care aprepitant containing regimens for prevention of CINV. With the current healthcare climate focusing on cost-savings, we are considering opening a large, multicenter study to look at non-inferiority of olanzapine-containing regimens.

In summary, olanzapine-containing antiemetic regimens were well tolerated and offered similar efficacy compared with the standard of care aprepitant-containing regimens in preventing CINV in patients receiving HEC. Larger studies are needed to evaluate non-inferiority, toxicity, and potential cost savings of olanzapine containing regimens.

ACKNOWLEDGMENTS

We would like to thank Robin S Howard, MA for her help with statistical analysis and use of SPSS software. The opinions or assertions contained herein are the private views of the authors and are not to be construed as official or reflecting the views of the US Army or the US Department of Defense. All of the other authors have no conflicts of interest relevant to the contents of this manuscript.

REFERENCES

[1] Cohen L, de Moor CA, Eisenberg P, Ming EE, Hu H. Chemotherapy-induced nausea and vomiting: incidence and impact on patient quality of life at community oncology settings. Support Care Cancer 2007;15(5):497-503.

[2] Richardson JL, Marks G, Levine A. The influence of symptoms of disease and side effects of treatment on compliance with cancer therapy. J Clin Oncol 1988;6(11):1746-52.

[3] Morran C, Smith DC, Anderson DA, McArdle CS. Incidence of nausea and vomiting with cytotoxic chemotherapy: a prospective randomised trial of antiemetics. BMJ 1979;1(6174):1323-4.

[4] Grunberg SM, Deuson RR, Mavros P, Geling O, Hansen M, Cruciani G, et al. Incidence of chemotherapy-induced nausea and emesis after modern antiemetics. Cancer 2004;100(10):2261-8.

[5] Poli-Bigelli S, Rodrigues-Pereira J, Carides AD, Julie Ma G, Eldridge K, Hipple A, et al. Addition of the neurokinin 1 receptor antagonist aprepitant to standard antiemetic therapy improves control of chemotherapy-induced nausea and vomiting. Results from a randomized, double-blind, placebo-controlled trial in Latin America. Cancer 2003;97(12):3090-8.

[6] Hesketh PJ, Grunberg SM, Gralla RJ, Warr DG, Roila F, de Wit R, et al. The oral neurokinin-1 antagonist aprepitant for the prevention of chemotherapy-induced nausea and vomiting: a multinational, randomized, double-blind, placebo-controlled trial in patients receiving high-dose cisplatin--the Aprepitant Protocol 052 Study Group. J Clin Oncol 2003;21(22):4112-9.

[7] Bateman DN, Rawlins MD, Simpson JM. Extrapyramidal reactions with metoclopramide. Br Med J (Clin Res Ed) 1985;291(6500):930-2.

[8] Herrstedt J, Sigsgaard T, Boesgaard M, Jensen TP, Dombernowsky P. Ondansetron plus metopimazine compared with ondansetron alone in patients receiving moderately emetogenic chemotherapy. N Engl J Med 1993;328(15):1076-80.

[9] Navari RM. Pharmacological management of chemotherapy-induced nausea and vomiting: focus on recent developments. Drugs 2009;69(5):515-33.

[10] Passik SD, Kirsh KL, Theobald DE, Dickerson P, Trowbridge R, Gray D, et al. A retrospective chart review of the use of olanzapine for the prevention of delayed emesis in cancer patients. J Pain Symptom Manage 2003;25(5):485-8.

[11] Passik SD, Lundberg J, Kirsh KL, Theobald D, Donaghy K, Holtsclaw E, et al. A pilot exploration of the antiemetic activity of olanzapine for the relief of nausea in patients with advanced cancer and pain. J Pain Symptom Manage 2002;23(6):526-32.

[12] Passik SD, Navari RM, Jung SH, Nagy C, Vinson J, Kirsh KL, et al. A phase I trial of olanzapine (Zyprexa) for the prevention of delayed emesis in cancer patients: a Hoosier Oncology Group study. Cancer Invest 2004;22(3):383-8.

[13] Navari RM, Einhorn LH, Passik SD, Loehrer PJ Sr, Johnson C, Mayer ML, et al. A phase II trial of olanzapine for the prevention of chemotherapy-induced nausea and vomiting: a Hoosier Oncology Group study. Support Care Cancer 2005;13(7):529-34.

[14] Navari RM, Einhorn LH, Loehrer PJ Sr, Passik SD, Vinson J, McClean J, et al. A phase II trial of olanzapine, dexamethasone, and palonosetron for the prevention of chemotherapy-induced nausea and vomiting: a Hoosier oncology group study. Support Care Cancer 2007;15(11):1285-91.

[15] Hesketh PJ, Kris MG, Grunberg SM, Beck T, Hainsworth JD, Harker G, et al. Proposal for classifying the acute emetogenicity of cancer chemotherapy. J Clin Oncol 1997;15(1):103-9.

[16] Cleeland CS, Mendoza TR, Wang XS, Chou C, Harle MT, Morrissey M, et al. Assessing symptom distress in cancer patients: the M.D. Anderson Symptom Inventory. Cancer 2000;89(7):1634-46.

[17] Warr DG, Grunberg SM, Gralla RJ, Hesketh PJ, Roila F, Wit Rd, et al. The oral NK(1) antagonist aprepitant for the prevention of acute and delayed chemotherapy-induced nausea and vomiting: Pooled data from 2 randomised, double-blind, placebo controlled trials. Eur J Cancer 2005;41(9):1278-85.

[18] Hesketh PJ. Chemotherapy-induced nausea and vomiting. N Engl J Med 2008;358(23):2482-94.

[19] Roila F, Rolski J, Ramlau R, Dediu M, Russo MW, Bandekar RR, et al. Randomized, double-blind, dose-ranging trial of the oral neurokinin-1 receptor antagonist casopitant mesylate for the prevention of cisplatin-induced nausea and vomiting. Ann Oncol. 2009 Nov;20(11):1867-73.

[20] Grunberg SM, Rolski J, Strausz J, Aziz Z, Lane S, Russo MW, et al. Efficacy and safety of casopitant mesylate, a neurokinin 1 (NK1)-receptor antagonist, in prevention of chemotherapy-induced nausea and vomiting in patients receiving cisplatin-based highly emetogenic chemotherapy: a randomised, double-blind, placebo-controlled trial. Lancet Oncol 2009;10(6):549-58.

[21] Navari RM. Antiemetic control: toward a new standard of care for emetogenic chemotherapy. Expert Opin Pharmacother 2009;10(4):629-44.

[22] Grunberg SM. Obstacles to the implementation of antiemetic guidelines. J Natl Compr Canc Netw 2009;7(5):601-5.

[23] Warr DG, Hesketh PJ, Gralla RJ, Muss HB, Herrstedt J, Eisenberg PD, et al. Efficacy and tolerability of aprepitant for the prevention of chemotherapy-induced nausea and vomiting in patients with breast cancer after moderately emetogenic chemotherapy. J Clin Oncol 2005;23(12):2822-30.

[24] Yeo W, Mo FK, Suen JJ, Ho WM, Chan SL, Lau W, et al. A randomized study of aprepitant, ondansetron and dexamethasone for chemotherapy-induced nausea and vomiting in Chinese breast cancer patients receiving moderately emetogenic chemotherapy. Breast Cancer Res Treat 2009;113(3):529-35.

[25] Rapoport BL, Jordan K, Boice JA, Taylor A, Brown C, Hardwick JS, et al. Aprepitant for the prevention of chemotherapy-induced nausea and vomiting associated with a broad range of moderately emetogenic chemotherapies and tumor types: a randomized, double-blind study. Support Care Cancer. 2010 Apr;18(4):423-31.

[26] Lordick F, Ehlken B, Ihbe-Heffinger A, Berger K, Krobot KJ, Pellissier J, et al. Health outcomes and cost-effectiveness of aprepitant in outpatients receiving antiemetic prophylaxis for highly emetogenic chemotherapy in Germany. Eur J Cancer 2007;43(2):299-307.

[27] Moore S, Tumeh J, Wojtanowski S, Flowers C. Cost-effectiveness of aprepitant for the prevention of chemotherapy-induced nausea and vomiting associated with highly emetogenic chemotherapy. Value Health 2007;10(1):23-31.

[28] Annemans L, Strens D, Lox E, Petit C, Malonne H. Cost-effectiveness analysis of aprepitant in the prevention of chemotherapy-induced nausea and vomiting in Belgium. Support Care Cancer 2008;16(8):905-15.

Submitted: May 20, 2015. *Revised:* June 25, 2015. *Accepted:* July 09, 2015.

In: Pain Management Yearbook 2015
Editor: Joav Merrick
ISBN: 978-1-63484-515-1

Chapter 27

SOCIAL DETERMINANTS OF QUALITY OF LIFE IN ADVANCED CANCER PATIENTS WITH BRAIN METASTASES UNDERGOING PALLIATIVE RADIOTHERAPY

Alvin Szeto[1], MD(C), Paul Cheon[1], MD(C), Liying Zhang[1], PhD, Natalie Pulenzas[1], MD(C), Marc Kerba[2], MD, Palmira Foro[3], MD, Brita Danielson[4], MD, Kinsey Lam[1], MD, Breanne Lechner[1], MD(C) and Edward Chow[1,*], MBBS

[1]Sunnybrook Odette Cancer Centre,
University of Toronto, Toronto, Ontario, Canada
[2]Division of Radiation Oncology, Department of Oncology,
Tom Baker Cancer Center, University of Calgary, Alberta, Canada
[3]Department of Radiation Oncology, Parc de Salut Mar, Barcelona Spain,
Universitat Pompeu Fabra, Barcelona, Spain
[4]Department of Oncology, Cross Cancer Institute,
University of Alberta, Alberta, Canada

Social determinants of health (SDOH) such as age, gender, marital status, education and employment may affect quality of life (QOL). This study analyzes SDOH in patients with brain metastases undergoing whole brain radiotherapy. Methods: The European Organization for Research and Treatment of Cancer Quality of Life Questionnaire brain module (EORTC QLQ-BN20+2) was administered to 156 patients from four centres (3 Canadian, 1 Spanish), at baseline and 1-month follow-up post-treatment. Univariate and multivariate analyses of variance were used to identify important factors at baseline. Wilcoxon rank-sum or Kruskal-Wallis tested scale changes of different variables between

[*] Correspondence: Professor Edward Chow MBBS, MSc, PhD, FRCPC, Department of Radiation Oncology, Odette Cancer Centre, Sunnybrook Health Sciences Centre, 2075 Bayview Avenue, Toronto Ontario, M4N 3M5, Canada. E-mail: edward.chow@sunnybrook.ca.

baseline and follow-up. Results: Median age was 61 years and 53% of participants were female. Median Karnofsky Performance Status (KPS) was 80. Primary cancer sites included lung (52%), breast (23%), and gastrointestinal (10%). At baseline, patient KPS > 80 predicted lower visual disorder ($p = 0.01$), motor dysfunction ($p < 0.0001$), drowsiness ($p = 0.045$), bladder dysfunction ($p=0.01$), and communication deficit ($p = 0.04$). Female gender predicted more difficulty remembering ($p = 0.02$) and higher communication deficit scales ($p = 0.02$). Age < 60 predicted fewer seizure-related issues ($p = 0.01$). Employment predicted lower visual disorder scales ($p = 0.001$). Marital status predicted less motor dysfunction ($p = 0.02$). Between baseline and follow-up, KPS >80 predicted greater decreases in pruritus ($p = 0.03$); female gender predicted greater decreases in future uncertainty ($p = 0.01$) and communication deficit scales ($p = 0.02$); age < 60 ($p = 0.03$) and employment ($p = 0.02$) predicted greater decreases in visual disorders. Conclusion: KPS had significant impacts on BN20+2 domain scores. SDOH had less importance across domains. Further defining these associations will help develop palliative strategies aimed to improve QOL.

Keywords: quality of life, social determinants, baseline factors, EORTC QLQ-BN20, brain metastases, advanced cancer

INTRODUCTION

Brain metastases are a cause of significant morbidity and mortality, where an estimated 25-40% of cancer patients will develop brain metastases at some point in the course of their illness (1). With improved imaging and screening, an increasing incidence of brain metastases will be observed (2). Patients with multiple brain metastases often face poor prognoses; median survival is only 3-6 months even with whole brain radiation therapy (WBRT) (3). Treatment for brain metastases is aimed at improving or preserving health-related quality of life (HRQOL) (4, 5). In addition to treatment, social determinants of health (SDOH) are also considered important and underexplored factors for affecting HRQOL (6). Patients with cancer have reported that unmet needs were primarily psychosocial and correlated with poorer HRQOL (7).

HRQOL is a multidimensional construct that involves both physical and psychosocial aspects; standardized questionnaires have been formulated to collect and analyze these subjective parameters (8). However, a recent comprehensive review of WBRT for treatments with multiple brain metastases identified that only a single randomized trial had included HRQOL as an endpoint (9). The European Organization for Research and Treatment of Cancer Core Quality of Life Questionnaire (EORTC QLQ) BN20+2 was developed as a supplementary module for patients with primary brain tumours (10). This questionnaire is completed in conjunction with the EORTC-QLQ-C30 which is a general questionnaire that assesses physical, functional, social and psychological domains (11).

The World Health Organization (WHO) has recognized the importance of the social determinants of health (SDOH), and there has since been a shift to identify these factors in the clinical setting and improve patient care (12). SDOHs identify a variety of social factors that predispose those of greater social and economic disadvantage at a greater risk of ill health. Social determinants, including but not limited to: income, education, class, gender, ethnicity, and occupation, play vital roles into population and individual health. Socioeconomic gradients and their link to cancer have been reviewed elsewhere (13).

Despite improvements and variety of possible therapies for single and multiple brain metastases, prognosis is still generally poor. Recursive partitioning analysis (RPA) Class I Patients (< 65 years of age with KPS > 70), have a median overall survival (OS) of 7.1 months. Class II patients (>65 years of age with KPS > 70) have median OS of 4.2 months, while Class 3 (KPS < 70) have a media OS of 2.3 months (14). Approximately 65% of patients present some form of cognitive impairment (2).

HRQOL can be seen as a balance between minimizing treatment side effects and maximizing benefits, including physical and psychosocial effects (15). Aside from clinical intervention, the socioeconomic aspect of a patients' life plays a vital role in their HRQOL. This study aimed to identify potential relationships between SDOH and HRQOL in this cohort of patients.

METHODS

Patients with advanced cancer and brain metastases received WBRT. Three Canadian sites and 1 Spanish site completed the EORTC QLQ-BN20+2 and the EORTC-QLQ-C15-PAL at baseline and at a one-month follow-up between October 2009 and July 2010. All research was conducted upon approval by the respective research ethics board at each institution. Patients over the age of 18 years with documented single or multiple brain metastases and who were able to provide written consent were eligible for the study. Patients completed the Mini Mental State Examination (MMSE) to ensure they were cognitively able to complete the assessment (16). A score of 23 or lower out of 30 was indicative of cognitive impairment. Patients who were not native speakers of the translated language of the EORTC QLQ-BN20+2 were not included.

The baseline collection demographic forms and EORTC QLQ-BN20+2 were administered to 156 patients with single or multiple brain metastases; and structured interviews were conducted with each patient individually after completion the questionnaire. Interviews were conducted in person by the trained research assistant (at the baseline assessment) and either by telephone or in person (if the patient was booked to return to the clinic) at the follow-up assessment.

Baseline data collection forms were used to collect demographic information (date of birth/age, gender, cohabitants, marital status, education level, and employment status), clinical data (primary cancer site, date of diagnosis of primary cancer, date of diagnosis of brain metastases, and previous local and systemic treatments), and current treatment (extent of known metastases, KPS at time of interview).

EORTC-QLQ-BN20+2 QUESTIONNAIRE

The EORTC-QLQ-BN20 is a HRQOL questionnaire developed for patients with primary brain tumours (10). This questionnaire consists of four scales (future uncertainty, visual disorder, motor dysfunction, and communication deficit), and seven individual items (headaches, seizures, drowsiness, hair loss, itchy skin, weakness of legs, and bladder control). The BN20+2 was developed by adding a two-item cognitive functioning scale (communication deficit and remembering difficulty), building upon the BN20 questionnaire that has been validated for use in patients with primary brain malignancies (17). Respondents rate each item on a Likert scale from 1 (not at all) to 4 (very much), with the exception of global health/HRQOL, which was rated from 1 (very poor) to 7 (excellent). All items are linearly transformed to a 0–100 scale. For the functioning scales and the global quality of life scales, a higher score represents a better level of functioning. A higher score for a symptom scale item represents greater symptom severity.

Statistical analysis

Summary statistics were calculated for eight patient groups based on baseline determinants: age (> 60 or ≤ 60), KPS (> 80 or ≤ 80), gender (female or male), married (Yes or No), education level (elementary school, high school, university, masters or PhD, or Other), employment (employed, unemployed, retired), cohabitant (spouse, spouse and child(ren), child(ren), alone, or other), and primary cancer site (breast, prostate, lung, gastrointestinal (GI), renal cell, other). Results were expressed as mean, standard deviation (SD), median and range for continuous variables and as proportions for categorical baseline determinants.

Simple univariate analysis of variance (ANOVA) was applied for detecting significant relationship between each BN20+2 scale and demographic factors at baseline. Natural log-transformation was applied for each BN20+2 scale to normalize the distribution. The outcome is natural log scale for each BN20+2 scale, and the independent variable was eight demographic covariates (age, KPS, gender, marital status, education level, employment status, cohabitants, primary cancer site).

After conducting univariate linear regression analysis, backward selection procedure was used to select the most significant items related to each BN20 scale. Multivariate analysis was performed on variables which were significant from univariate ($p<0.10$). P-value< 0.05 was considered as statistical significance. To compare baseline and follow-up scores, Wilcoxon Signed rank test was used. To compare BN20+2 changes from baseline to follow-up in patients with different demographics, Wilcoxon rank-sum test was used for comparing patients with different age group, KPS, gender, and marital status. Kruskal-Wallis nonparametric test was used for comparing patients with different education level, employment status, cohabitant, and primary cancer site. All analyses were conducted using Statistical Analysis Software (SAS version 9.3 for Windows).

RESULTS

One hundred fifty-six patients from two countries (four sites) completed the EORTC QLQ-BN20+2 at baseline, of whom data were available for 100 at follow-up (Table 1). Female patients made up 53.2% of the study population patients, while 46.8% were male. Median age was 61 years (range: 22-86) and median KPS was 75.6 (range: 40-100). Of these patients, 74.7% were married and 84.5% of them lived with a spouse, child or other cohabitant. The most common primary cancer sites were lung (51.5%), breast (22.6%), gastrointestinal (10.3%), melanoma (5.8%) and renal cell (3.2%). At follow-up, three EORTC QLQ-BN20+2 domain scales (future uncertainty, visual disorder, and concentrating difficulty) and three item scales (drowsiness, hair loss, itchy skin) demonstrated significant changes from baseline.

Table 1. Baseline demographics

	BN (N = 156)
Age at baseline (years)	
n	156
Mean (SD)	60.3 (11.4)
Median (range)	61 (22-86)
> 60 years	80
≤ 60 years	76
KPS at baseline	
n	153
Mean (SD)	75.6 (14.4)
Median (range)	80 (40-100)
> 80	46
≤ 80	107
Gender	
Female	83
Male	73
Education level	
Elementary School	14
High School	64
University	50
Masters or PhD	5
Others	18
Employment status	
Retired	72
Employed	48
Unemployed	32
Cohabitants	
Spouse	64
Spouse and child(ren)	42
Alone	24
Child(ren)	13
Others	12
Married	
Yes	115
No	39
Primary cancer site	
Lung	80
Breast	35
Gastrointestinal	16
Melanoma	9
Renal Cell	5
Other	10
No. of Brain metastases	
1	43
2 to 3	54
>3	51

At baseline (see Table 2)

At baseline, patient KPS >80 predicted lower visual disorder (p = 0.01), motor dysfunction (p < 0.0001), drowsiness (p = 0.045), bladder dysfunction (p = 0.01), and communication deficit (p = 0.04) scales. Female gender predicted more difficulty remembering (p = 0.02) and higher communication deficits scales (p = 0.02). Age < 60 predicted fewer seizure-related issues (p = 0.01). Employment predicted lower visual disorder scales (p = 0.001). Marital status predicted less motor dysfunction (p = 0.02).

Table 2. EORTC-QLQ-BN20+2 domain scores changes at baseline. P-value < 0.005 was considered as statistical significance

Domain	Demographic Covariates	Coefficient	SE	p-value
Visual Disorder	KPS > 80 (1 = Y, 0 = N)	-0.697	0.275	0.0124
	Employment Status (Overall Effect)			0.0052
	Employed vs. Unemployed	1.166	0.357	0.0014
	Retired vs. Unemployed	0.566	0.332	0.0904
Motor Dysfunction	KPS > 80 (1 = Y, 0 = N)	-1.003	0.247	<.0001
	Married (1 = Y, 0 = N)	-0.637	0.259	0.0152
	Intercept = 0.093; MSE = 1.098			
Seizure	Age > 60 years (1 = Y, 0 = N)	0.451	0.169	0.0085
Drowsiness	KPS > 80 (1 = Y, 0 = N)	-0.657	0.327	0.0454
Itchy Skin	Married (1 = Y, 0 = N)	-0.885	0.259	0.0009
Weakness of Legs	Educational level (Overall Effect)			0.0391
	Elementary School vs. University, Masters or PhD	0.617	0.552	0.2652
	High School vs. University, Masters or PhD	0.527	0.342	0.1260
	Other Education vs. University, Masters or PhD	1.437	0.501	0.0048
Bladder Control	KPS > 80 (1 = Y, 0 = N)	-0.762	0.283	0.0079
Communication Deficit	KPS > 80 (1 = Y, 0 = N)	-0.684	0.333	0.0428
	Gender (1 = F, 0 = M)	0.800	0.324	0.0151
Remembering Difficulty	Gender (1 = F, 0 = M)	1.006	0.412	0.0164
	Primary Cancer Site (Overall Effect)			0.0267
	Lung vs. Breast	-1.079	0.510	0.0367
	Gastrointestinal vs. Breast	0.384	0.818	0.6400
	Other vs. Breast	-0.267	0.690	0.7001

Table 3. EORTC QLQ-BN20+2 domain score changes between baseline and follow-up. P-value <0.05 was considered as statistical significance

BN20+2 Changes (Follow-up – Baseline)	Demographic Covariates	p-value
Concentrating difficulty	Age > 60 years (1 = Y, 0 = N)	0.2975
	KPS > 80 (1 = Y, 0 = N)	0.2735
	Gender (1 = F, 0 = M)	0.9876
	Married (1 = Y, 0 = N)	0.9964
	Education	0.7700
	Employment Status	0.4967
	Cohabitant	0.8590
	Primary Cancer Site	0.8511
Future uncertainty	Age > 60 years (1 = Y, 0 = N)	0.1695
	KPS > 80 (1 = Y, 0 = N)	0.5018
	Gender (1 = F, 0 = M)	**0.0096** *
	Married (1 = Y, 0 = N)	0.2889
	Education	0.0796
	Employment Status	0.8919
	Cohabitant	0.8577
	Primary Cancer Site	0.6365
Visual disorder	**Age > 60 years (1 = Y, 0 = N)**	**0.0284** *
	KPS > 80 (1 = Y, 0 = N)	0.2694
	Gender (1 = F, 0 = M)	0.5009
	Married (1 = Y, 0 = N)	0.4844
	Education	0.0527
	Employment Status	**0.0150** *
	Cohabitant	0.1694
	Primary Cancer Site	0.1220
Motor dysfunction	Age > 60 years (1 = Y, 0 = N)	0.4194
	KPS > 80 (1 = Y, 0 = N)	0.5583
	Gender (1 = F, 0 = M)	0.7503
	Married (1 = Y, 0 = N)	0.8962
	Education	0.4104
	Employment Status	0.1713
	Cohabitant	0.0854
	Primary Cancer Site	0.9878
Headaches	Age > 60 years (1 = Y, 0 = N)	0.8236
	KPS > 80 (1 = Y, 0 = N)	0.6700
	Gender (1 = F, 0 = M)	0.0542
	Married (1 = Y, 0 = N)	0.5558
	Education	0.6855
	Employment Status	0.6558
	Cohabitant	0.8681
	Primary Cancer Site	0.0688
Seizures	Age > 60 years (1 = Y, 0 = N)	0.1529
	KPS > 80 (1 = Y, 0 = N)	0.7907
	Gender (1 = F, 0 = M)	0.8753
	Married (1 = Y, 0 = N)	0.8937
	Education	0.8018
	Employment Status	0.3560
	Cohabitant	0.7850
	Primary Cancer Site	0.8081
Drowsiness	Age > 60 years (1 = Y, 0 = N)	0.2283
	KPS > 80 (1 = Y, 0 = N)	0.8958
	Gender (1 = F, 0 = M)	0.6357

Table 3. (Continued).

BN20+2 Changes (Follow-up – Baseline)	Demographic Covariates	p-value
	Married (1 = Y, 0 = N)	0.2792
	Education	0.2779
	Employment Status	0.2690
	Cohabitant	0.2582
	Primary Cancer Site	0.6559
Hair loss	Age > 60 years (1 = Y, 0 = N)	0.2689
	KPS > 80 (1 = Y, 0 = N)	0.1976
	Gender (1 = F, 0 = M)	0.9473
	Married (1 = Y, 0 = N)	0.0528
	Education	0.2768
	Employment Status	0.8963
	Cohabitant	0.4799
	Primary Cancer Site	**0.0313** *
Itchy skin	Age > 60 years (1 = Y, 0 = N)	0.2487
	KPS > 80 (1 = Y, 0 = N)	**0.0254** *
	Gender (1 = F, 0 = M)	0.5074
	Married (1 = Y, 0 = N)	0.9382
	Education	0.5527
	Employment Status	0.8606
	Cohabitant	0.9196
	Primary Cancer Site	0.1397
Weakness of legs	Age > 60 years (1 = Y, 0 = N)	0.1379
	KPS > 80 (1 = Y, 0 = N)	0.7983
	Gender (1 = F, 0 = M)	0.3449
	Married (1 = Y, 0 = N)	0.2841
	Education	0.6182
	Employment Status	0.7992
	Cohabitant	0.2084
	Primary Cancer Site	0.5175
Bladder control	Age > 60 years (1 = Y, 0 = N)	0.5874
	KPS > 80 (1 = Y, 0 = N)	0.1630
	Gender (1 = F, 0 = M)	0.8493
	Married (1 = Y, 0 = N)	0.6825
	Education	0.2391
	Employment Status	0.2817
	Cohabitant	0.6484
	Primary Cancer Site	0.3925
Communication deficit	Age > 60 years (1 = Y, 0 = N)	0.6040
	KPS > 80 (1 = Y, 0 = N)	0.4845
	Gender (1 = F, 0 = M)	**0.0171** *
	Married (1 = Y, 0 = N)	0.4165
	Education	0.4237
	Employment Status	0.3678
	Cohabitant	0.3647
	Primary Cancer Site	0.3585
Remembering difficulty	Age > 60 years (1 = Y, 0 = N)	0.7660
	KPS > 80 (1 = Y, 0 = N)	0.8670
	Gender (1 = F, 0 = M)	0.6216
	Married (1 = Y, 0 = N)	0.7224
	Education	0.9920
	Employment Status	0.9586
	Cohabitant	0.8867
	Primary Cancer Site	0.3466

Between baseline and follow-up between different demographics (see Table 3)

There were significant changes in females from baseline in future uncertainty ($p = 0.0096$) and communication deficit ($p = 0.0171$) compared to males. Females had less uncertainty about the future compared to males (mean: -13.74 in females vs. -0.06 in males). Furthermore, females reported less communication deficit compared to males (mean: -6.14 in females vs. +7.78 in males). Patients with age > 60 had significant improvements from baseline in visual disorder ($p = 0.0284$) compared to patients with age ≤ 60. However, younger patients (age ≤ 60) experienced greater overall improvements in vision (mean change: -11.1 for age ≤ 60 vs. -1.7 for age > 60).

Patients with different employment statuses had significant changes from baseline in visual disorder ($p = 0.015$). Patients who were employed report the most improvement in visual disorder compared to retired or unemployed (mean: -9.58 in employed, -2.20 in retired, -0.62 in unemployed). Patients with different primary cancer sites had significant changes from baseline in hair loss ($p = 0.0313$). Patients with lung primary cancer site had the greatest degree of improvement in hair loss compared to other cancer sites (mean: 6.48 in lung, 27.78 in breast, 33.33 in GI or Other).

DISCUSSION

The current study examined the relationship between sociodemographic, medical factors and HRQOL as assessed by BN20+2 in cancer patients with brain metastases. The BN20+2 has been previously validated for use along with the EORTC-QLQ-C15-PAL as a universal assessment tool for patients with brain metastases (17). A recent longitudinal analysis using the BN20 as a preliminary HRQOL assessment found more negative responses with the recurrence group compared to patients with primary brain tumours, including leg weakness, coordination difficulties, and unsteady gait (18). Other studies assessing HRQOL in patients with palliative brain metastases suggest that baseline QOL is prognostic of survival (19).

As the aim of palliative treatments for these patients is to improve overall HRQOL, certain criteria may help decide whether radiotherapy is appropriate for a patient given their pre-treatment cognitive status. A recent systematic review found that radiosurgery and WBRT may improve local control, but neurocognitive outcomes may be better with radiosurgery alone in patient with poorer outcomes (3). Additionally, WBRT may negatively impact HRQOL (e.g., global health status, physical functioning, cognitive functioning, and fatigue) for at least 1-year post-treatment (20). Interim data from an RCT comparing optimal supportive care (OSC) and WBRT vs. OSC alone indicates that there is no early evidence of detriment to quality of life, overall survival or quality-adjusted life years (QALYs) from OSC alone (21). Therefore, consideration of social determinants and cognitive functions prior to radiotherapy may help in the clinical decision making while always being mindful of HRQOL.

At baseline, patients with better KPS (>80) reported lower visual disorder, motor dysfunction, drowsiness, bladder dysfunction, and communication deficit scales. At follow-up, patients with better KPS reported more decreases in pruritus scores. This correlation between KPS and the scales are consistent with previous findings by our group in a similar patient population where the C15 and BN20 were administered: patients with a lower KPS at baseline reported greater symptom burden in communication deficit and motor dysfunction and headache (22). Also, study of advanced cancer patients undergoing various treatments using the FACT-G questionnaire identified performance status to be a strong determinant of HRQOL (23).

At baseline, patients under the age of 60 predicted fewer seizure-related issues. At follow-up, these patients experienced more improvements in visual disorder. A validation study by the Radiation Therapy Oncology Group (RTOG) validated age and performance status as survival prognostic factors in clinical trials involving patients with brain metastases (14). A study by Fossa et al. showed that general HRQOL was significantly influenced by any cancer diagnosis (24). Furthermore, a significant impairment of HRQOL was seen in cancer patients with comorbidities (hypertension, diabetes mellitus and/or psychological distress) (24). A comparison of self-reported QOL scores in old and young patients with metastatic cancer using EORTC QLQ-C15-PAL questionnaire showed that elderly patients have a different QOL profile (25).

At baseline, female gender predicted more difficulty remembering and more communication deficit. Between baseline and follow up, females reported less future uncertainty and communication deficit compared to males. Similarly, in a study assessing psychological sequelae and QOL in patients with primary brain tumours, there were statistically significant differences with higher levels of psychological and sexual dysfunction in females (26). Other studies have shown that women generally experience lower HRQOL compared to men (5, 27–29), though there is little evidence in current literature to explain these differences. It was found in the literature that females had a lower QOL compared to males at 1-year post-surgical removal of primary brain tumours (30). Patients with brain tumours were found to have high depressive symptoms, which correlate with poor QOL (31). It has also been proposed that depressive females withdraw from their social support network during their cancer crisis, which may cause lowered QOL in conjunction with increased emotional reactivity and decreased tolerance for stressful situations in patients with brain tumours (26, 32).

Employment predicted lower level of visual disorder. However, even survivors of brain tumours found difficulty in completing cognitive tasks, though work rehabilitate programs were shown to be effective depending on their physical impairment if enough time is available (33, 34). In general, unemployment has been correlated with lower HRQOL when assessed with the EORTC-QLQ-C30 questionnaire (5, 23, 35).

The current study suggests that marital status correlates with less motor dysfunction. As neurological and physical decline continues, there may be a role for more aggressive palliative care depending on the social support available to that patient (33). Clinical decisions may also be based on interventions to reduce patient and caregiver distress (36).

Study limitations

We were unable to analyze cultural factors in this study. Though marital status was found to be significant for some scales, the quality and nature of the relationships were not assessed. Furthermore, financial burden, accessibility to healthcare, and number of dependents were not investigated. It was found that baseline HRQOL scores did not profoundly add to clinical factors to predict survival in their statistical models (8). Thus, it is important to find clinically important factors to effectively adjust care for this cohort of patients (22). Though the BN20+2 and associated questionnaires have been found useful in assessing patients with brain metastases, it has been suggested that in addition to HRQOL scores, proxy measures such as independent activities of daily living could complement measures of patient function (37).

Additionally, we did not extend the analysis on cultural differences, especially with respect to marriages; dependents and treatment of the elderly were not qualitatively or quantitatively analyzed. Variations of cultural differences between the 3 Canadian and 1 Spanish site were also not directly assessed. Future prospective studies may address for these possible confounders, such as health policy and cultural attitudes.

Though the primary cancer sites and number of metastases were assessed, this study did not assess the depth and location of the brain tumours, which may have influenced the reported scales. In previous studies, patients with deep tumours reported more bladder control problems compared to cortical tumours. It was also noted that CNS tumour location, post-operative radiation, and tumour recurrence also consistently associated with poorer QOL (38). The variation in primary sites may also vary the degree of change in HRQOL (5).

Future studies may investigate specific cultural factors and the effectiveness of individualized interventions. A more qualitative approach may help elucidate key clinical and modifiable factors for these patients.

Acknowledgments

We thank the generous support of Bratty Family Fund, Michael and Karyn Goldstein Cancer Research Fund, Joey and Mary Furfari Cancer Research Fund, Pulenzas Cancer Research Fund, Joseph and Silvana Melara Cancer Research Fund, and Ofelia Cancer Research Fund.

References

[1] Lukas R V, Gabikian P, Garza M, Chmura SJ. Treatment of Brain Metastases. Oncology 2014;87(6):321–9.

[2] Eichler AF, Loeffler JS. Multidisciplinary management of brain metastases. Oncologist 2007;12(7):884–98.

[3] Tsao M, Lloyd N, Wong R, Chow E, Rakovitch E, Laperriere N, et al. Whole brain radiotherapy for the treatment of newly diagnosed multiple brain metastases. Cochrane Database Syst Rev 2012;4:3869.

[4] Kirkbride P, Tannock IF. Trials in palliative treatment-have the goal posts been moved. Lancet Oncol 2008;9(3):186–7.

[5] Lam K, Chow E, Zhang L, Wong E, Bedard G, Fairchild A, et al. Determinants of quality of life in advanced cancer patients with bone metastases undergoing palliative radiation treatment. Support Care Cancer 2013;21(11):3021–30.

[6] Kivits J, Erpelding M-L, Guillemin F. Social determinants of health-related quality of life. Rev Epidemiol Sante Publique 2013;61:S189–94.

[7] Santin O, Murray L, Prue G, Gavin A, Gormley G, Donnelly M. Self-reported psychosocial needs and health-related quality of life of colorectal cancer survivors. Eur J Oncol Nurs 2015 [Epub ahead of print].

[8] Mauer ME, Bottomley A, Taphoorn MJB. Evaluating health-related quality of life and symptom burden in brain tumour patients: instruments for use in experimental trials and clinical practice. Curr Opin Neurol 2008;21(6):745–53.

[9] Tsao MN, Rades D, Wirth A, Lo SS, Danielson BL, Gaspar LE, et al. Radiotherapeutic and surgical management for newly diagnosed brain metastasis(es): An American Society for Radiation Oncology evidence-based guideline. Pract Radiat Oncol 2012;2(3):210–25.

[10] Osoba D, Aaronson NK, Muller M, Sneeuw K, Hsu M a, Yung WK, et al. The development and psychometric validation of a brain cancer quality-of-life questionnaire for use in combination with general cancer-specific questionnaires. Qual Life Res 1996;5(1):139–50.

[11] Aaronson NK, Ahmedzai S, Bergman B, Bullinger M, Cull A, Duez NJ, et al. The European Organization for Research and Treatment of Cancer QLQ-C30: a quality-of-life instrument for use in international clinical trials in oncology. J Natl Cancer Inst 1993;85(5):365–76.

[12] Marmot M, Friel S, Bell R, Houweling T a J, Taylor S. Closing the gap in a generation: health equity through action on the social determinants of health. Lancet 2008;372(9650):1661–9.

[13] Hiatt R a, Breen N. The social determinants of cancer: a challenge for transdisciplinary science. Am J Prev Med 2008;35(2 Suppl):S141–50.

[14] Gaspar L, Scott C, Rotman M, Asbell S, Phillips T, Wasserman T, et al. Recursive partitioning analysis (RPA) of prognostic factors in three radiation therapy oncology group (RTOG) brain metastases trials. Int J Radiat Oncol 1997;37(4):745–51.

[15] Wong J, Hird A, Kirou-Mauro A, Napolskikh J, Chow E. Quality of life in brain metastases radiation trials: a literature review. Curr Oncol 2008;15(5):25–45.

[16] Folstein F, Folstein S, McHugh P. Mini-mental state: A practical method for grading the cognitive state of patients for the clinician. J Psychatric Res 1975;12(3):189–98.

[17] Caissie A, Nguyen J, Chen E, Zhang L, Sahgal A, Clemons M, et al. Quality of life in patients with brain metastases using the EORTC QLQ-BN20+2 and QLQ-C15-PAL. Int J Radiat Oncol Biol Phys 2012;83(4):1238–45.

[18] Shields LBE, Choucair A, Choucair AK. Quality of life measures as a preliminary clinical indicator in patients with primary brain tumors. Surg Neurol Int 2013;4:48.

[19] Steinmann D, Paelecke-Habermann Y, Geinitz H, Aschoff R, Bayerl A, Bölling T, et al. Prospective evaluation of quality of life effects in patients undergoing palliative radiotherapy for brain metastases. BMC Cancer 2012;12:283.

[20] Soffietti R, Kocher M, Abacioglu UM, Villa S, Fauchon F, Baumert BG, et al. A European Organisation for Research and Treatment of Cancer phase III trial of adjuvant whole-brain radiotherapy versus observation in patients with one to three brain metastases from solid tumors after surgical resection or radiosurgery: quality-of-life. J Clin Oncol 2013;31(1):65–72.

[21] Langley RE, Stephens RJ, Nankivell M, Pugh C, Moore B, Navani N, et al. Interim data from the Medical Research Council QUARTZ Trial: does whole brain radiotherapy affect the survival and quality of life of patients with brain metastases from non-small cell lung cancer? Clin Oncol (R Coll Radiol) 2013;25(3):23–30.

[22] Wong E, Zhang L, Kerba M, Foro Arnalot P, Danielson B, Tsao M, et al. Minimal clinically important differences in the EORTC QLQ-BN20 in patients with brain metastases. Support Care Cancer 2015 [Epub ahead of print].

[23] Zimmermann C, Burman D, Swami N, Krzyzanowska MK, Leighl N, Moore M, et al. Determinants of quality of life in patients with advanced cancer. Support Care Cancer 2011;19(5):621–9.

[24] Fosså SD, Hess SL, Dahl AA, Hjermstad MJ, Veenstra M. Stability of health-related quality of life in the Norwegian general population and impact of chronic morbidity in individuals with and without a cancer diagnosis. Acta Oncol 2007;46(4):452–61.

[25] Koo K, Zeng L, Chen E, Zhang L, Culleton S, Dennis K, et al. Do elderly patients with metastatic cancer have worse quality of life scores? Support Care Cancer 2012;20(9):2121–7.

[26] Harrison J, Maguire P, Pitceathly C. Confiding in crisis: gender differences in pattern of confiding among cancer patients. Soc Sci Med 1995;41(9):1255–60.

[27] Jordhøy MS, Fayers P, Loge JH, Saltnes T, Ahlner-Elmqvist M, Kaasa S. Quality of life in advanced cancer patients: the impact of sociodemographic and medical characteristics. Br J Cancer 2001;85(10):1478–85.

[28] Peuckmann V, Ekholm O, Rasmussen NK, Møller S, Groenvold M, Christiansen P, et al. Health-related quality of life in long-term breast cancer survivors: Nationwide survey in Denmark. Breast Cancer Res Treat 2007;104(1):39–46.

[29] Taechaboonsermsak P, Kaewkungwal J, Singhasivanon P, Fungladda W, Wilailak S. Causal relationship between health promoting behavior and quality of life in cervical cancer patients undergoing radiotherapy. Southeast Asian J Trop Med Public Health 2005;36(6):1568–75.

[30] Mainio A, Hakko H, Niemelä A, Koivukangas J, Räsänen P. Gender difference in relation to depression and quality of life among patients with a primary brain tumor. Eur Psychiatry 2006;21(3):194–9.

[31] Pelletier G, Verhoef MJ, Khatri N, Hagen N. Quality of life in brain tumor patients: The relative contributions of depression, fatigue, emotional distress, and existential issues. J Neurooncol 2002;57(1):41–9.

[32] Taphoorn MJ, Heimans JJ, Snoek FJ, Lindeboom J, Oosterink B, Wolbers JG, et al. Assessment of quality of life in patients treated for low-grade glioma: a preliminary report. J Neurol Neurosurg Psychiatry 1992;55(5):372–6.

[33] Gofton TE, Graber J, Carver A. Identifying the palliative care needs of patients living with cerebral tumors and metastases: A retrospective analysis. J Neurooncol 2012;108(3):527–34.

[34] Rusbridge SL, Walmsley NC, Griffiths SB, Wilford PA, Rees JH. Predicting outcomes of vocational rehabilitation in patients with brain tumours. Psychooncology 2013;22(8):1907–11.

[35] Michelson H, Bolund C, Nilsson B, Brandberg Y. Health-related quality of life measured by the EORTC QLQ-C30--reference values from a large sample of Swedish population. Acta Oncol 2000;39(4):477–84.

[36] Bruera E, Bush SH, Willey J, Paraskevopoulos T, Li Z, Palmer JL, et al. Impact of delirium and recall on the level of distress in patients with advanced cancer and their family caregivers. Cancer 2009;115(9):2004–12.

[37] Dirven L, Reijneveld JC, Aaronson NK, Bottomley A, Uitdehaag BMJ, Taphoorn MJB. Health-related quality of life in patients with brain tumors: Limitations and additional outcome measures. Curr Neurol Neurosci Rep 2013;13(7):359.

[38] Nwachukwu CR, Youland RS, Chioreso C, Wetjen N, NageswaraRao A, Keating G, et al. Health related quality of life (HRQOL) in long-term survivors of pediatric low grade gliomas (LGGs). J Neurooncol 2014;121(3):599–607.

Submitted: June 9, 2015. *Revised:* July 8, 2015. *Accepted:* July 14, 2015.

In: Pain Management Yearbook 2015
Editor: Joav Merrick

ISBN: 978-1-63484-515-1

Chapter 28

BONE METASTASIS TO THE MANDIBLE IN RECTAL CANCER AND A REVIEW OF THE LITERATURE

Aaron Woo[1], MBBS(C), Breanne Lechner[1], BSc(C), Linda Probyn[2], MD, Natalie Pulenzas[1], BSc(C), Terence Fu[1], MD(C), Hany Soliman[1], MD, Tracy Shum[1], MBBS, Edward Chow[1], MBBS and C Shun Wong[1,*], MD

[1]Rapid Response Radiotherapy Program, Department of Radiation Oncology, Odette Cancer Centre, Sunnybrook Health Sciences Centre, University of Toronto, Toronto, Canada

[2]Department of Medical Imaging, Sunnybrook Health Sciences Centre, University of Toronto, Toronto, Ontario, Canada

Bone metastases are a common occurrence in patients with advanced cancer. The most common sites where bone metastases are found include the spine, pelvis, ribs and skull. Bone metastases from colorectal cancer are less common and cases where colorectal cancer has metastasized to the jaw bones are even more infrequently found in literature. Mandibular metastases are often found as a late complication of advanced cancer when there are already extensive metastatic lesions. Management offered to the patients are usually palliative in nature aiming to reduce the pain and preserve oral function to improve the quality of life of the patients. Treatment options include local surgical excision, chemotherapy or radiotherapy. We present the case of a 59-year-old female patient with primary rectal cancer with extensive metastatic lesions in multiple sites including the mandible.

Keywords: colorectal cancer, bone metastases, mandible

* Correspondence: Professor C Shun Wong, MD, FRCPC, Department of Radiation Oncology, Odette Cancer Centre, Sunnybrook Health Sciences Centre, 2075 Bayview Avenue, Toronto, Ontario, Canada M4N 3M5. E-mail: Shun.Wong@sunnybrook.ca.

INTRODUCTION

Bone metastases are conditions that are typically present in patients with advanced cancer, with the prevalence highest in breast and prostate cancer accounting for more than 80% of cases of bone metastases (1). Bone metastases are not commonly found in patients with colorectal cancer, which typically spreads to the liver, lung, adrenal glands and ovaries (2).

Colorectal cancer metastasizing to the jaw bones is even more infrequently found in the literature. In this report, we present the case of a 59-year-old female patient with primary rectal cancer with extensive metastatic lesions in multiple sites including the mandible.

CASE REPORT

A 59-year-old female patient was diagnosed with rectal cancer and a solitary liver metastasis in August 2011. This was managed by neoadjuvant chemoradiation, FOLFOX chemotherapy, right hepatic lobectomy and low anterior resection. Unfortunately, in December 2012, she suffered a recurrence of the disease involving her liver, lung and adrenal metastases. The patient was treated with chemotherapy consisting of FOLFIRI and Avastin.

A bone scan in January 2014 showed multiple bone metastases in her ribs and spine. She was managed by kyphoplasty, radiation to her ribs and lumbar spine.

In June 2014, the patient presented with increasing pain over the left temporo-mandibular joint and difficulty swallowing. Her previous bone scan did reveal increased activity in the left mandible near the temporo-mandibular joint. A CT scan showed a lytic lesion involving the left mandible with pathological fractures. The patient was given a single dose of 8Gy to her left face. Additional palliative radiation was administered to other sites of painful bone metastases, and the patient subsequently died.

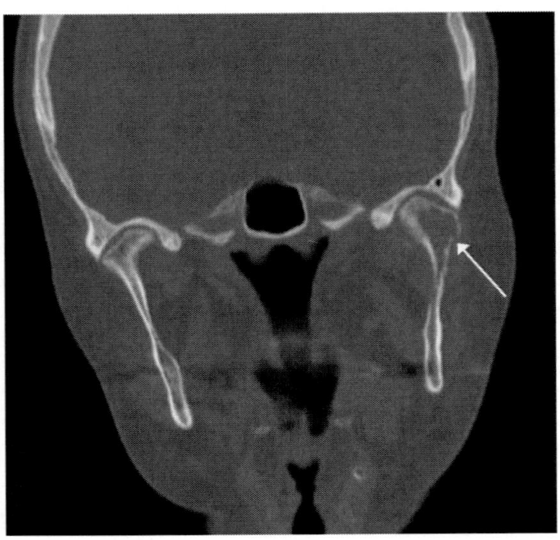

Figure 1. Bone window.

Figures 1-3 (Figure 1. Bone window, Figure 2. Soft tissue window and Figure 3. Soft tissue window) show the CT findings of the metastatic lesion in the mandible. There was a lytic destructive process involving the left mandibular condyle, neck and upper ramus with a pathological fracture in the lateral condylar head. There was an extraosseous soft tissue component measuring 16 by 18 by 20mm that abutted the subarticular surface of the condyle but did not extend into the temporo-mandibular joint.

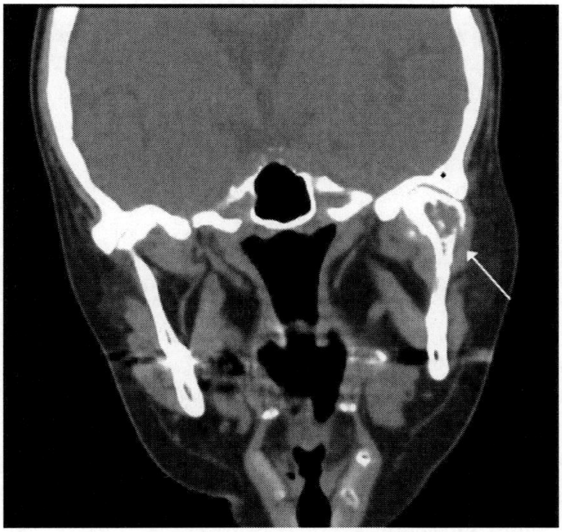

Figure 2. Soft tissue window.

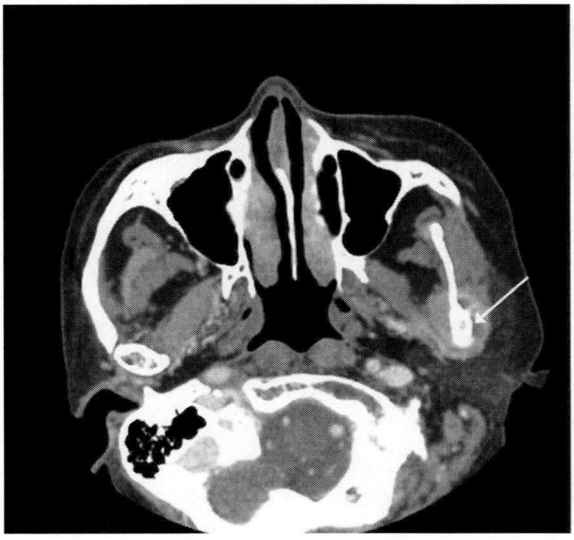

Figure 3. Soft tissue window.

DISCUSSION

Colorectal cancer is the fourth most common cancer in men and the third most common cancer in women worldwide (3). Typically, two-thirds of the tumors occur in the colon and one-third in the rectum. Metastases are common in patients with advanced colorectal cancer, and frequently occur in the liver, lung, adrenal glands, ovaries and less commonly in bone (2). Colorectal metastases in the oral and maxillofacial region are rare. Hirshberg et al. (4) reviewed 673 cases of metastatic tumors of the oral cavity and reported that only 40 cases (6%) originated from a colorectal primary. Of these 40 cases, 28 involved the mandible and the other 12 involved the oral soft tissues.

Only 1% of oral neoplasms are metastatic cancers (5). Common primary sites of oral metastases in men include lung, kidney and prostate, while common sites in women include the breast, genital organs and kidney (6). Metastases to skeletal bones are typically observed in bones with hematopoietically active marrow such as the vertebral column. The mandible or the maxilla is not a site of active hematopoiesis in adults, particularly in older individuals (7). Bone metastases in the face preferentially affect the mandible over the maxilla, and more often are located in the posterior molar area of the mandible (4). In general, symptoms of oral metastases include pain, difficulty in chewing and swallowing, bleeding and facial disfigurement (8). In this present case, the patient suffered from dysphagia and severe pain over the left mandible near the temporo-mandibular joint.

Patients with colorectal cancer with a solitary metastasis are usually managed by surgical resection with the goal of long term tumor control. However, most bone metastases are unresectable (9). Mandibular metastatic lesions are often associated with advanced cancer as a late complication when there are already extensive distant metastases present (8). Similarly, in the presented case, the metastatic lesion in the left mandible was identified when the patient was suffering from widespread metastases to her liver, lungs, adrenals as well as diffuse bone metastases. Given the extent of cancer spread in these cases, the prognosis is typically poor with an average survival of about seven months (4). Management options for mandibular metastases are primarily based on the extent of metastatic spread (8). Aggressive therapy should be considered if the colorectal cancer is responding to systemic therapy or there are low volume metastases and the patient's medical condition permits. In Hirshberg's review, surgical resection was associated with improvement in the prognosis in cases of a solitary metastasis in the oral cavity (4). However, if there is evidence of widespread metastases, the jaw lesion should be managed conservatively. In these cases, palliative options include pain management, radiotherapy, chemotherapy or local surgical excision. Palliative radiotherapy was commonly used in reported series and case reports (7-12) and was also used in the case we presented. The ultimate goal of palliative treatment is to control the patient's pain and to preserve oral function.

CONCLUSION

While metastases to bone from colorectal cancer are not uncommon, the presentation of a metastasis to the mandible is quite rare. Only 1% of all oral neoplasms are metastatic tumors. Metastases to the oral cavity, while quite rare, are reported in the mandible in 80-90% of cases (8). Unfortunately, mandibular metastases are often found with advanced recurrent cancer with extensive metastatic lesions when definitive treatments are no longer options. Such tumors are usually debilitating and portend a poor prognosis. The case report highlights the importance of early recognition of mandibular metastases to optimize the quality of life of patients with these rare lesions.

ACKNOWLEDGMENTS

We thank the generous support of the Bratty Family Fund, Michael and Karyn Goldstein Cancer Research Fund, Joey and Mary Furfari Cancer Research Fund, Pulenzas Cancer Research Fund, Joseph and Silvana Melara Cancer Research Fund, and Ofelia Cancer Research Fund.

REFERENCES

[1] Coleman RE. Metastatic bone disease: clinical features, pathophysiology and treatment strategies. Cancer Treat Rev 2001;27(3):165-76.

[2] August DA, Ottow RT, Sugarbaker PH. Clinical perspective of human colorectal cancer metastasis. Cancer Metastasis Rev 1984;3:303-24.

[3] Center MM, Jemal A, Ward E. International trends in colorectal cancer incidence rates. Cancer Epidemiol Biomarkers Prevent 2009;18(6):1688-94.

[4] Hirshberg A, Shnaiderman-Shapiro A, Kaplan I, Berger R. Metastatic tumours to the oral cavity - pathogenesis and analysis of 673 cases. Oral Oncol 2008;44:743-52.

[5] Meyer HL, Shklar G. Malignant tumours metastatic to mouth and jaws. Oral Surg Oral Med Oral Pathol 1965;20:350-6.

[6] Gomes A, Neto PJ, de Oliveria e Silva ED, Savio E, Neto IC. Metastatic adenocarcinoma involving several bones of the body and the cranio-maxillofacial region: a case report. J Can Dent Assoc 2009;75:211-4.

[7] Mason AC, Azari KK, Farkas LM, Duvvuri U, Myers EN. Metastatic adenocarcinoma of the colon presenting as a mass in the mandible. Head Neck 2005;27(8):729-32.

[8] Kumar GS, Manjunatha BS. Metastatic tumors to the jaws and oral cavity. J Oral Maxillofac Surg 2013;17(1):71.

[9] Soda H, Doi K, Kinoshita T, Yamamoto H, Nagata M, Takiguchi N, et al. Mandibular bone metastasis of rectal cancer: report of a case. Surgery today 2010;40(12):1188-91.

[10] Coad FHGS, Thayalasekaran S, Booth J. An unusual presentation of metastasis from a rectal adenocarcinoma. Q J Med 2012 Jun 29. Doi: http://doi.org/10.1093/qjmed/hcs122.

[11] Lipa B, Sion-Vardy N, Geffen DB, Nash M. Metastatic tumors to the jaws: a report of eight new cases. Med Oral Patol Oral Cir Bucal 2006;11(2):132-5.

[12] Tamiolakis D, Tsamis I, Thomaidis V, Lambropoulou M, Alexiadis G, Venizelos I, et al. Jaw bone metastases: four cases. Acta Dermatovenerol Alp Pannonica Adriat 2007;16(1):21-5.

Submitted: April 20, 2015. *Revised:* May 15, 2015. *Accepted:* May 21, 2015.

In: Pain Management Yearbook 2015
Editor: Joav Merrick

ISBN: 978-1-63484-515-1

Chapter 29

SOLITARY BONE METASTATIC LESION TO THE CUBOID IN ENDOMETRIAL CANCER AND A REVIEW OF THE LITERATURE

Aaron Woo[1], MBBS(C), Breanne Lechner[1], BSc(C), Linda Probyn[2], MD, Natalie Pulenzas[1], BSc(C), Terence Fu[1], MD(C), Hany Soliman[1], MD, C Shun Wong[1], MD, Tracy Shum[1], MBBS, Edward Chow[1], MBBS, Ida Ackerman[1], MD and Eric Leung[1,*], MD

[1]Rapid Response Radiotherapy Program, Department of Radiation Oncology, Odette Cancer Centre, Sunnybrook Health Sciences Centre, University of Toronto, Toronto, Canada

[2]Department of Medical Imaging, Sunnybrook Health Sciences Centre, University of Toronto, Toronto, Ontario, Canada

Advanced malignant tumors frequently metastasize to bone. Types of primary cancer that are often reported to develop metastases to bone include breast, lung and prostate carcinoma. However, acrometastasis or secondary cancer in the hand or foot is extremely rare. Metastases to the feet are even more uncommon and have been reported to be half to one-third the incidence of hand metastases. Foot metastases are generally associated with advanced cancer where there are extensive metastases. Given the poor prognosis, management options are usually palliative with the aim of relieving pain and preserving the motor function; these options include local surgical excision, chemotherapy, radiotherapy or combinations of the above. We present the case of a 78-year-old female patient with primary endometrial cancer and a solitary bone metastatic lesion to the cuboid and a review of the literature of acrometastases in the foot.

* Correspondence: Eric Leung, MD, FRCPC, Department of Radiation Oncology, Odette Cancer Centre, Sunnybrook Health Sciences Centre, 2075 Bayview Avenue, Toronto, Ontario, Canada M4N 3M5. E-mail: Eric.Leung@sunnybrook.ca.

Keywords: endometrial cancer, bone metastases, cuboid

INTRODUCTION

Advanced malignant tumors frequently metastasize to bone. Previous study has reported that prostate and breast cancers have the highest prevalence of bone metastases, contributing more than 80% of the cases (1). However, acrometastases, the spread of cancer to the hand or foot are extremely rare (2, 3). The first case of metastasis to the foot was reported in 1920 by Bloodgood. He described a patient with multiple metastases to the foot from primary prostate cancer (4). This rarity is surprising considering that small bones of the hands and feet comprise more than half (106 of 206) of all the bones in the human body. Metastases to the feet are even more uncommon and have been reported to be half to one-third the incidence of hand metastases (2, 3). In this report, we present a rare case of a 78-year-old female patient with primary endometrial carcinoma with a solitary metastasis in the cuboid bone.

CASE REPORT

A 78-year-old woman was diagnosed with stage IIIc serous endometrial carcinoma in February 2013. In April 2013, she underwent Total abdominal hysterectomy and bilateral salpingo-oophorectomy, and post-operative chemotherapy with carboplatin that was completed in October 2013. She declined adjuvant radiation. She remained well but recurred in May 2014 with a lower vaginal metastatic lesion. Biopsy confirmed a high-grade adenocarcinoma. Imaging demonstrated no extrapelvic disease and she received external beam radiation therapy. There was no obvious persistent disease detected in August 2014.

In November 2014, she had new onset of vaginal bleeding which clinical examination and magnetic resonance imaging (MRI) showed evidence of a mass within the urethra extending to the neck of the bladder without invasion. The mass also involved the anterior portion of the lower vagina and was associated with a fistula between the vagina and urethra. As the recurrent lesion was situated in the previous radiated field, interstitial brachytherapy was being considered for palliation. However, restaging imaging demonstrated new metastases in the lungs, liver and inguinal lymph nodes. Brachytherapy was abandoned and a single fraction of palliative external beam radiation of 8 Gy was given in January 2015 to control her bleeding. The patient went on to receive palliative doxorubicin chemotherapy.

Independent of her cancer, the patient had progressive spinal stenosis causing back pain and significant weakness in her right leg. This required laminectomy in January 2015. Despite surgery, she had pain radiating from the right inguinal region down to her right leg and the sole of her foot. MRI of the pelvis demonstrated a mass adherent to the right obturator nerve leading to a denervation edema of right pelvic musculature. MRI of the lumbar spine showed no bone metastasis but a new right-sided hydronephrosis.

As the pain in the plantar aspect of the right foot remained particularly significant, a computed tomography (CT) was done which identified an extensive lytic destructive metastatic lesion in the medial part of the cuboid bone. A single dose of radiation of 8Gy was given in April 2015 to the cuboid as well as the right obturator nerve to control the progressing pain. Repeated radiation was planned because of the persistent pain in the right foot.

Figures 1-3 show the lytic lesion in the medial cuboid with a poorly defined medial margin and it appeared to cross the joint with the lateral cuneiform. It was measured to be approximately 1.5cm.

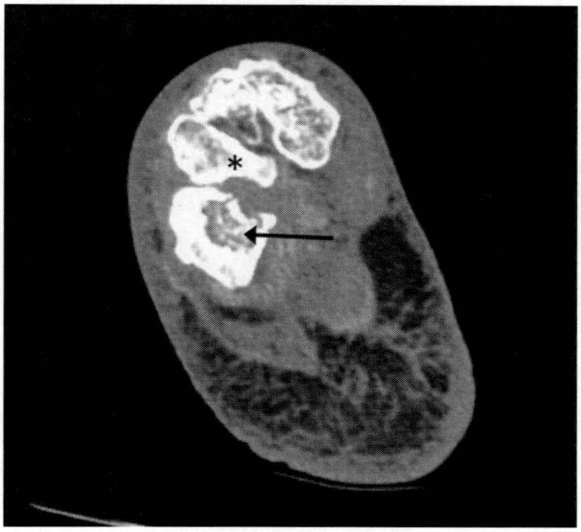

Figure 1. Soft tissue window.

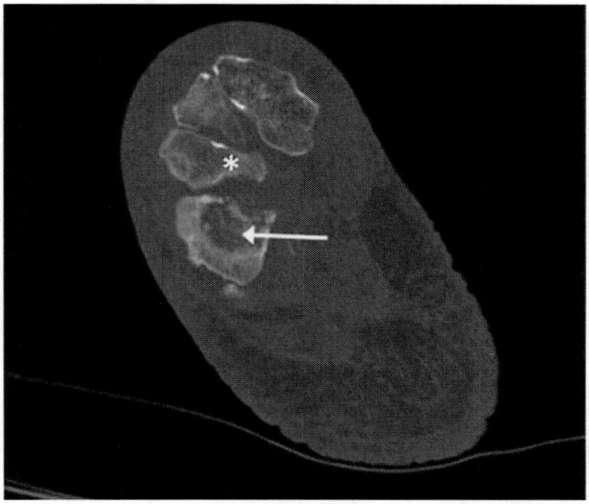

Figure 2. Bone window.

Figures 1-3 are axial (Figure 1 is soft tissue window and Figure 2 bone window) and sagittal (Figure 3 bone window) CT images of the foot which showed a lytic destructive lesion in the medial cuboid with a poorly defined medial margin destroying the cortex with extraosseous soft tissue crossing the joint to the lateral cuneiform. (Measuring approximately 1.5cm.) Arrows indicate the lesion in the cuboid and asterisks indicate the lateral cuneiform.

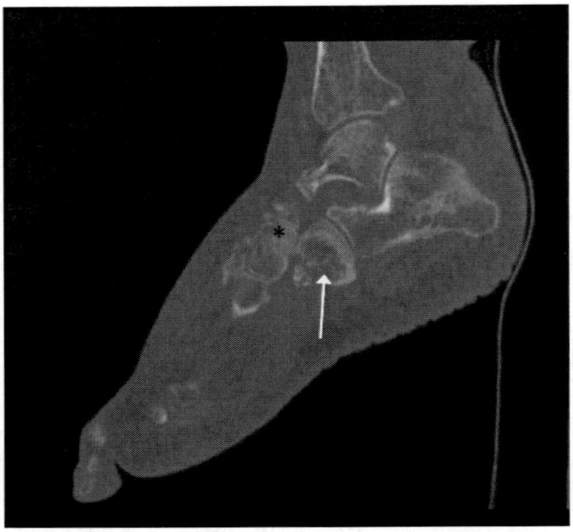

Figure 3. Bone window.

Discussion

Although malignant tumors frequently metastasize to bone, it is rare for cancer to metastasize distal to the elbow or knee (5). Typically, bone metastases develop in sites including the vertebrae, pelvis, ribs and skull. Acrometastases or secondary cancers in the hand or foot are very rare, contributing less than 1% of all the cases of bone metastasis (2, 3). Endometrial cancer is one of the most common malignancies in females together with cervical cancer (6). Endometrial cancer frequently metastasizes to nearby structures such as the ovaries, fallopian tubes and cervix. The most common site of recurrence of endometrial cancer is either local in the pelvis, intra-abdominal or lung. Bone metastases are uncommon and have an incidence of only 1% (7).

Maheshwari et al. (8) reviewed 278 cases of metastatic lesions of the foot including 229 cases which the primary malignancy was specified. They reported that the genitourinary system was the most common primary site comprising more than half the cases. Previous reviews of literature by Zindrick et al. (9) and Libson et al. (3) reported the same finding. Within the genitourinary system, the urinary bladder and the uterus are the most common primary sites of origin. Other than the genitourinary system, lungs and kidneys are the most common single organ sites of cancer to metastasize to the foot. The hind part of the foot was most common area involved in foot metastases. The hind foot is composed of 2 of the 7 tarsal bones, the calcaneus and talus. Metastatic lesions involving the calcaneus contributed 31.1% of the cases reviewed. Apart from the tarsal bones, phalangeal and metatarsal involvement are the second and third most common sites for foot metastases. In the case we presented, the patient had a metastatic lesion in the medial part of the cuboid and the lesion was starting to cause destruction to the lateral margin of the neighboring lateral cuneiform bone. In Maheshwari's review, metastatic lesions involving cuboid contributed 9.5% of the cases reviewed and cases involving the lateral cuneiform were very rare (8).

Foot metastases are usually associated with advanced cancer when there are already widespread metastases. In the case we presented, the patient had extensive and progressive metastatic lesions in her lungs, liver and inguinal lymph nodes. What is of particular interest in the case we reported is that the metastasis to the cuboid was the only bone metastatic site, and all other metastatic lesions involved the viscera. Management options offered to the patients are usually palliative with the aim of relieving pain and preserving the motor function. Treatment options include local surgical excision if possible, chemotherapy, radiotherapy or combinations of the above (10-13).

CONCLUSION

Bone metastases are relatively uncommon in endometrial cancer, and acrometastases to the cuboid bone are particularly rare. This report describes a patient with a rare cuboid metastasis in the absence of any other skeletal disease from a primary endometrial carcinoma. Although metastatic lesions involving the foot are rare, they should be considered in the differential diagnosis of patients with cancer presenting with a painful foot especially in the setting of known metastatic genitourinary cancers. Treatment is usually palliative with the aim of relieving pain and improving quality of life.

ACKNOWLEDGMENTS

We thank the generous support of the Bratty Family Fund, Michael and Karyn Goldstein Cancer Research Fund, Joey and Mary Furfari Cancer Research Fund, Pulenzas Cancer Research Fund, Joseph and Silvana Melara Cancer Research Fund, and Ofelia Cancer Research Fund.

REFERENCES

[1] Coleman RE. Metastatic bone disease: clinical features, pathophysiology and treatment strategies. Cancer Treat Rev 2001;27(3):165-76.

[2] Healey JH, Turnbull AD, Miedema B, Lane JM. Acrometastases. A study of twenty-nine patients with osseous involvement of the hands and feet. J Bone Joint Surg Am1986;68:743-6.

[3] Libson E, Bloom RA, Husband, JE, Stoker DJ. Metastatic tumours of bones of the hand and foot. A comparative review and report of 43 additional cases. Skeletal Radiol 1987;16:387-92.

[4] Bloodgood JC. Bone tumors, benign and malignant: a brief review of the salient features, based on a study of 370 cases. Am J Surg 1920;16:387.

[5] Leeson MC, Makley JT, Carter JR. Metastatic skeletal disease distal to the elbow and knee. Clin Orthop 1986;206:94.

[6] Siegel, Rebecca, Jiemin Ma, Zhaohui Zou, and Ahmedin Jemal. Cancer statistics, 2014. CA Cancer J Clin 2014;64(1):9-29.

[7] Uccella S, Morris JM, Bakkum-Gamez JN, Kenney GL, Podratz KC, Mariani A. Bone metastases in endometrial cancer: report on 19 patients and review of the medical literature. Gynecologic Oncol 2013;130(3):474-82.

[8] Maheshwari AV, Chiappetta G, Kugler CD, Pitcher JD, Temple HT. Metastatic skeletal disease of the foot: case reports and literature review. Foot Ankle Int 2008;29(7):699-710.

[9] Zindrick MR, Young MP, Daley RJ, Light TR. Metastatic tumors of the foot: case report and literature review. Clin Orthop Relat Res 1982;170:219-25.

[10] Soda H, Doi K, Kinoshita T, Yamamoto H, Nagata M, Takiguchi N, et al. Mandibular bone metastasis of rectal cancer: report of a case. Surgery today 2010;40(12):1188-91.

[11] Allman LM. Metastatic bone involvement of the hallux distal phalanx and cuboid in an elderly patient with non-Hodgkin lymphoma. Foot Ankle Spec 2008;1(6):355-8.

[12] Zindrick MR, Young MP, Daley RJ, Light TR. Metastatic tumors of the foot: case report and literature review. Clin Orthop Relat Res 1982;170:219-25.

[13] Hattrup SJ, Amadio PC, Sim FH, Lombardi RM. Metastatic tumors of the foot and ankle. Foot Ankle Int 1988;8(5):243-7.

Submitted: April 22, 2015. *Revised:* May 17, 2015. *Accepted:* May 21, 2015.

SECTION FOUR: SOCIAL WORK, CANCER AND END OF LIFE ISSUES

In: Pain Management Yearbook 2015
Editor: Joav Merrick

ISBN: 978-1-63484-515-1

Chapter 30

THE ROLE OF PERCUTANEOUS VERTEBRAL AND PELVIC AUGMENTATION IN THE PALLIATION OF PAINFUL BONE METASTASES

Sagi Kaduri, MDCM, FRCPC
and Elizabeth David, MD, FRCPC*
Interventional Radiology, Sunnybrook Health Sciences Centre,
University of Toronto, Ontario, Canada

Radiologically guided vertebral and pelvic augmentation via vertebroplasty and osteoplasty are safe and effective in the palliation of bone metastases. The techniques are complimentary to standard treatments such as external beam radiotherapy and can enhance traditional treatments by providing rapid pain relief through mechanical stabilization of pathological fractures. The technique is readily adopted into clinical practice and has a low risk of major complications. The minimally invasive approach has the added benefit of not requiring general anesthesia in an already medically frail population. Radiofrequency ablation can be used to enhance pain relief and improve the control of cement injection.

Keywords: vertebroplasty, osteoplasty, radiofrequency ablation, bone metastases, palliation

INTRODUCTION

Percutaneous vertebral augmentation in the form of vertebroplasty (VP) or kyphoplasty (KP) with or without radiofrequency ablation (RFA) is an accepted form of palliation in bone metastases and is often used as an adjunct to external beam radiotherapy. The advantage of this technique over others is the rapidity in which it can produce pain relief and the minimally invasive nature of the technique. Quality of life is an important component of care in this subset of patients so rapid pain relief is crucial in providing optimal palliative care. Patients

* Correspondence: Elizabeth David, MD, FRCPC, Interventional Radiology, Sunnybrook Health Sciences Centre, 2075 Bayview Avenue, Toronto, ON Canada. Email: Elizabeth.david@sunnybrook.ca.

with bone metastases are often in advanced stages of their disease and although life expectancy has increased with advanced techniques, it is still limited. The median overall survival of patients with spinal metastases is reported to be less than 1 year (1). Given this, the quality of life at this stage becomes increasingly important. Bone metastases can be a significant source of disability and pain. Rapid relief of pain and maintaining mobility becomes an essential goal when treating these patients. Lesions that have metastasized to the bone can result in fractures, instability and considerable discomfort. Conservative strategies to manage these pathological fractures usually involve analgesics, often in the form of opioids and bed rest; this can be effective but can decrease the quality of life parameters for the patient. Often radiotherapy is given concurrently but this treatment requires time to achieve optimal efficacy. During this period, the patient can suffer a great deal. Multiple studies have established that percutaneous vertebral and pelvic augmentation is a safe and effective form of palliation in this population (2-5). It can provide rapid pain relief and enhanced stability with minimal side effects. Pain relief is often immediate; in most studies within 24-48 hours. Objective measures of reduction in pain intensity are often noted by a decrease in analgesic requirement. Patient satisfaction with the treatment in most studies exceeded 60%.

Vertebral and Pelvic Augmentation

Vertebral augmentation, also known as vertebroplasty, is a minimally invasive, radiologically guided procedure that consists of percutaneous injection of surgical cement (polymethylmethacrylate or PMMA) into the vertebral body. The term "osteoplasty" is often used when cement injection is extraspinal. Vertebroplasty has been most heavily studied in the context of osteoporotic fractures. More recent studies, however, have consistently shown benefit of vertebral augmentation when used in spinal bone metastases (6-8). A joint position statement supported by multiple interventional radiology and neurosurgical societies acknowledges the growing body of evidence supporting this procedure and stated that "percutaneous vertebroplasty remains medically appropriate therapy for treatment of painful vertebral compression fractures refractory to nonoperative medical therapy and for vertebrae weakened by neoplasia when performed for medical indications outlined in the published standards" (2).

Cement injected into the vertebral body (VP) or pelvic bone (Osteoplasty) provides structural stability to the treated bone and solidifies pathologic fractures, if present. The manner in which pain relief is obtained is thought to be from closure of fracture clefts and enhanced stability. Other mechanisms of pain relief have been hypothesized; one other possible mechanism is the destruction of nerve ending of pain fibers as a result of the exothermic reaction associated with the hardening of Polymethylmethacrylate (*PMMA*). The cytotoxicity of PMMA may also be related to vascular or chemical effects (9).

Complication rates related to vertebroplasty vary greatly in the literature. Major complications are uncommon especially with proper intraprocedural imaging. The complication rate per level treated ranges from 0 to 17%, whereas it is 0-33% per patient, as many patients have a few vertebral body levels treated (9). Most of these complications are minor. The majority of complications are due to cement leakage or extravasation outside of the target, either the vertebral body or pelvic bone. Most cement leaks are inconsequential

(10, 11). Rare neurological complications have been described (12, 13). In one series, Cotton et al. (14) described 1 case out of 258 who developed spinal cord compression requiring surgical decompression. Other rare complications include rib or pedicle fractures, pneumothorax, discitis and pulmonary or fat emboli.

RADIOFREQUENCY ABLATION

Vertebral and pelvic augmentation have more recently been done following ablative therapy of the lesions treated. Ablative treatment in bone was first used in benign primary bone tumors, namely osteoid osteomas, more than 20 years ago. Percutaneous ablation has since become well established as the primary approach to treat osteoid osteomas (15, 16). More recently, ablative treatment has been used in the treatment of painful bone metastases, usually in combination with percutaneous augmentation (vertebroplasty in the spine or osteoplasty in extraspinal sites). RFA is the most commonly used ablative modality that has been used in combination with osteoplasty; this combined procedure has been shown to be safe and effective in the treatment of painful bone metastases (17, 18). It remains unclear if there is a synergistic effect when RFA is combined with vertebroplasty or osteoplasty (19-21). Different factors that may contribute to the therapeutic effect of RFA prior to osteoplasty or vertebroplasty include the reduction of interleukins and TNF responsible for a sensitization of nerve endings and the inhibition of osteoclasts. Direct destruction of sensitive nerve endings within the periosteum may also play a role (17).

It has been anecdotally noted that the use of RFA prior to vertebroplasty or osteoplasty improves the control of cement injection (17, 22-25). Radiofrequency ablation may diminish tumor bulk prior to cement deposition. It is postulated that ablation of the lesion changes the consistency of the tumor, which can shrink the tumor and destroy the "cohesion" of the tumor cells (17). This creation of a "thermal cavity" allows for a more controlled injection of cement, and we believe that it limits the rate of posterior cement leaks when used prior to vertebroplasty (unpublished data). Furthermore, the use of RFA prevents theoretical displacement of tumor cells by the cement into adjacent vascular spaces and should therefore increases the safety of cement injection.

One of the concerns when using RFA is the possibility of thermal injury to adjacent structures. This is particularly relevant in the spine due to proximity to the neural structures. Injury to adjacent structures has been described in the past (18). The insulative nature of cortical bone gives a measure of safety especially for structures in the epidural space. The risk of injury can be further reduced with bipolar design of the RFA probe. Most conventional RFA devices use a monopolar probe. Newer designs are bipolar in nature, limiting deposition of energy outside the desired field. One such system has been used at our institution with good success (OsteoCool, Baylis Medical) (26, 27).

Patient Selection

Patient selection is key in obtaining optimal and durable results. The pain should localize to the region of pathology as seen on imaging studies, and there should be a reasonable temporal relationship between the development of new pathology and onset of symptoms. Pain should be limited to one or few sites. In diffuse disease, it can be difficult to identify the source of maximal pain. Multiple levels can be treated in a staged fashion to optimize pain relief. However, patients with numerous lesions and diffuse rather than focal pain are better treated with systemic therapy rather than a focused approach (28).

The degree and nature of the pain are also important factors in patient selection. Patients with mild pain may benefit from the use of analgesics alone, which are often effective. As for the nature of the pain, it is important to note that this intervention provides little benefit in treatment of nerve root or radicular pain.

Finally, the structural integrity of weight bearing or axial loading regions in the skeleton, namely lesions in the spine and peri-acetabular region, is another important consideration. Patients with lesions in these regions are therefore often good candidates for cement augmentation.

The procedure is complimentary to radiation therapy, and can be performed either before or after radiotherapy. It can be done on an outpatient basis, under local anesthesia and conscious sedation, and in most centers does not require a general anesthetic. The minimally invasive nature of the procedure is advantageous in this population as they are often in the advanced stages of disease and may not tolerate a more aggressive approach.

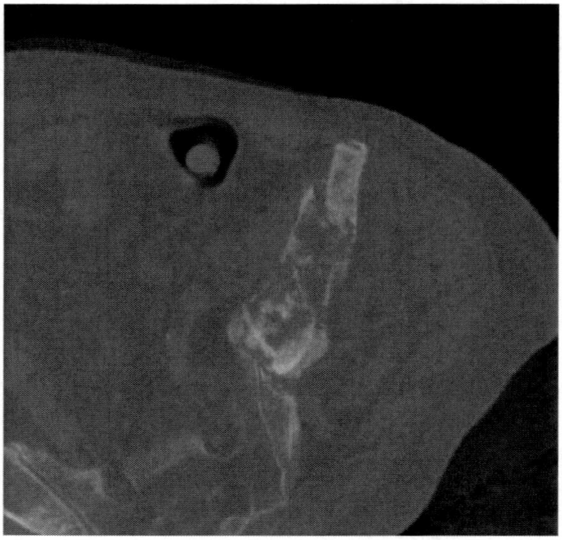

Figure 1. Pre procedure CT shows multiple mixed lytic/sclerotic metastases in left iliac wing, with a subacute pathologic displaced fracture through the iliac wing.

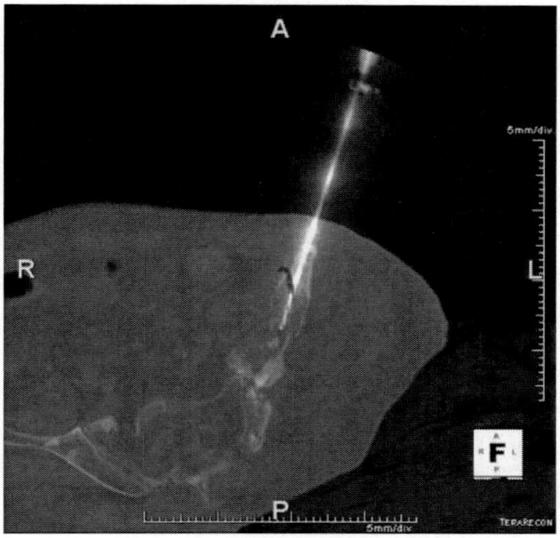

Figure 2. A bone needle is being inserted under CT guidance into the iliac bone via the iliac crest, and a bone drill is used for advancement across the pathologic fracture.

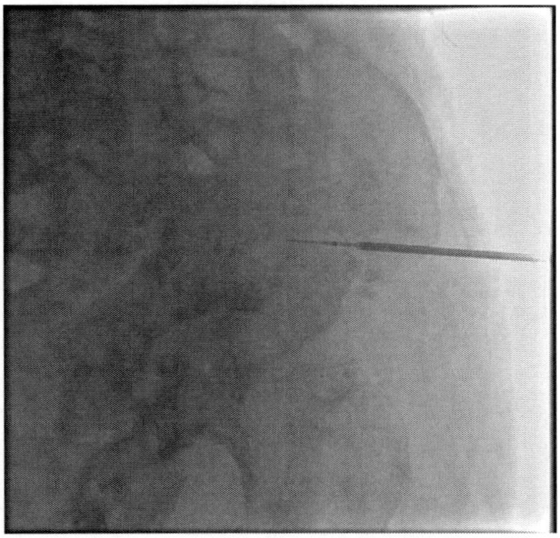

Figure 3. The bone drill has been removed, and the RFA probe has been inserted. The end of the active tip of probe is denoted by a radiopaque marker. With the bipolar design, no heating occurs posterior to this marker.

ILLUSTRATIVE CASES

Case 1

88 year old male with metastatic prostate cancer with multiple lytic and sclerotic bone metastases, recently developed a pathologic fracture of the left iliac wing (see Figure 1). He was experiencing severe left pelvic pain (rated at 10 out of 10). Under conscious sedation and local anesthesia, and under CT guidance, a 11 gauge bone needle was inserted into the left

iliac wing. A 13 gauge bone drill was needed to get across sclerotic regions of the bone, and across the pathologic fracture (Figure 2). Under fluoroscopic guidance, the RFA probe was inserted (Figure 3) and RFA was performed. Live monitoring of the temperature achieved, as well as of the power used and measured impedance was done, as per routine (Figure 4). A temperature of 70 degree Celsius is achieved and kept constant for 15 minutes.

Once done, the RFA probe is removed and cement (Kyphon – PMMA) injection is done through the same needle under fluoroscopic guidance (Figure 5). Post procedure CT shows filling of the fracture cleft (Figure 6). The patient had near immediate pain relief (down to 4 out of 10). Follow up CT over a year after the procedure showed interval stable appearance without progression of the fracture.

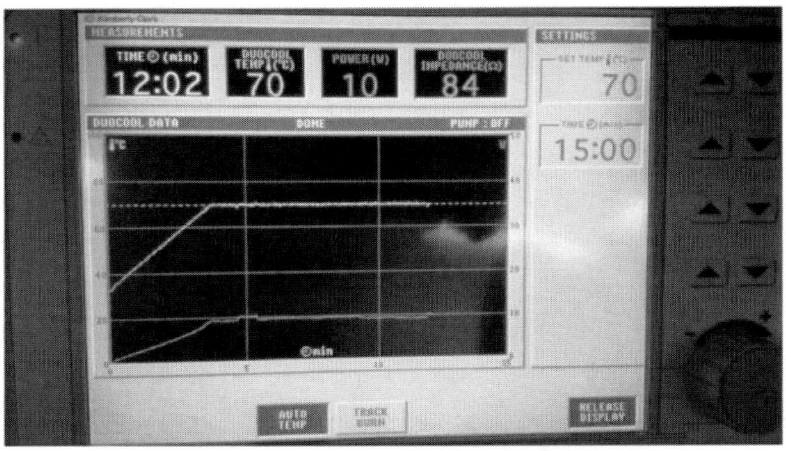

Figure 4. Live monitoring of the RF ablation, showing the measured temperature, power and impedance used. Temperature of 70 degrees is achieved and then kept constant for 15 minutes. This achieves an ablation zone of 2 by 3 cm.

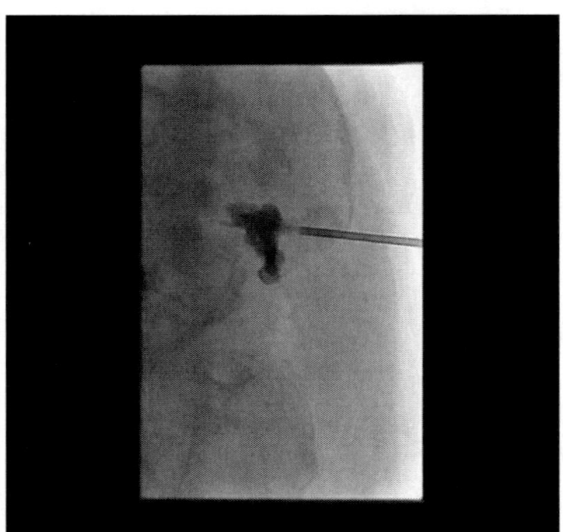

Figure 5. Following RFA, cement is injected via the same needle, and is seen filling the fracture cleft.

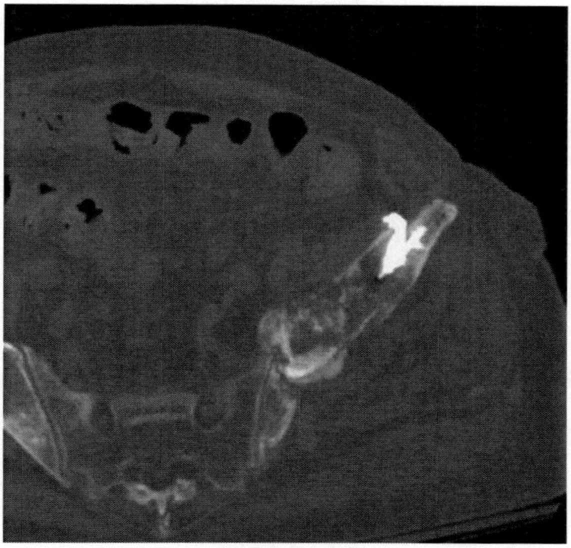

Figure 6. Post procedure confirms good cement filling of the fracture cleft. A small amount of contrast extends through the cleft anterior to the bone, of no consequence.

Case 2

A 69 year old male with metastatic prostate cancer was found to have a new painful lytic right acetabular lesion, at risk for fracture (see Figure 7). Under conscious sedation and local anesthesia, a 13 gauge Cook M1M Osteo Site needle was inserted into the acetabular lesion by an anterior approach, using *XperCT* guide (Figure 8).

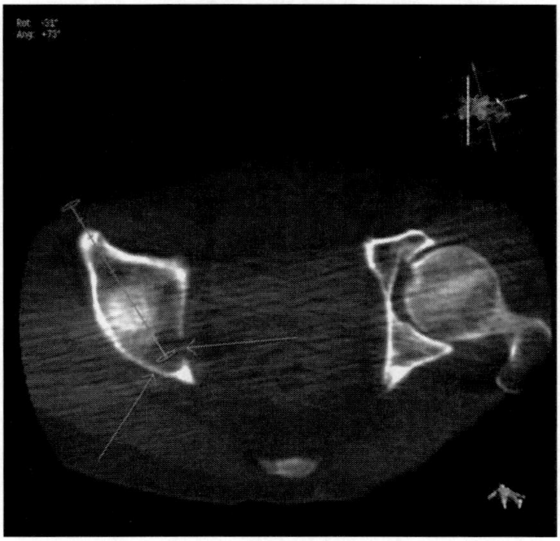

Figure 7. A preliminary CT shows a lytic right acetabular lesion, at risk of fracture.

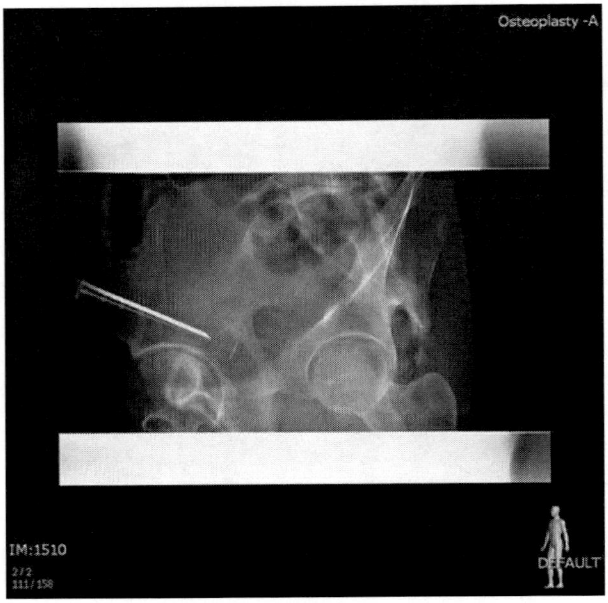

Figure 8. XperCT guidance of needle into the lytic lesion.

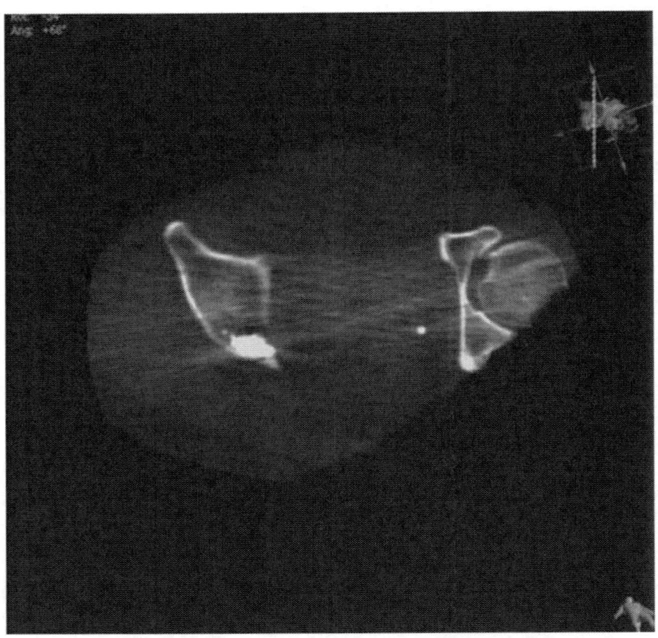

Figure 9. CT done post cement delivery into the lesion.

A bipolar RFA probe was then used to perform a 12 minute ablation. This was followed by cement injection using the *Duro-Ject* system, achieving good filling of the lytic lesion (Figure 9). Though not immediate, the patient experienced improvement in right hip pain following the procedure.

Case 3

An 83 year old male with metastatic prostate cancer who developed a pathologic, painful metastasis at L2 was referred for treatment. RFA-assisted vertebroplasty was performed at L2, using a left unipedicular approach. Needle placement for vertebroplasties is done under biplanar fluoroscopy. Once in place, The RFA probe is inserted and a 15 minute ablation takes place. Following this, cement (PMMA) is injected. This patient had pain rated at 9.5 out of 10 prior to the procedure, which improved to 5 out of 10, at the end of the procedure (see Figures 10-12).

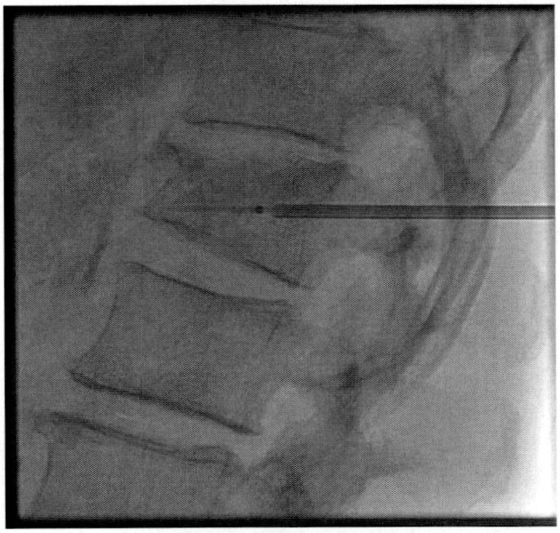

A

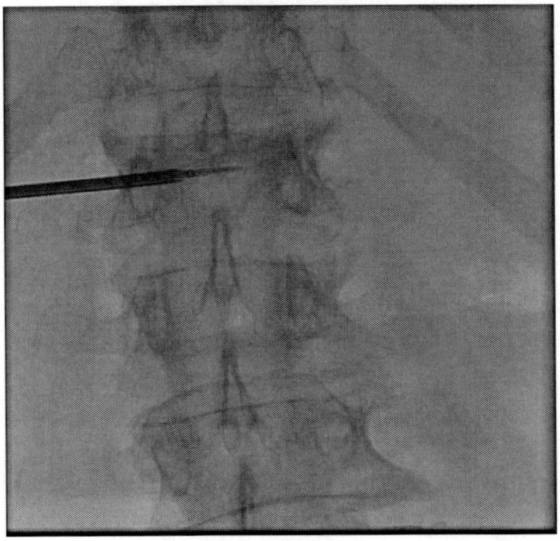

B

Figure 10. (A: lateral, B: frontal). A pathologic fracture is seen at L2. Needle placement was done under fluoroscopic guidance and using a unipedicular approach. The needle is placed just beyond the midline in order to optimize cement distribution. The RFA probe has been placed; its radiopaque marker has been uncovered by the outer needle. Ablation can now be performed.

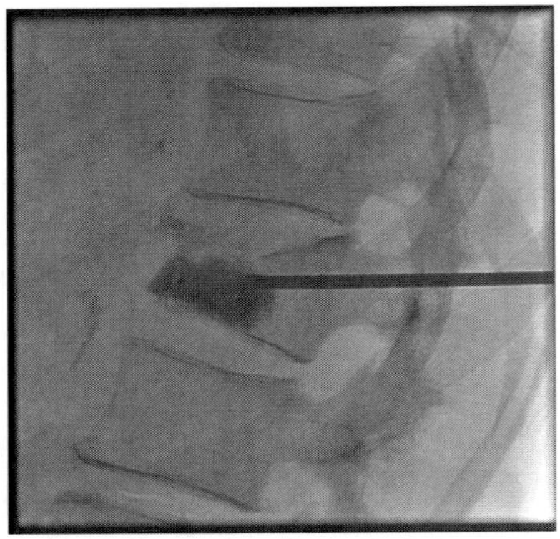

Figure 11. Cement filling of the anterior 2/3 of the vertebral body can be seen.

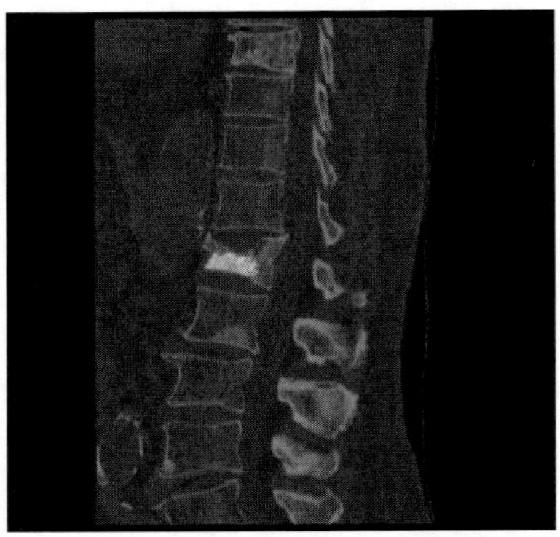

A

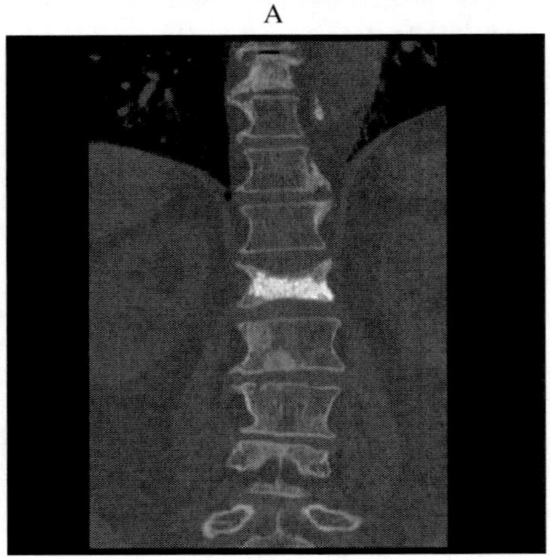

B

Figure 12. Post procedure CT (A: Sagittal); (B: Coronal): There is good cross filling laterally. There is no leak.

Case 4

A 73 year old male with metastatic renal cell carcinoma was found to have a painful lytic bone metastasis in the T12 vertebral body. Pre procedure CT and MRI are shown in Figures 13 and 14. Pain was rated at 6 out of 10 prior to the procedure. An RFA-assisted vertebroplasty was done using a unipedicular access from the left pedicle (Figure 15). Good cement filling of the majority of the lesion was achieved as seen fluoroscopically (Figure 16) and on post procedure CT (Figure 17) and MRI (Figure 18). Pain was alleviated down to 2.5 out of 10 following the procedure.

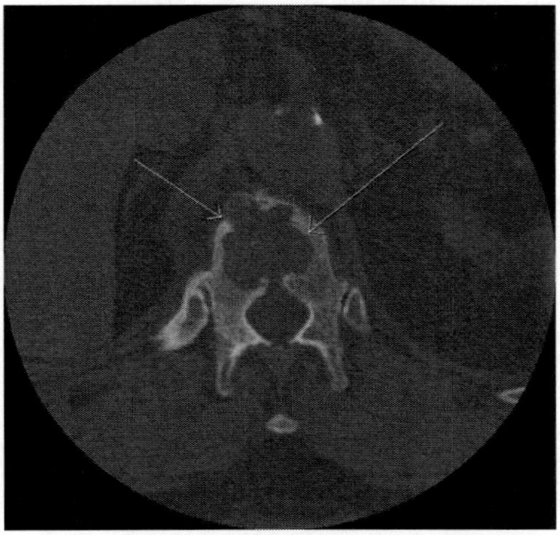

A

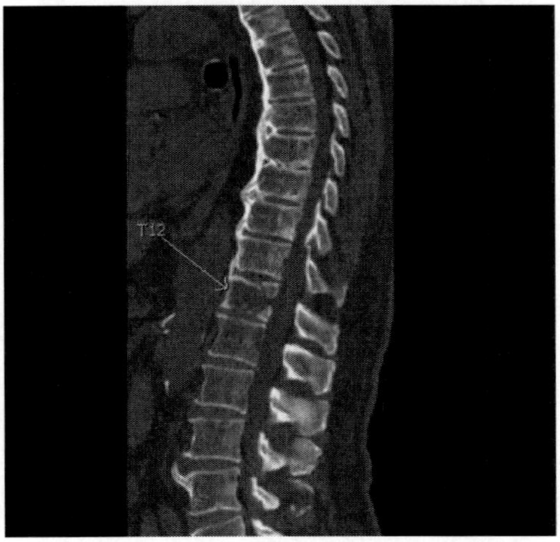

B

Figure 13. Pre-procedure CT; A: axial and B: Sagittal- B. A lytic lesion is seen at T12. There is breech of the posterior cortex. There is a superior endplate fracture posteriorlym.

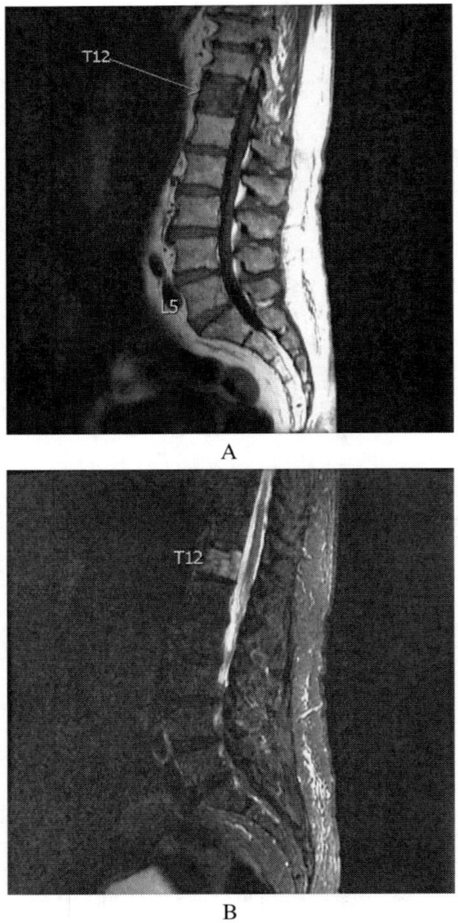

Figure 14. Pre-procedure MRI; A: T1 sagittal and B: STIR sagittal. A metastatic lesion replaces the normal bright fatty marrow by dark signal on T1. The lesion is hyperintense on STIR.

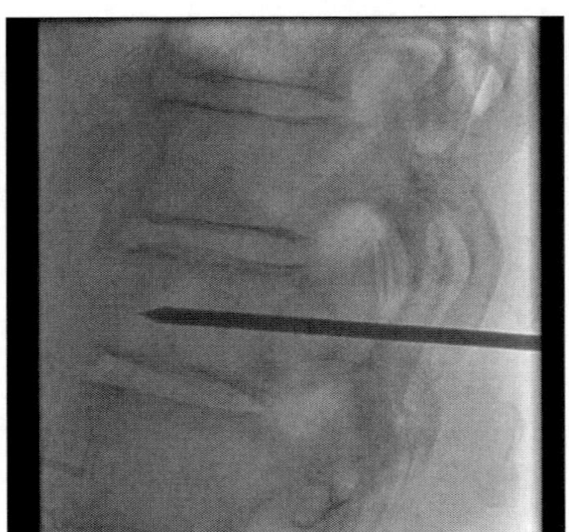

Figure 15. Fluoroscopic guidance of the bone needle into the T12 vertebral body. The lytic lesion is only faintly appreciated.

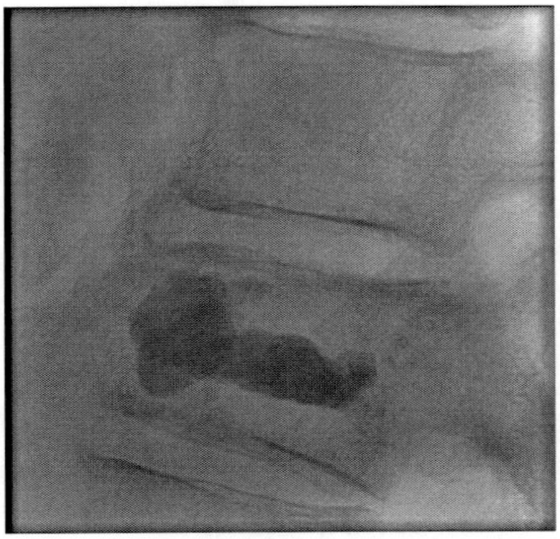

A

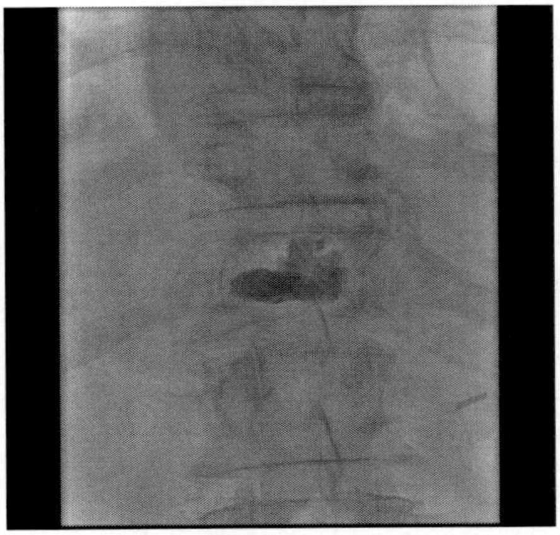

B

Figure 16. Following RF ablation, cement has been injected and fills the majority of the lesion.

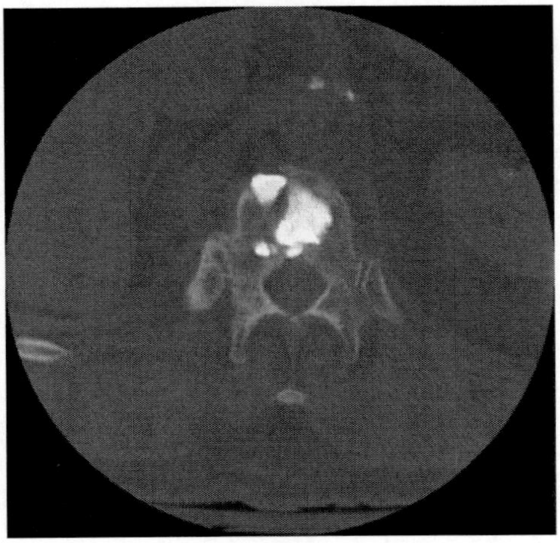

A

Figure 17. (Continued).

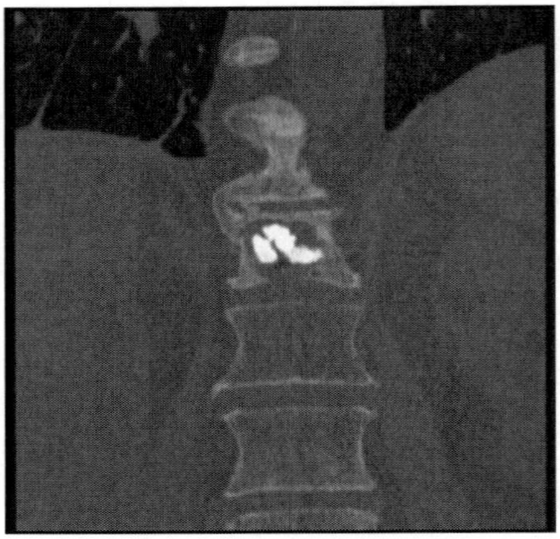

B

Figure 17. Post procedure CT. Cement fills the majority of the lesion.

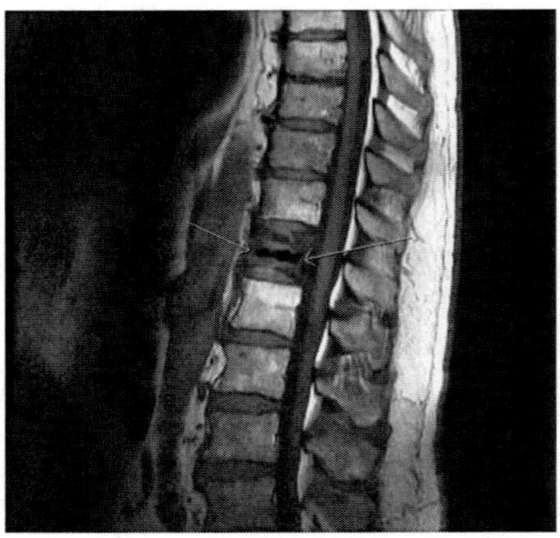

A

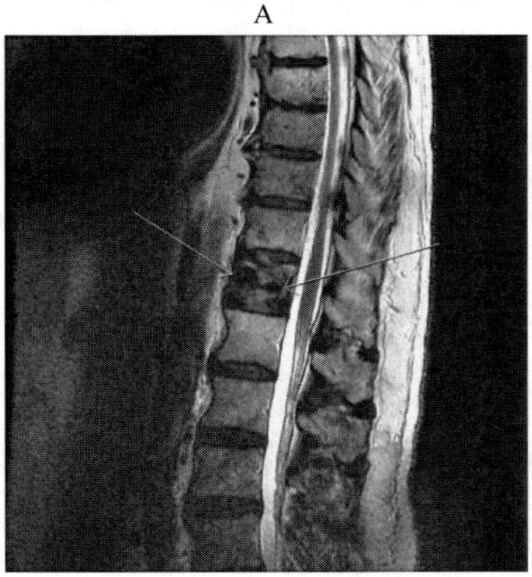

B

Figure 18. Post procedure MRI. Cement (dark signal) is seen within the T12 vertebral body.

Case 5

A 77 year male with multiple myeloma was admitted with a significant pain crisis due to multiple compression fractures in the lumbar spine. He was bed bound, and heavily dependent on narcotic medications. He required CADD pump during admission. He underwent conventional (no RFA used prior to cement injection) vertebroplasty at L1, L2 and L3 (Figure 19).

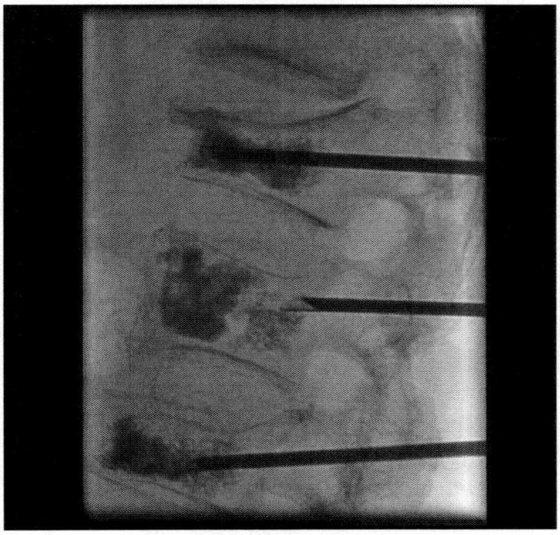

A

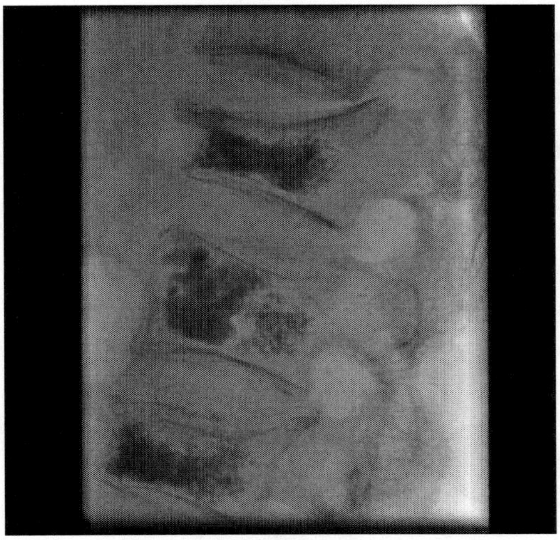

B

Figure 19. A: Lateral fluoroscopic image shows needle placement into the L1, L2 and L3 vertebral bodies. The L2 and L3 needles have already been retracted. B: Cement has been placed and the needles were removed.

He had tremendous pain relief almost immediately following the procedure and was able to move around much better, and required lesser doses of narcotics. On follow up 18 days following the procedure he only had mild residual lower back pain. 6 weeks after the procedure he had essentially no residual pain. Post procedure CT (Figure 20) and MRI (Figure 21) are shown. Note this patient's diffuse disease, best appreciated on the MRI (Figure 21).

This is a good example of a patient with diffuse disease but whose pain was more focal and localized to the treated levels. He therefore benefited from treatment of these levels.

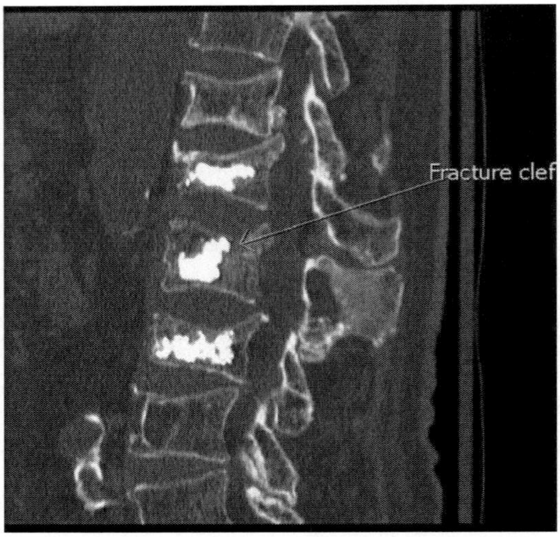

Figure 20. Post procedure CT shows good filling of L1, L2, and L3 vertebral bodies, including into the superior end plate fracture at L2.

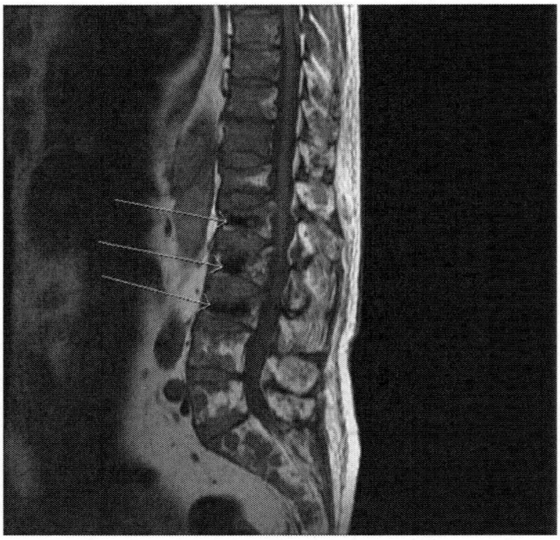

Figure 21. Post procedure MRI (T1 sagittal) shows cement delivery into the compressed L1, L2 and L3 vertebral bodies. Note that the majority of the spine is infiltrated by tumor (low signal has replaced the majority of visualized bones), except for a few islands of normal residual fatty (bright) marrow, as seen in the posterior aspect of L4 and L5.

Conclusion

In summary, percutaneous vertebral and pelvic augmentation can provide rapid, durable pain relief without the need for major surgery and is an effective adjunct to radiotherapy in palliating bone metastases.

References

[1] Ellsworth S, Alcorn S, Hales R, McNutt T, DeWeese T, Smith T. Patterns of care among patients receiving radiation therapy for bone metastases at a large academic institution. Int J Radiat Oncol Biol Phys 2014;89(5):1100-5.

[2] Barr J, Jensen M, Hirsch J, McGraw J, Barr R, Brook A et al. Position Statement on percutaneous vertebral augmentation: A consensus statement developed by the Society of Interventional Radiology (SIR), American Association of Neurological Surgeons (AANS) and the Congress of Neurological Surgeons (CNS), American College of Radiology (ACR), American Society of Neuroradiology (ASNR), American Society of Spine Radiology (ASSR), Canadian Interventional Radiology Association (CIRA), and the Society of NeuroInterventional Surgery (SNIS). J Vasc and Interv Radiol 2014;25(2):171-81.

[3] Chi J, Gokaslan Z. Vertebroplasty and kyphoplasty for spinal metastases. Curr Opin Support Palliat Care 2008;2(1):9-13.

[4] Cai Z. A preliminary study of the safety and efficacy of radiofrequency ablation with percutaneous kyphoplasty for thoracolumbar vertebral metastatic tumor treatment. Med Sci Monit 2014;20:556-3.

[5] Voormolen M, Lohle P, Lampmann L, van den Wildenberg W, Juttmann J, Diekerhof C et al. Prospective clinical follow-up after percutaneous vertebroplasty in patients with painful osteoporotic vertebral compression fractures. J Vasc Interv Radiol 2006;17(8):1313-20.

[6] Kaemmerlen P, Thiesse P, Bouvard H, Biron P, Mornex F, Jonas P. Vertebroplastie percutanee dans le traitement des metastases: technique et resultats. J Radiol 1989;70(10):557-62.

[7] Weill A, Chiras J, Simon J, Rose M, Sola-Martinez T, Enkaoua E. Spinal metastases: indications for and results of percutaneous injection of acrylic surgical cement. Radiology 1996;199(1):241-7.

[8] Fourney D, Schomer D, Nader R, Chlan-Fourney J, Suki D, Ahrar K et al. Percutaneous vertebroplasty and kyphoplasty for painful vertebral body fractures in cancer patients. J Neurosurg 2003;98(1):21-30.

[9] Halpin R, Bendok B, Liu J. Minimally invasive treatments for spinal metastases: Vertebroplasty, kyphoplasty, and radiofrequency ablation. Support Oncol 2004;2(4):339-55.

[10] Zoarski G, Snow P, Olan W, Stallmeyer M, Dick B, Hebel J et al. Percutaneous vertebroplasty for osteoporotic compression fractures: Quantitative prospective evaluation of long-term outcomes. J Vasc Intervent Radiol 2002;13(2):139-48.

[11] Cotten A, Dewatre F, Cortet B, Assaker R, Leblond D, Duquesnoy B et al. Percutaneous vertebroplasty for osteolytic metastases and myeloma: effects of the percentage of lesion filling and the leakage of methyl methacrylate at clinical follow-up. Radiology 1996;200(2):525-30.

[12] Lee B, Lee S, Yoo T. Paraplegia as a complication of percutaneous vertebroplasty with polymethyl methacrylate. Spine 2002;27(19):419-22.

[13] Harrington K. Major neurological complications following percutaneous vertebroplasty with polymethylmethacrylate: a case report. J Bone Joint Surg Am 2001;83(7):1070-3.

[14] Cotten A, Boutry N, Cortet B, Assaker R, Demondion X, Leblond D et al. Percutaneous vertebroplasty: state of the art. RadioGraphics 1998;18(2):311-20.

[15] Rosenthal D, Callstrom M. Critical review and state of the art in interventional oncology: Benign and metastatic disease involving bone. Radiology 2012;262(3):765-80.

[16] Rosenthal D, Alexander A, Rosenberg A, Springfield D. Ablation of osteoid osteomas with a percutaneously placed electrode: a new procedure Radiology. 1992;183(1):29-33.

[17] Hoffmann R, Jakobs T, Trumm C, Weber C, Helmberger T, Reiser M. Radiofrequency ablation in combination with osteoplasty in the treatment of painful metastatic bone disease. J Vasc Intervent Radiol 2008;19(3):419-25.

[18] Munk P, Rashid F, Heran M, Papirny M, Liu D, Malfair D et al. Combined cementoplasty and radiofrequency ablation in the treatment of painful neoplastic lesions of bone. J Vasc Intervent Radiol 2009;20(7):903-11.

[19] Anselmetti G, Manca A, Ortega C, Grignani G, DeBernardi F, Regge D. Treatment of Extraspinal Painful Bone Metastases with Percutaneous Cementoplasty: A Prospective Study of 50 Patients. CardioVasc Intervent Radiol 2008;31(6):1165-73.

[20] Kojima H, Tanigawa N, Kariya S, Komemushi A, Shomura Y, Sawada S. Clinical assessment of percutaneous radiofrequency ablation for painful metastatic bone tumors. CardioVasc Intervent Radiolm2006;29(6):1022-6.

[21] Proschek D. Prospective pilot-study of combined bipolar radiofrequency ablation and application of bone cement in bone metastases. Anticancer Res. 2009;29(7):2787-92.

[22] Halpin R, Bendok B, Sato K, Liu J, Patel J, Rosen S. Combination treatment of vertebral metastases using image-guided percutaneous radiofrequency ablation and vertebroplasty: a case report. Surg Neurol 2005;63(5):469-74.

[23] Schaefer O, Lohrmann C, Herling M, Uhrmeister P, Langer M. Combined radiofrequency thermal ablation and percutaneous cementoplasty treatment of a pathologic fracture. J Vasc Intervent Radiol 2002;13(10):1047-50.

[24] Georgy B. Bone cement deposition patterns with plasma-mediated radio-frequency ablation and cement augmentation for advanced metastatic spine lesions. Am J Neuroradiol 2009;30(6):1197-1202.

[25] Lane M, Le H, Lee S, Young C, Heran M, Badii M et al. Combination radiofrequency ablation and cementoplasty for palliative treatment of painful neoplastic bone metastasis: experience with 53 treated lesions in 36 patients. Skeletal Radiol 2010;40(1):25-32.

[26] Gofeld M, Yee A, Whyne C, Akens M, Pezeshki P, Woo J. New palliative intervention for painful metastatic bone disease: The OsteoCool™ system. Eur Cells and Mater 2012;23(3):11.

[27] Woo J, Pezeshki P, Yee A, Whyne C, Akens M, Won E et al. Validation of a novel bone tumor RF ablation system: Physics and animal data. Boston: Group de recherche interdisciplinaire sur les biomatériaux ostéo-articulaires injectable (GRIBOI), 2011.

[28] Nicholas Kurup A, Callstrom M. Ablation of musculoskeletal metastases: Pain palliation, fracture risk reduction, and oligometastatic disease. Tech Vasc Interv Radiol 2013;16(4):253-61.

Submitted: June 10, 2015. *Revised:* July 03, 2015. *Accepted:* July 15, 2015.

In: Pain Management Yearbook 2015
Editor: Joav Merrick

ISBN: 978-1-63484-515-1

Chapter 31

SUPERIOR VENA CAVA SYNDROME

Cyril Danjoux*[*], MD, Breanne Lechner, BSc(C), Natalie Pulenzas, BSc(C), May Tsao, MD, Elizabeth Barnes, MD and Edward Chow, MBBS

Rapid Response Radiotherapy Program, Department of Radiation Oncology, Odette Cancer Centre, Sunnybrook Health Sciences Centre, University of Toronto, Toronto, Ontario, Canada

Superior vena cava syndrome (SVCS) is a well-recognized manifestation of obstruction of the superior vena cava. It is clinically striking but rarely requires emergency treatment. Nowadays SVCS is most commonly due to external compression by malignancy or intrinsic thrombus due to an indwelling catheter. A tissue diagnosis is needed to guide diagnosis and treatment. An aggressive multimodality approach to investigation, support and treatment is indicated. Radiotherapy and intravascular stents are effective methods of achieving immediate symptom relief. The presence of SVCS does not reduce the probability of cure of the underlying malignancy and should not compromise the choice of appropriate treatment. A significant proportion (10-20%) survives over 2 years.

Keywords: superior vena cava, radiotherapy, stent

INTRODUCTION

Superior vena cava syndrome (SVCS) results from obstruction of blood flow through the thin walled superior vena cava (SVC). The superior vena cava is the major venous drainage from the head, neck, arms and upper thorax to the right atrium. It is located in the upper chest, surrounded by rigid structures which include the sternum, trachea, bronchi and mediastinal nodes and is vulnerable to compression. If this vein is compressed by outside structures, or if blocked by a thrombus or clot within it, the flow of blood to the heart is compromised leading

[*] Correspondence: Cyril Danjoux MD, FRCPC, Odette Cancer Centre, Sunnybrook Health Sciences Centre, 2075 Bayview Ave. Toronto, ON, M4N 3M5, Canada. E-mail: Cyril.Danjoux@sunnybrook.ca.

to increased pressure and swelling of the veins of the head, face, neck and arms. When the SVC is obstructed, blood flows through collateral vessels to the lower body and inferior vena cava or azygos vein. Several weeks are needed for collaterals to dilate sufficiently to accommodate the blood flow (1, 2). The severity of symptoms depends on the degree and speed of narrowing of the SVC. Symptoms may improve as collateral circulation develops.

ETIOLOGY

William Hunter first described the syndrome in 1757 in a patient with syphilitic aortic aneurysm (3). In 1954, Schechter reviewed 274 well documented cases of SVCS reported in the literature; 40% of them were due to syphilitic aneurysms or tuberculous mediastinitis (4).

Nowadays obstruction of the SVC is caused by malignancies in 50% of cases, with lung cancer at the top of the list, followed by lymphoma as seen in Table 1 (5-10). Thrombosis or non-malignant conditions account for 35% of cases.

Table 1. Malignant causes of SVCS

Tumour Type	Percentage (Range)
Non-small cell lung cancer	50 (43-59)
Small-cell lung cancer	**22 (7-39)**
Lymphoma	12 (1-25)
Metastatic cancer	**9 (1-15)**
Germ cell cancer	3 (0-6)
Thymoma	**1 (0-1)**

Data from Wilson et al. (5), Armstrong et al. 6, Bell et al. (7), Schraufnagel et al. (8), Yellin et al. (9), Parish et al. (10).

Table 2. Signs and symptoms of SVCS

Symptoms	Frequency (%)
Dyspnea	63
Facial swelling or head fullness	**50**
Cough	24
Arm swelling	**18**
Chest Pain	15
Dysphagia	**9**
Signs	
Venous distension of neck	66
Venous distension on chest wall	**54**
Facial Edema	46
Cyanosis or facial plethora	**19**
Arm edema	14

Data from Armstrong et al. (6), Bell et al. (7), Schraufnagel et al. (8), Yellin et al. (9).

SYMPTOMS AND SIGNS

SVCS has an insidious onset. Symptoms develop over two weeks in a third of patients and over longer periods in other cases (6, 8, 9, 11, 12). Shortness of breath on lying down, facial swelling and a sensation of fullness in the head are the most common symptoms. Cough and hoarseness are other possible presentations. Common clinical findings are neck and chest vein distention, with typical collateral venous drainage over the upper thorax and swollen puffy face, eyelids, and arm edema (see Table 2) (7-9). Serious effects of obstruction of the SVC are rare. Only one death was documented in 1986 patients with SVCS (13).

ASSESSMENT AND DIAGNOSIS

Clinical recognition of SVCS is relatively straightforward since the signs and symptoms are usually typical. Once SVCS is recognized, prompt clinical attention is important. A chest X-ray usually shows the presence of mediastinal widening, pleural effusion or right hilar mass (10, 14). Contrast Computer tomography (CT) of the chest is the most useful imaging study. It provides information about the SVC, collateral circulation, the presence of SVC thrombosis, mediastinal nodes, and involvement of surrounding structures.

Diagnostic procedures include sputum cytology, which provides a clue in half of the patients. Pleural effusion drainage for cytology or supraclavicular nodal biopsy is usually helpful. Other procedures include bronchoscopy, mediastinoscopy or bone marrow biopsy for diagnosis and staging.

MANAGEMENT

Traditionally SVCS was considered as an emergency. However recent data suggests that in most cases the course is relatively benign, and often improves without any active treatment (5, 8). In most cases symptoms are generally progressive over several weeks and then improves over time. (5).

The aims of treatment are to relieve symptoms and cure potentially curable primary malignancies such as Hodgkin's, germ cell tumors and small cell lung cancer. Treatment can be considered as supportive or definitive therapy. Supportive therapeutic maneuver include bed rest, elevation of the patient's head to decrease the hydrostatic pressure and thereby the edema, bronchodilators, and oxygen supplement. There are no data documenting the effectiveness of these maneuvers, but it is simple and with little risk. Short term steroids may help reduce symptoms associated with tumour necrosis, inflammation, and oedema although there are no controlled clinical trials to quantify their efficacy. Dexamethasone, (4 mg every 6 h) is commonly prescribed, although its effects have not been well studied. Diuretics are also commonly used, but it is unclear whether venous pressure distal to the obstruction is affected by small changes in right atrial pressure. Anticoagulation and thrombotic therapy may be of benefit if the underlying cause is due to a thrombus and an indwelling catheter. One study reported an overall 84% rate of clinical improvement to be similar among patients receiving steroids, diuretics, or neither (8).

A histological diagnosis is essential. Treatment prior to definitive diagnosis is not justified. SVCS is rarely a true emergency. Cancer patients diagnosed with SVCS do not die of the syndrome itself but from the extent of their underlying disease. Only those presenting with severe airway compromise, cardiovascular collapse, or significantly elevation of intracranial pressure are at risk of immediate morbidity and require emergency treatment. Expandable intravascular stents insertion by interventional radiologist can provide rapid relief of symptoms in those with severe respiratory distress who require immediate urgent intervention. This can facilitate subsequent tissue diagnosis or radiotherapy or can also be considered for those after maximum tolerance of radiotherapy. The optimal timing of stent insertion is not well defined.

Definitive therapy includes radiotherapy, chemotherapy and surgery. There are no good randomized controlled studies to guide the selection of treatment modality. It is recommended that a multi-disciplinary approach, involving radiation oncologist, medical oncologist, surgeon, respirologist, be used to decide on an overall plan and the most appropriate modality to use in treatment of SVCS for each individual patient. The optimal decision will depend on the histology, stage, prognosis (independent of SVCS), the patient general condition and expected response and side effects of the treatment options.

Surgical options are reserved for those with a benign cause such as granulomatous disease, aortic aneurysm or retrosternal goiter. In cases of thrombosis due to indwelling catheter, removal of the catheter with anticoagulant therapy is recommended.

Radiotherapy is often used for malignant SVCS, as the majority of tumour types respond well to radiotherapy. Complete symptomatic relief is reported in nearly 80% of small cell lung cancer, 60% of NSCLC at 2 weeks. Clinical improvement often occurs within 72 hours (6, 8, 9, 12, 13, 15, 16-20). Objective complete relief of SVCO as seen on serial venogram was reported in 31% with partial relief in 23% despite reported 85% symptom relief, suggesting that development of collateral circulation may play unimportant part in symptomatic relief. Depending on the underlying pathology, stage and condition of the patient radiotherapy can be given as a short 1-2 week course of palliative of RT or as part of a combined modality approach combined with chemotherapy.

The majority of SVCS due to small cell lung cancer or non-Hodgkin's lymphoma are chemo sensitive. Following chemotherapy complete relief of symptoms of SVCS is reported in 80% of non-Hodgkin's lymphoma or small cell lung cancer (8, 15, 21, 22). Combined chemo-radiation often results in better cure rates and longer survival than radiation alone.

Rowell reported no clinically significant difference on SVCS relief whether chemotherapy radiotherapy or chemotherapy with radiotherapy was used (22). In two randomized trials there was no difference in symptom relief, relapse or survival with initial chemotherapy alone compared to either sequential or concurrent chemo-radiotherapy among NSCLC (15, 18).

The results of stent insertion were reported in 23 studies (24). Overall, the procedure helped improve the effects of narrowing or blockage in 151 out of 159 patients (95%). During follow-up to 8 months after the procedure, in 146 patients (92%), the vena cava remained open. However obstruction recurred in 17 patients. In comparison, the response following chemotherapy, radiotherapy or both was reported in 377 out of 487 patients (77%) (23). The role of radiotherapy post stent insertion has not been well studied.

General recommendation supporting radiotherapy, stent placement, or both for symptomatic SVCS due to lung cancer has been made by the National Institute for Health and

Clinical Excellence NICE (23) the American College of Chest Physicians (24) the National Comprehensive Cancer Network (NCCN) (25) and the Cardiovascular and Interventional Radiological Society of Europe CIRSE (26).

Following various treatment modalities the duration of relief of SVCS appear to be similar. Symptomatic recurrence of SVCS occurred in about 20% of patients with lung cancer after chemotherapy, radiotherapy or both (15). The optimal management of recurrent SVCS is still controversial as there are no good randomized trials comparing the use of various treatment modalities.

Prognosis depends on the underlying cause, stage, performance status co-morbidity and appropriate management. One year survival, range from less than 1% in advanced NSCLC, to over 40% in non-Hodgkin's lymphoma (6). The average life expectancy for patients who present with malignancy associated SVCS is 6-9 months. Overall 10-20% survives over 2 years. In the absence of distant metastases aggressive management and support are indicated.

Conclusion

There is no good classification scheme to grade the severity of symptoms of SVCS and guide treatment. Yu et al. (27) proposed a classification system based on the Common Terminology Criteria for Adverse Events (CTCAE) of the National Institutes of Health and divided into mild, moderate, severe, life threatening and fatal and proposed a treatment algorithm based on the presence or absence of potential life threatening symptoms, performance status and histology. Both await further validation and refinement.

References

[1] Kim HJ, Kim HS, Chung SH. CT diagnosis of superior vena cava syndrome: importance of collateral vessels. Am J Roentgenol 1993;161:539-42.

[2] Trigaux JP, Van Beers B. Thoracic collateral venous channels: normal and pathologic CT findings. J Comput Assist Tomogr 1990;14:769-73.

[3] Hunter W. The history of an aneurysm of the aorta with some remarks on aneurysms in general. Med Observ Inq 1957;1:323.

[4] Schechter MM. The superior vena cava syndrome. Am J Med Sci 1954;227(1):46-56.

[5] Wilson LD, Detterbeck FC, Yahalom J. Clinical practice Superior vena cava syndrome with malignant causes. N Eng J Med 2007;356:18:1862-1869.

[6] Armstrong BA, Perez CA, Simpson JR, Hederman MA. Role of irradiation in the management of superior vena cava Syndrome. Int J Radiat Oncol Biol Phys 1987;13:531-9.

[7] Bell DR, Woods RLI, Levi JA. Superior vena caval obstruction: A 10-year experience. Med J Aust 1986;145:566.

[8] Schraufnagel DE, Hill R, Leech JA, Pare JAP. Superior Vena cava obstruction. Is it an emergency? Am J Med 1981;70:1169-74.

[9] Yellin A, Rosen A, Rweichert N, Lieberman Y. Superior vena cava syndrome: The myth-the facts. Am Rev Respir Dis 1990;141:1114-8.

[10] Parish JM, Marschke RF, Dines DE, Lee RE. Etiologic considerations in Superior vena cava syndrome. Mayo Clin Proc 1981;56:407-10.

[11] Abner A. Approach to the patient who presents with superior vena cava obstruction. Chest 1993;103: Suppl 4:394-7S.

[12] Ostler PJ, Clarke DP, Watkinson AF, Gaze MN. Superior vena cava obstruction: a modern management strategy. Clin Oncol (R Coll Radiol) 1997;9:83-9.

[13] Ahmann FR. A reassessment of the clinical implications of the superior vena cava syndrome. J Clin Oncol 1984;2:961-9.

[14] Chow E, Danjoux C, Andersson L. Superior vena cava syndrome. Patient Care Canada 1999;10(7):57-61.

[15] Spiro SG, Shah S, Harper PG, Tobias JS, Geddes DM, Souhami RL. Treatment of obstruction of the superior vena cava by combination chemotherapy with and without irradiation in small-cell carcinoma of the bronchus. Thorax 1983;38:501.

[16] Nicholson AA, Ettles DF, Arnold A, Greenstone M, Dyet JF. Treatment of malignant superior vena cava obstruction: metal stent or radiotherapy. J Vasc Interv Radiol 1997;8:781-8.

[17] Anderson PR, Coia LR. Fractionation and outcomes with palliative radiotherapy. Semi Radiot Oncol. 2000;10:191-9.

[18] Pereira JR, Martins SJ, Ikari FK, Nikaedo SM, Gampel O. Neoadjuvant chemotherapy vs radiotherapy alone for superior vena cava syndrome (SVCS) due to non-small cell lung cancer (NSCLC): preliminary results of randomized phase II trial. Eur J Cancer 1999;35 Suppl 4:260.

[19] Wurschmidt F, Bunemann H, Heilmann HP. Small cell lung cancer with and without superior vena cava syndrome: a multivariate analysis of prognostic factors in 408 cases. Int J Radiat Oncol biol Phys 1995;33:77-82.

[20] Chan RH, Dar AR, Yu E, Stitt LW, Whiston F, Truong P, et al. Superior vena cava obstruction in small cell lung cancer. Int J Radiat Oncol Biol Phys 1997;38:513-20.

[21] Sculier JP, Evans WK, Feld R, DeBoer G, Payne DG, et al. Superior vena cava obstruction syndrome in small cell lung cancer. Cancer 1986;57:847-51.

[22] Rowell NP, Gleeson FV. Steroids, radiotherapy, chemotherapy and streets for superior vena caval obstruction in carcinoma of the bronchus: a systematic review. Colin Oncol (R Coll Radiol) 2002;14:338-51.

[23] Stent placement for superior vena caval obstruction. The National Institute for Health and Clinical Excellence (NICE). Accessed 2015 May 14. URL: www.nice.org.uk/IPG079guidance.

[24] Kvale PA, Simoff M, Prakash UBS. Lung cancer: Palliative care. Chest 2003; 123 Suppl 1:284S-284S.

[25] NCCN clinical Practice Guidelines in Oncology: non-small cell lung cancer. National Comprehensive Cancer Network. Accessed 2015 May 14. 2006 URL: http://www.nccn. org/professionals/physician_gls/pdf/nscl.pdf.

[26] Uberoi R, Moran R. Quality assurance guidelines for superior vena cava stenting in malignant disease. The cardiovascular and interventional Radiological Society of Europe (CIRSE). Cardiovasc Intervent Radiol 2006;29:319-22.

[27] Yu JB, Wilson LD, Detterbeck F. Superior Vena Cava Syndrome – A proposed classification system and algorithm for management. J Thoracic Oncology 2008;3(8): 811-4.

Submitted: June 15, 2015. *Revised:* July 31, 2015. *Accepted:* August 15, 2015.

In: Pain Management Yearbook 2015
Editor: Joav Merrick

ISBN: 978-1-63484-515-1

Chapter 32

A REVIEW OF MEDICAL HUMANITIES CURRICULUM IN MEDICAL SCHOOLS

Michael Lam, BMSc(C), Breanne Lechner, MD(C), Ronald Chow, Leonard Chiu, BSc(C), Nicholas Chiu, MD(C), Henry Lam, MLS, Marko Popovic, MD(C), Milica Milakovic, BSc(C), Carlo DeAngelis, PharmD, Edward Chow, MBBS and Blair Henry, MTS (Bioethics) *

Sunnybrook Health Sciences Centre,
University of Toronto, Toronto, Ontario, Canada

This paper reviews the current status of medical humanities courses in Canadian undergraduate medical school curricula as a foundation for ethics and professionalism training. It studies relevant literature and compares the course offerings of the 17 Canadian medical schools as presented on the official school websites and course calendars. It discusses how medical humanities courses have grown to become an integral part of the medical education syllabus in many schools. Programs specifically dedicated to humanities are also reviewed.

Keywords: humanities, medical humanities, ethics, medical school, medical student, medical training, medical education, curriculum

INTRODUCTION

'Medical humanities' is a field that utilizes a multidisciplinary approach to integrate knowledge and skills of non-natural-sciences into medical practices. It includes language arts, written literature, history, philosophy, religious studies, jurisprudence, anthropology,

* Correspondence: Mr. Blair Henry MTS (Bioethics), Sunnybrook Health Sciences Centre, 2075 Bayview Avenue, Toronto, Ontario, M4N 3M5, Canada. Phone: 416-480-6100x 7178, Fax: 416-480-6899, E-mail: blair.henry@sunnybrook.ca.

sociology and psychology (1). Fine arts including music, visual arts and performing arts are also included by some authors (2). Although the natural sciences are the foundation of medical knowledge, it has been recognized since the early 20th century that the practice of medicine as the care of the patient requires more than scientific knowledge (3), and that facts alone are unable to manage medical problems in the context of the entire human experience (4). Medical students and clerks reported that many of their professors did not behave as humanistic caregivers or were poor role models in teaching the physician-patient relationship (5). At the beginning of the new millennium it was suggested by the results of a randomized controlled trial that the integration of humanities subject areas into the medical school curriculum could have a long term positive effect on the practice of medical school graduates in terms of managing patients with psychosocial issues, establishing holistic views of patients' predicaments, and assisting to communicate, listen, and accept different perspectives in a team setting (19). For instance, 40% of NP students eventually pursued primary practice or psychiatry, compared to a mere 18% for non NP students (19).

Efficient diagnosis and treatment of disease in our modern multicultural society requires understanding of the complex socioeconomic, ethnic and religious backgrounds of patients and their families (6). It involves genuine empathy in addition to attentive listening skills (7). For instance, a primary care physician must take into consideration the fasting tradition of a religious patient when the latter complains of headache and dizziness. At the same time, they must acknowledge the fact that fasting practices vary among different faiths and that each possesses a unique overall influence on the health of individuals (8). Moreover, peculiar skills seemingly unrelated to science, such as the art of magic performance, might also ameliorate clinical situations. A family physician could use magic tricks to calm and hearten a crying child into an intrigued, cooperative patient, thereby facilitating a thorough clinical examination (9). These are all considered humanities-based 'soft' skills outside the realm of natural sciences training.

The increasing awareness of the importance of medical humanities is evident throughout this past decade. Recently, the Association of American Medical Colleges (AAMC) made changes to the content of the Medical College Admission Test (MCAT) to cover humanities and social sciences (10). The 2015 MCAT will include a section entitled "Psychological, Social, and Biological Foundations of Behaviour" (11). This ensures that students have a better understanding of the psychosocial aspects of health and diseases, which will allow them to perform better as a clinician overall. The purpose of this paper is to examine the current circumstances involving medical humanities curricula in medical training by analyzing results from published literature and online.

Methods

A literature search was conducted in Ovid Medline (1946-July week 1 2015) and Ovid Embase (1947-2015 week 28) to retrieve relevant studies. The subject headings and keywords used included 'humanities', 'medical humanities', 'humanism', 'humanizing', 'humanistic', 'ethics', 'medical ethics', 'medical school' and 'undergraduate medical education'. Results were limited to English or French language. There were 45 articles found in Medline and 97 from Embase. After removal of duplicates and screening, a total of 45 papers were reviewed.

Papers were excluded if the full text could not be obtained or if abstracts were not available. Official websites and online course calendars of the 17 medical schools in Canada were also examined to derive knowledge on whether medical humanities components were present in their curricula.

RESULTS

It is evident from the literature and the official websites reviewed that many medical schools have been gradually introducing humanities components into their syllabus, either as an integral part of their core medical courses, or as required or elective courses. Results are discussed below by geographical location.

Canada

We reviewed the official websites and/or online course calendars of all 17 Canadian medical schools. Results are summarized in Table 1. Out of the 17 Canadian schools, 3 show no humanities-related courses in their curriculum on their online calendar (Montreal, Queens, Sherbrooke) (44, 48, 50). University of Manitoba, on the other extreme, offers different medical humanities subjects in all three categories: as a component of a clinical course, a required course, and as electives (41). McMaster University, known for its eminence in medical education, has a special program focusing on psychological and social mechanisms of illness (43). Dalhousie University features a medical humanities program for similar purposes (39). With 15 distinct courses geared towards humanities and social sciences, the University of Alberta is the leader among Canadian schools in terms of medical humanities course offerings (36).

Out of 45 results, the literature search yielded only one relevant Canadian article that documented medical humanities curricula in medical schools. The article detailed the Human Values Program at the University of Manitoba. First introduced in 1986, this required medical humanities module intermingles literary arts, social psychology, and spirituality into medical practice. Students became better equipped, and excelled marvelously in the 2002 ethics qualifying examinations. They went on to apply their social skills in the Canadian health care system (12). Notably, there is no Canadian survey analyzing this subject from the perspectives of students.

United States

The United States, as one of the leaders in medical education in the last century, has long recognized the importance of humanities education. In 2011, 69 of the 133 accredited medical schools in the country required students to take a course in the medical humanities (13). The literature is filled with reports on many such programs. The University of Texas at San Antonio and at Galveston (14, 15) reported a longitudinal and integrated humanities curriculum including the history of ethics and the establishment of the Institute for Medical

Humanities in 1973. Another paper from 1973 mentioned that the incorporation of "humanistic aspects of medicine" into medical education did not progress with much momentum at that time (16). In 1978, the East Caroline University School of Medicine decided to make their medical humanities courses mandatory in the preclinical curriculum (17). By the 1980s, the American medical education system began to receive feedback pointing out its failure to provide adequate training in the areas of ethics, morality, and spirituality/religion and hence called for improvement (18).

Of particular interest was an aforementioned randomized controlled trial conducted at Harvard Medical School in 1998 in regards to the New Pathway (NP) Program which had a significant humanistic medicine component (19). Results showed that NP candidates felt more confident in their ability to handle psychosocial problems, and that they succeeded in developing decent communication and collaboration assets (19). A 1999 study examined the perspectives of patients as opposed to medical students or professors. Interestingly, some physicians were reported to be seen as "unfeeling technicians" as opposed to "humane caregivers" from patients' points of view. (36). The paper further suggested that weaving the study of philosophy into other facets of medical training would allow students to develop not merely empathy, but also a more open view and a connection to the ideas and backgrounds of patients (20).

By the twenty-first century, the addition of humanities programs into medical curricula grew significantly. For instance, Dr. S. C. Weiss from Duke University began to conduct seminars in medical humanities on a biweekly basis, arguing it was necessary for physicians to engage in "productive dialogue with the patient" (21). According to a 2003 paper, the medical ethics course at the University of Arkansas College of Medicine is compulsory for all 2nd year students (22). The year 2000 saw the arrival of the Arts and Humanities Medical Scholars (AMHS) branch at the Stanford University School of Medicine. This enhancement promoted the enthusiasm of students towards streams of medical humanities including but not limited to literature, music, and history (22). Furthermore, the establishment of the Department of Anthropology, History, and Social Medicine at the University of California in 1930, along with 10 other medical humanities programs at American institutions were outlined in the same study (22).

In 2015, Haidet et al. suggested that arts trigger imagination and emotions while improving students' overall skills, insights, and outlooks towards illness (23). In the same year Hildebrandt proposed that more measures should be taken in directing the study of anatomical dissection towards a more ethics-based approach (24). With the second most medical schools worldwide, the United States has undoubtedly made an effort to expand the domain of humanities within the curriculum of medicine. It is a prominent example of a nation whose transition from passivity to awareness and promotion of this area in the past few decades is clearly presented in this literature review.

Europe

Of the 5 articles retrieved on European programs (8, 41, 44, 45, 46), 3 highlighted the outcomes of the inclusion of literary arts in medical education (8, 41, 46). Prominent ideas presented included that literature and theatre expose students to personal suffering (7), and that the former aids in the communication and expression of emotions (25). Indeed, fine arts are shown to improve the overall quality of medical education. A 2003 study analyzed the programs of medical schools across Europe. It revealed the fact that Croatia and Italy led the continent with the highest amount of humanistic studies in their syllabus. On the other hand, there was a general "lack of uniform curriculum", implying that European faculties must strive to establish more standardized curricula in order that future health care professionals be capable of communicating and performing with a common foundation (26).

The need for medical students to express themselves with creativity and assertiveness and to boost their comprehension of society and culture is summarized in a 2004 paper (27). Two articles stressed the significance of the role of medical ethics and philosophy in aiding students to recognize ethical situations in health care (28, 29). An Italian study from 2013 showed that despite being limited, Italian literature is in favour of having medical humanities as an essential component of the training of health care professionals (30).

Asia

One article documented the ethics and humanities course, first offered in 2003, for premedical students at Weill Cornell Medical College in Qatar (31). Designed with the intention to help students adapt to and be prepared for the global health care system, the course was found to greatly foster students' ethical reasoning, familiarity with philosophy and written literature, and to improve their verbal skills. A 2008 paper focused on the contribution of humanism and ethics to Japanese society. It mentioned that such qualities and skills as altruism, excellence, integrity, and duty needed to be practiced by health care professionals. A survey of 3993 faculty members of Japanese medical schools showed that 60% was in favour of the introduction of a new, refined medical school system that would include humanities and social sciences. A special emphasis was placed on the notion that arts and sciences are equally important in the profession of medicine (31). The most recent article in this group is a 2014 survey study from India (32). It discovered that although the Medical Council of India does incorporate ethics in its syllabus, less than one-third of medical students believed ethical principles could assist in the avoidance of legal issues in health care. This study called for additional programs and workshops to be established in order for knowledge of ethics to be sufficient among medical students.

Australia

A 1977 article from the University of Melbourne focused on physician-patient interactions being studied in literary works mandatory for the curriculum. It argued this familiarized them with the psychosocial scopes of medicine and made them more comfortable in handling ethical dilemmas (33). The rise of humanities in medical curricula was defended by a paper published by Milligan et al. in 2009. A mention was made about how the fine arts, including poetry, music, and written literature could augment clinicians' understanding of illness. It added that science and humanities should not be approached as "polar opposites" but rather "complementary disciplines" (34).

South America

A 1976 paper from Argentina described how humanities became part of the medical curriculum at the University of La Plata in Buenos Aires, Argentina, but was not compulsory. Among included branches were history, anthropology, and philosophy. After two decades, the Department of Medical Humanities gained popularity and demonstrated enhancement in the overall quality of medical training. The author also emphasized his preference for the term "alleviating art" as opposed to "healing art" when describing medicine (35), implying that physicians should relieve the emotional stress of patients as opposed to merely improving their physical condition.

Discussion

A rising number of American medical schools are at the very least recognizing the importance of, if not experimenting, with the incorporation of such subfields as cultural/community studies, anthropology, written literature, theatre, film, and visual arts into their agendas (22). Although merely one report from this search documented the use of humanities in Canadian medical schools, 14 out of 17 Canadian medical schools have humanities components in their curricula to various degrees. We anticipate that those 3 which lack such courses will eventually incorporate them in their syllabi. Additionally, this paper focuses merely on the curricula of medical schools. It does not discuss extracurricular activities.

In terms of limitations, this review only reports on information published in academic literature and online. Of the 27 full-text articles reviewed from the US, 18 focused on one specific medical school or program. Although this paper is not a systematic review, it is apparent that the majority of the varied literature either focused on the benefits of broadening the curriculum to include medical humanities, or promoted future action that would allow such success to be achieved.

In the past, reliance on a strong science background was regarded as a primary criterion for acceptance into medical school. Currently, motives involve a more holistic approach to the selection of medical students, and in many cases spaces have been set aside for candidates with prior training in humanities. It is true that the main duty of a physician is to recognize a patient's health problems and to resolve them.

Nonetheless, countless sociological factors are changing nowadays. For instance, the world population is augmenting at an accelerating pace. Contemporary society is simply unable to thrive without health care professionals who have strong backgrounds in medical humanities. Therefore, the ability to communicate well, to demonstrate professionalism, and to tackle psychosocial and ethical issues is essential for physicians. Because these aspects are all integrated in the disciplines of humanities and social sciences, it is crucial to promote the inclusion of these 'soft' subjects into medical and premedical training.

As clinicians often need to treat patients with diverse cultural backgrounds and living habits, knowledge of medical humanities becomes essential for cross-cultural sensitivity in this era. Though consensus on the need for more humanities training seems to have been reached, our report identified a definitive lack of uniformity and standardization of humanities programming overall. It is unsurprising that the new 2015 version of the MCAT evaluates students on humanities.

The notion of medicine as an art and a social service must no longer be ignored. Given the abundant literature discussing the merits of humanities, it is important that medical humanities be incorporated into medical school curricula locally as well as globally. In our review, no articles reported negative outcomes as a result of the incorporation of medical humanities into the curriculum. To fully assess the impact of student selection and curriculum development, a long term longitudinal study will be required in order to reveal whether today's new practices have in fact assisted in the making of a 'good doctor'.

Table 1. Medical humanities courses offerings in all 17 Canadian medical schools

Medical School	Name of course(s) (year)
Alberta, University of (36)	*Independent elective course:* Arts and Humanities in Health and Medicine (AHHM) Program • Art in Medicine (1st, 2nd) • Designing Health: A Collaborative Project with the Health Humanities and the Community (1st, 2nd) • Directed Studies in Medical/Health Humanities (1st, 2nd) • Communicating Care: A Theatre-Based Approach (1st, 2nd) – study of theatre • Maladjusted: Engaging in Community-based Dialogue about Mental Health through Forum Theatre (1st, 2nd) • Shadowing Artists on the Wards: Promoting Patient-Centeredness through an Arts-based Medical Elective (1st, 2nd) • Spiritual Screening and Assessment: A Communication Skills Workshop (1st, 2nd) • Spirituality and Health: Spiritual Care Shadowing Elective (1st, 2nd) • The Art of Observation Elective (1st, 2nd) – study of art • Medical Ethics: An Introduction (1st, 2nd) • Art in Medicine (AIM) Project: Clinical Elective (3rd, 4th) • Designing Health: A Collaborative Project with the Health Humanities and the Community (3rd, 4th) • Directed Studies in Medical/ Health Humanities: Clinical Elective (3rd, 4th) • An Experience in Bioethics (3rd, 4th) *Integral part of a required medical course:* • Physicianship I, II, III (1st, 2nd, 3rd) – study of ethics, public health, health equity
British Colombia, University of (37)	*Integral part of a required medical course:* • Doctor Patient and Society (1st, 2nd) – study of social determinants of health, ethics, multiculturalism
Calgary, University of (38)	*Integral part of a required medical course:* • Medical Skills (1st, 2nd) • Ethics • Physicianship
Dalhousie University (39)	*Integral part of a required medical course:* • Professional Competencies I (1st) – study of ethics, social / historic elements of medicine *Independent elective Course:* • special medical humanities program: Healing and Education through the Arts and Life-Skills (HEALS) – includes visual arts, performing arts, creative writing, history of medicine

Table 1. (Continued).

Medical School	Name of course(s) (year)
Laval University (40)	*Independent elective course* • Ethique médicale et bioethique (1st)
Manitoba, University of (41)	*Integral part of a required medical course:* • Clinical Skills (1st, 2nd) – study of ethics *Independent required course:* • Medical Ethics and Humanities (1st, 2nd) *Independent elective course:* • Psychotherapy (4th) Co-occurring Disorders Initiative (4th) – study of mental health
McGill University (42)	*Integral part of a required medical course:* • Community Health Alliance Project (2nd) – study of social diversity, determinants of health, community • Basic Science, Medicine and Society (4th) – study of family, culture, politics
McMaster University (43)	*Independent elective course:* • special program known as COMPASS (optional) – involves the study of psychological and social mechanisms
Montréal, Université de (44)	N/A
Newfoundland, Memorial University of (45)	*Integral part of a required medical course:* • The Healthy Person (1st) – study of family, community
Northern Ontario School of Medicine (46)	*Integral part of a required medical course:* • Social and Population Health (1st, 2nd, 3rd, 4th) – study of culture, society • Personal and Professional Aspects of Medical Practice (1st, 2nd, 3rd, 4th) – study of ethics
Ottawa, University of (47)	*Integral part of a required medical course:* • Link Period (3rd) – study of community, ethics
Queen's University (48)	N/A
Saskatchewan, University of (49)	*Independent required course:* • Medicine and Society (1st, 2nd)
Sherbrooke, Université de (50)	N/A
Toronto, University of (51)	*Integral part of a required medical course:* • Art and Science of Clinical Medicine • Community, Population and Public Health-1 (1st) – study of social determinants of health • Determinants of Community Health 2 (2nd) – study of society, community, social justice
Western Ontario, University of (52)	*Independent required course:* • Medical Ethics and Humanities (1st, 2nd)

ACKNOWLEDGMENTS

We thank the generous support of Bratty Family Fund, Michael and Karyn Goldstein Cancer Research Fund, Joey and Mary Furfari Cancer Research Fund, Pulenzas Cancer Research Fund, Joseph and Silvana Melara Cancer Research Fund, and Ofelia Cancer Research Fund.

REFERENCES

[1] Cole TRC, Carlin NS, Carson, R.A. Medical humanities: and introduction: Cambridge University Press, 2014.

[2] Rodenhauser P, Strickland MA, Gambala CT. Arts-related activities across U.S. medical schools: A follow-up study. Teach Learn Med 2004;16(3):233-9.

[3] Peabody FW. THe care of the patient. JAMA Intern Med 1927;88(12):877-82.

[4] Cooper RA, Tauber AI. Viewpoint: New physicians for a new century. Acad Med 2005;80(12):1086-8.

[5] Maheux B, Beaudoin C, Berkson L, Cote L, Des Marchais J, Jean P. Medical faculty as humanistic physicians and teachers: The perceptions of students at innovative and traditional medical schools. Med Educ 2000;34(8):630-4.

[6] Tucker CM, Herman KC, Pedersen TR, Higley B, Montrichard M, Ivery P. Cultural sensitivity in physician-patient relationships: perspectives of an ethnically diverse sample of low-income primary care patients. Med Care 2003;41(7):859-70.

[7] Baum M. Teaching the humanities to medical students. Clin Med 2002;2(3):246-9.

[8] Trepanowski JF, Bloomer RJ. The impact of religious fasting on human health. Nutr J 2010;9:57. Doi:10.1186/1475-2891-9-57.

[9] Reynolds M. Making medicine magical. Med Post 2010;46(6):16.

[10] Geller G. Tolerance for ambiguity: An ethics-based criterion for medical student selection. Acad Med 2013;88(5):581-4.

[11] Colleges AoAM. What's on the MCAT2015 Exam? 2015 Accessed 2015 July 16. URL: https://www.Acad Med.org/students/services/343550/mcat2015.html.

[12] Magwood B, Casiro O, Hennen B. The Medical Humanities Program at the University of Manitoba, Winnipeg, Manitoba, Canada. Acad Med 2003;78(10):1015-9.

[13] Banaszek A. Medical humanities courses becoming prerequisites in many medical schools. Can Med Assoc J 2011;183(8):E441-E2.

[14] Jones T, Verghese A. On becoming a humanities curriculum: The Center for Medical Humanities and Ethics at the University of Texas Health Science Center at San Antonio. Acad Med 2003;78(10):1010-4.

[15] Jones AH, Carson RA. Medical Humanities at the University of Texas Medical Branch at Galveston. Acad Med 2003;78(10):1006-9.

[16] Kepler MO. Human values in medicine: Some helping organizations. JAMA Intern Med 1973;223(3):305-7.

[17] Kopelman LM. Development of the medical humanities program at East Carolina University. Acad Med 1989;64(12):730-4.

[18] Patel K. Physicians for the 21st century. Challenges facing medical education in the United States. Eval Health Prof 1999;22(3):379-98.

[19] Peters AS, Greenberger-Rosovsky R, Crowder C, Block SD, Moore GT. Long-term outcomes of the new pathway program at Harvard Medical School: A randomized controlled trial. Acad Med 2000;75(5):470-9.

[20] Stempsey WE. The quarantine of philosophy in medical education: why teaching the humanities may not produce humane physicians. Med Health Care Philos 1999;2(1):3-9.

[21] Weiss SC. Humanities in medical education: revisiting the doctor-patient relationship. Med Law 2000;19(3) :559-67.
[22] Hackler C. University of Arkansas College of Medicine, division of medical humanities. Acad Med 2003;78(10):1059.
[23] Haidet P, Jarecke J, Adams N, Green M, Stuckey H, Shapiro D, et al. Concepts underlying effective use of the arts in medical education: A qualitative synthesis of the literature. J Gen Intern Med 2015;30:S126-S7.
[24] Hildebrandt S. A proposal for ethical guidelines in anatomical education. FASEB J 2015;29(1 Suppl 547):1.
[25] Smith BH. Literature in our medical schools. Br J Gen Pract 1998;48(431):1337-40.
[26] Dusek T, Bates T. Analysis of European Medical Schools' teaching programs. Croat Med J 2003;44(1):26-31.
[27] McCombs PR. Crossing the Rubicon. Preparing residents for professional life after residency. Eur J Dermatol 2004;14(6):371-4.
[28] Meakin R. Editorial: Philosophy in the undergraduate medical curriculum - Beyond medical ethics. Med Humanit 2004;30(1):53.
[29] Parker M. Medical ethics and the undergraduate curriculum. Clin Med 2009;9(6):512-3.
[30] Fieschi L, Matarese M, Vellone E, Alvaro R, De Marinis MG. Medical humanities in healthcare education in Italy: a literature review. Annali Dell'Istituto Superiore di Sanita 2013;49(1):56-64.
[31] del Pozo PR, Fins JJ. The globalization of education in medical ethics and humanities: evolving pedagogy at Weill Cornell Medical College in Qatar. Acad Med 2005;80(2):135-40.
[32] Tokuda Y, Hinohara S, Fukui T. Introducing a new medical school system into Japan. Ann Acad Med Singapore 2008;37(9):800-2.
[33] Moore AR. Medical humanities: an aid to ethical discussions. J Med Ethics 1977;3(1):26-32.
[34] Milligan E, Woodley E. Creative expressive encounters in health ethics education: Teaching ethics as relational engagement. Teach Learn Med 2009;21(2):131-9.
[35] Acuna LE. Don't cry for us Argentinians: two decades of teaching medical humanities. Med Humanit 2000;26(2):66-70.
[36] Faculty of Medicine and Dentistry UoA. MD Program Curriculum: Edmonton: University of Alberta 2015. Accessed 2015 July 16. URL: https://www.med.ualberta.ca/programs/md/curriculum.
[37] Faculty of Medicine UoBC. MD Undergraduate Program: Vancouver: University of British Colombia 2015. URL: https://mdprogram.med.ubc.ca/program-information/curriculum-educational-programs/.
[38] Cumming School of Medicine UoC. Undergraduate Medical Education 2015. URL: www.ucalgary.ca /mdprogram/current-student/introduction-curriculum.
[39] Faculty of Medicine DU. Undergraduate Medical Education 2015. Accessed 2015 July 16. URL: www.dal.ca/academics/programs/professional/Medicine/what_will_i_learn.html.
[40] Faculté de Médecine UL. Répertoire des Cours offerts à l'UL 2015. Accessed 2015 July 16. URL: https://www2.ulaval.ca/les-etudes/cours/repertoire.html?matierecours=127&page=4.
[41] College of Medicine UoM. UGME Program Overview: Winnipeg: University of Manitoba 2015. Accessed 2015 July 16. URL: http://umanitoba.ca/faculty/health_sciences/medicine/education/ undergraduate/program_overview.html.
[42] Faculty of Medicine MU. M.D., C.M. - Doctor of Medicine and Master of Surgery Program Requirements 2015. Accessed 2015 July 16. URL: http://www.mcgill.ca/study/ 2015-2016/faculties/medicine/undergraduate/programs/mdcm-%E2%80%93-doctor-medicine-and-master-surgery.
[43] Michael G. DeGroote School of Medicine MU Overview 2015. Accessed 2015 July 16. URL: http://fhs.mcmaster.ca/main/medschool.html.
[44] Faculté de Médecine UdM. Programmes d'études 2015. Accessed 2015 July 16. URL: https://admission.umontreal.ca/programmes-detudes/filtres/cycle_1/cycle _2/faculte_12/niveau_5/.
[45] Faculty of Medicine MUoN. Undergraduate Medical Education Curriculum Map Overview 2015. Accessed 2015 July 16. URL: www.med.mun.ca/ugmecurriculum /default.aspx?cmd=change Cohort&cohort=59B.

[46] Northern Ontario School of Medicine LU. Undergraduate Courses 2015. Accessed 2015 July 16. URL: http://navigator.lakeheadu.ca/Catalog/ViewCatalog.aspx?pageid=viewcatalog&catalogid=18&chapterid=2414&loaduseredits=False.

[47] Faculty of Medicine UoO. Undergraduate Medical Education (MD Program) 2015. Accessed 2015 July16]. URL: www.uottawa.ca/academic/info/regist/calendars/programs/1098.html.

[48] School of Medicine QsU. MD Program Curriculum 2015. Accessed 2015 July 16. URL: www.queensu.ca/calendars/medicine/MD_Program___Curriculum.html.

[49] College of Medicine UoS. UGME Curriculum Summary 2015. Accessed 2015 Julyu 16]. URL: www.medicine.usask.ca/education/medical/undergrad/about-us/md-program/md-program/md-program-curriculum-summary.php.

[50] Santé FdMedSdl. Université de Sherbrooke 2015. Accessed 2015 July 16. URL: https://www.usherbrooke.ca/doctorat-medicine/programme/diagramme-schematique-du-programme/.

[51] Faculty of Medicine UoT. Undergraduate Medical Education 2015. Accessed 2015 July 16. URL: www.md.utoronto.ca/program.htm.

[52] Schulich School of Medicine and Dentistry UoWO. Undergraduate Medical Education - Curriculum Overview 2015. Accessed 2015 July 16. URL: www.schulich.uwo.ca/medicine/undergraduate/about_us/curriculum/overview.html#.

Submitted: June 18, 2015. *Revised:* July 31, 2015. *Accepted:* August 15, 2015.

In: Pain Management Yearbook 2015
Editor: Joav Merrick

ISBN: 978-1-63484-515-1

Chapter 33

SURVIVAL BENEFIT FROM PALLIATIVE TREATMENT IN PATIENTS WITH ADVANCED PROSTATE CANCER: A SELECTED REVIEW

Gordon Fu, Arnav Agarwal, Marko Popovic, Michael Lam, Milica Milakovic, Wayne Fu, Stephanie Cheon, Julia DiGiovanni, Ronald Chow, Terence Fu, Henry Lam, Breanne Lechner, Natalie Pulenzas and Edward Chow [*]

Sunnybrook Odette Cancer Centre, University of Toronto,
Toronto, Ontario, Canada

There is promising but limited data suggesting a survival benefit of palliative care in prostate cancer. We performed a selected review of randomized controlled trials examining the impact of various palliative treatments on overall survival among patients with advanced prostate cancer. A search was conducted in Ovid MEDLINE, EMBASE, and Cochrane Central. Using Review Manager Version 5.3, the results of overall one-year and five-year mortalities were expressed as risk ratios (RR), alongside of their corresponding confidence intervals (CIs). Our search strategy identified 1,108 studies. Of these, we included 8 studies containing 4,699 patients for analysis. Palliative treatments included androgen deprivation or other hormonal-therapy (n = 4), radiotherapy (n = 3), radio-pharmaceuticals (n = 2), bisphosphonates (n = 2), and glucocorticoids (n = 1). Multiple studies (n = 5) combined treatments. Our meta-analysis showed that palliative interventions significantly improved one-year mortality (RR = 0.79, 95% CI 0.73-0.86; p < 0.00001), but did not significantly improve five-year mortality (RR = 0.87, 95% CI 0.6-1.22; p = 0.41), when compared to control cohorts. One-year and five-year mortality were the lowest in patients who received radiotherapy combined with hormonal-therapy. In closing, palliative interventions may improve short-term survival in patients with advanced prostate cancer. Due to the limited number of studies examining survival in advanced prostate cancer patients receiving palliative care, more studies with longer

[*] Corresponding author: Professor Edward Chow MBBS, MSc, PhD, FRCPC, Department of Radiation Oncology, Odette Cancer Centre, Sunnybrook Health Sciences Centre, 2075 Bayview Avenue, Toronto Ontario, M4N 3M5, Canada. E-mail: edward.chow@sunnybrook.ca.

follow-up are needed to fully assess the potential long-term survival benefit of palliative interventions.

Keywords: prostate cancer, prostatic neoplasm, advanced cancer, palliative care, survival benefit, mortality

INTRODUCTION

Prostate cancer is the second most common form of cancer and third most common cause of cancer death in North American men (1). The most common complaint amongst prostate cancer patient is urinary retention secondary to bladder outlet obstruction (2). Late symptoms such as bone pain, weight loss, fatigue, anemia, spinal cord injury and compression are often due to metastases and cause potentially debilitating disease-specific morbidity (3).

Treatment of prostate cancer depends on the stage of the disease (4). Active surveillance is often considered in early stage disease or among older asymptomatic men, especially if natural life expectancy is less than a decade (3). Localized disease is potentially curable with radical prostatectomy or radiotherapy; in certain cases, adjuvant hormonal or androgen-deprivation therapy is indicated (5). Advanced stage disease is typically managed with palliative surgery, radiation therapy, or hormonal-therapy, in addition to pain control with opioid analgesics, bisphosphonates, and glucocorticoids (6-9). In addition to significant physical symptoms, prostate cancer and its associated treatment are often associated with reduced quality of life and psychiatric conditions such as depression and anxiety (10).

Palliative care is an inter-disciplinary approach to prevent and relieve suffering in patients whose disease is non-responsive to curative treatment (11). Caregivers focus not only on physical symptoms but also social, spiritual, and psychiatric problems to help establish the best possible quality of life in their patients (11). Although not limited to advanced illness, there is a wealth of literature that advocates for palliative care at any time in the clinical course of an illness (11). Numerous randomized trials have highlighted the benefits of palliative care in terms of lower health-care costs, less aggressive end-of-life-care, and improved patient satisfaction and symptom-management (1-8). However, these trials are limited by small sample size and evaluate a wide range of palliative treatments (5, 7-8). In light of the promising but limited data examining the impact of palliative care on survival in prostate cancer, we performed a selected review of randomized controlled trials assessing palliative treatments among patients with advanced prostate cancer.

METHODS

A literature search was conducted in Ovid MEDLINE, EMBASE, and the Cochrane Central Register of Controlled Trials from 2000-2015. We used the following search strategy to elicit relevant literature: ("exp prostate cancer/ and ((terminal* or advanced or "stage IV") adj2 (cancer or neoplasm* or carcinoma or disease)).mp.") and ("exp cancer survival/") and ("exp metastasis/" or "metastat*.mp.") We also reviewed the reference lists of included articles to identify additional studies.

Inclusion and exclusion criteria

We included randomized controlled trials that reported survival outcome(s) after palliative treatment(s) in patients with advanced (i.e., stage III or IV) prostate cancer. We only included studies in which stage III or IV patients comprised at least 50% of the cohort. Studies were excluded if they were duplicates, not written in English, reviews or did not report survival outcomes. Studies reporting the TNM (T – primary tumor, N – regional lymph nodes, M – distant metastasis) classification of malignant tumors were converted to clinical staging (10). For our selected review, studies reporting on the following treatments were included: androgen deprivation or hormonal-therapy, radiotherapy, radio-pharmaceuticals, bisphosphonates and glucocorticoids. When multiple studies were published by a single institution with updated patient follow-up data, only the most recent publication was included to minimize redundancy.

Data collection and statistical analysis

Extracted variables included sample size, study design, baseline mean age, Gleason score, prior history, Karnofsky Performance Status (KPS), serum prostate specific antigen (PSA), clinical cancer stage, intervention received, mean follow-up, number of deaths during follow-up, hazard ratios, one-year probability of survival, and five-year probability of survival. The primary endpoints, one-year and five-year probabilities of survival, were obtained directly from the study if available, or estimated using Adobe Illustrator (Adobe Systems Incorporated, San Jose, California) on published Kaplan-Meier curves.

Statistical analyses were performed using Review Manager (RevMan 5.3) by the Cochrane Collaboration. Risk ratios (RR) and their accompanying 95% confidence interval (95% CI) were generated using the Mantel-Haenszel method and a random effects model for one-year and five-year overall mortality comparing patients receiving palliative treatment(s) versus control. The statistical significance was set at 0.05 for the test of overall effect and p-values less than 0.05 were deemed statistically significant. Due to the variety of palliative treatment options, the Cochrane Q statistic was used to assess heterogeneity and the proportion of variation among our studies was measured with the I-squared statistic.

RESULTS

Our search strategy and review of reference lists identified a total of 1,108 articles (Figure 1), from which 8 studies (1-8) containing 4,699 patients were eligible for the review. These studies were conducted in Sweden (n = 3), Canada (n = 1), United Kingdom (n = 2), Greece (n = 1), and the Netherlands (n = 1).

A total of 2,703 patients were randomized to palliative intervention, and 1,996 were randomized to controls. Mean age for the intervention and control groups across three studies (1, 5, 8) were 66 years (range 65 to 72) and 66 years (range 66 to 73) respectively. The aggregated median age of five studies (2-4, 6, 7) for intervention and control groups was 73.2 years (range 68 to 78) and 70 years (range 66 to 78) respectively. Control groups received either placebo (3, 4, 6, 7) or standard oncologic care without palliative treatment (1, 2, 5, 8). The proportion of stage III and IV patients, as reported in two studies, was 80% and 81%, and 4% and 5% in intervention and control groups, respectively (1, 2). The remaining patients across these two same studies were diagnosed with stage I or II prostate cancer.

All studies included overall survival curves (Table 1). Median probability of one-year survival in patients receiving palliative interventions and control was 0.66 and 0.54, respectively, while median probability of five-year survival was 0.82 and 0.75, respectively. Only four studies (1, 2, 4, 5) reported five-year overall survival probability. Four studies detailed the median duration of survival, which was 15.4 months (range 5.5 to 15.9) and 11.2 months (range 9 to 12) for the intervention and control groups, respectively (3, 6, 7, 9). Five studies (2-4, 6, 7) reported hazard ratios comparing the risk of death between palliative and control groups. Hazard ratios for overall survival in the palliative intervention group ranged from 0.47 to 0.77 with a median of 0.70.

Palliative interventions and survival benefits

Palliative interventions included in our review were androgen deprivation or hormonal-therapy (n = 4) (1-3, 5), radiotherapy (n = 3) (1, 2, 5), radio-pharmaceuticals (n = 2) (6, 8), bisphosphonates (n = 2) (4, 9), and glucocorticoids (n = 1) (3). Multiple studies (n = 5) (1-3, 5, 8) combined treatments. Androgen-deprivation treatments that were used included leuprorelin (n = 2) (1, 2), flutamide (n = 1) (1), orchiectomy (n = 1) (5), and abiraterone acetate (n = 1) (3). Radio-pharmaceuticals used included radium-223 (n = 2) (6, 8). Bisphosphonates included zoledronate (n = 1) (8) and sodium-clodronate (n = 1) (4). Of the eight studies (1-8) that reported overall survival, one study comparing sodium clodronate to a placebo did not report any survival benefit (HR = 0.80, 95% CI = 0.62 to 1.03; $p = 0.066$) (4). Of the studies reporting median duration of overall survival, radium-223 had the greatest benefit (7). Median overall survival was 16 months in the radium-223 group versus 11 months in the placebo group (log-rank $p = 0.056$) (7). One-year and five-year mortality were the lowest in patients who received radiotherapy combined with hormonal-therapy (1).

Meta-analysis

Meta-analysis showed that palliative interventions significantly improved one-year mortality (RR = 0.79, 95% CI 0.73-0.86; $p < 0.00001$), but did not significantly improve five-year mortality (RR = 0.87, 95% CI 0.6-1.22; $p = 0.41$) when compared to the control group (Figures 2, 3). The risk ratio for one-year overall mortality could not be estimated in one study (1) because there were no events in the treatment and control groups.

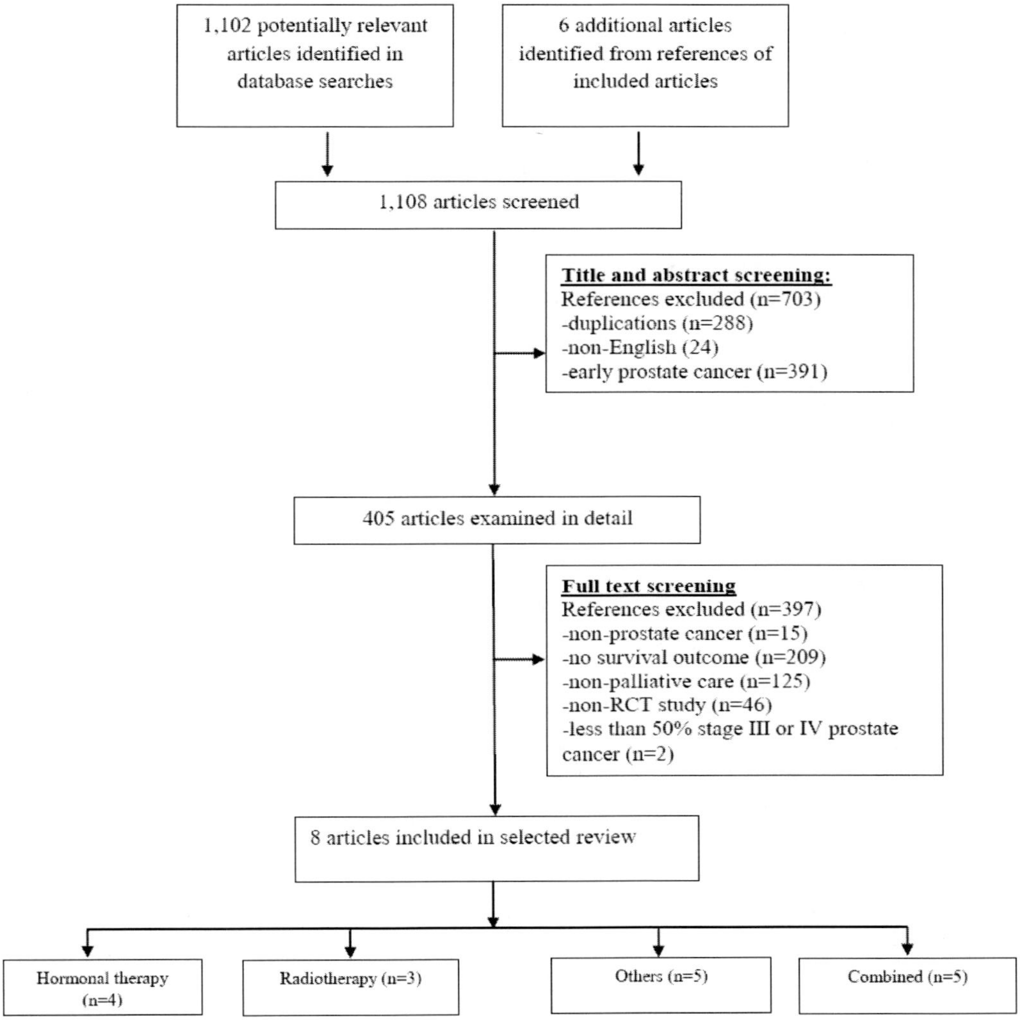

Figure 1. Flowchart of study inclusions from title and abstract and full text screening.

	Palliative intervention		Placebo or control			Risk Ratio
Study or Subgroup	Events	Total	Events	Total	Weight	M-H, Fixed, 95% CI
Dearnaley et al 2003	42	155	59	156		Not estimable
Granfors et al 2005	0	45	1	46		Not estimable
Mitsiades et al 2006	10	20	15	18	72.4%	0.60 [0.37, 0.97]
Mulders et al 2013	327	797	214	397		Not estimable
Nilsson et al 2013	14	33	17	31		Not estimable
Parker et al 2013	340	614	204	307		Not estimable
Warde et al 2011	12	603	6	602	27.6%	2.00 [0.75, 5.29]
Total (95% CI)		**623**		**620**	**100.0%**	**0.98 [0.62, 1.58]**
Total events	22		21			

Heterogeneity: Chi² = 6.04, df = 1 (P = 0.01); I² = 83%
Test for overall effect: Z = 0.06 (P = 0.95)

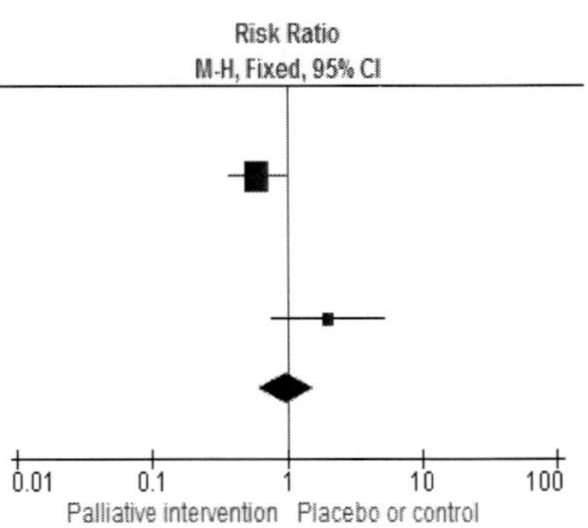

Figure 2. Palliative intervention compared to control for one year overall mortality in advanced prostate cancer.

Table 1. Baseline demographic characteristics and outcomes of included trials

			Staging		Palliative intervention		1 year survival rate		5 year survival rate		
First Author	**Sample-size**	**Baseline age**	**Treatment**	**Control**	**Treatment**	**Control**	**Treatment**	**Control**	**Treatment**	**Control**	**HR (95%CI)**
Dearnaley et al. 2003	Total: 311 PT*: 155 PC*: 156	PT*: 71 (median) PC*: 71	Metastatic	Metastatic	Sodium clodronate	Placebo	72%	62%	5%	7%	0.7
Granfors et al. 2005	Total: 91 PT*: 45 PC*: 46	PT*: 68.8 (median) PC*: 68.8	Metastatic	Metastatic	Orchiectomy, radiotherapy	Radiotherapy	100%	98%	80%	71%	NR
Mitsiades et al. 2006	Total: 38 PT*: 20 PC*: 18	PT*: 69.7 (median) PC*: 69.7	Metastatic	Metastatic	Dexamethasone, octreotide, zoledronate	Zoledronate	48%	15%	NR	NR	NR
Mulders et al. 2013	Total: 1194 PT*: 797 PC*: 397	PT*: 78 (median) PC*: 72	Metastatic	Metastatic	Abiraterone acetate, low dose prednisone	Placebo plus low dose prednisone	59%	46%	NR	NR	0.71
Nilsson et al. 2013	Total: 64 PT*: 33 PC*: 31	PT*: 65 (mean) PC*: 66	Metastatic	Metastatic	Radium-223	Placebo	57%	45%	NR	NR	0.476
Parker et al. 2013	Total: 921 PT*: 614 PC*: 307	PT*: 71 (median) PC*: 71 (median)	Metastatic	Metastatic	Radium-223	Placebo	44%	33%	NR	NR	0.7
Warde et al. 2011	Total: 1205 PT*: 603 PC*: 602	PT*: 69.7 (median) PC*: 69.7 (median)	Stage 2 (12%) Stage 3 (83%) Stage 4 (5%)	Stage 2 (13%) Stage 3 (83%) Stage 4 (4%)	Hormonal-therapy[A], and radiotherapy	Hormonal-therapy[A]	98%	99%	84%	80%	0.77
Widmark et al. 2009	Total: 875 PT*: 436 PC*: 439	PT*: 66.2 (mean) PC*: 65.7 (mean)	Stage 1 (2.6%) Stage 2 (19.7%) Stage 3 (76.8%)	Stage 1 (1.8%) Stage 2 (18.9%) Stage 3 (79%)	Hormonal-therapy[B] and radiotherapy	Hormonal-therapy[B]	100%	100%	89%	87%	NR

Legend: PT*: palliative treatment group. PC*: control group. Hormonal-therapy[A]: orchiectomy or luteinizing hormone-releasing hormone agonist. Hormonal-therapy B: leuprorelin. HR: hazard ratio 95% CI: 95% confidence interval.

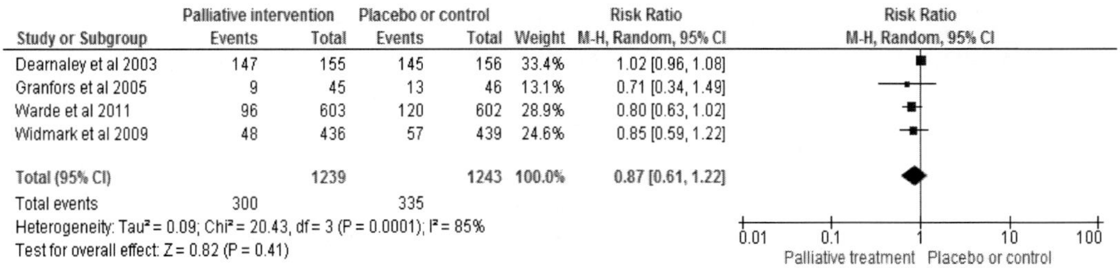

Figure 3. Palliative intervention compared to control for five year overall mortality in advanced prostate cancer.

Four studies (3, 6, 7, 8) were excluded from our analysis of five-year overall mortality because follow-up was less than five years (Figure 3).

Discussion

Palliative treatment options for advanced prostate cancer include radiotherapy, androgen-deprivation or hormonal-therapy, pain control, bisphosphonates, and glucocorticoids (11). Radiotherapy is the most common first line option for palliation of metastatic prostate cancer and is sub-divided into localized external-beam radiation, hemi-body irradiation, and systemic radionuclides (11). The most common symptom in metastatic prostate cancer is pain, and palliative radiotherapy has been shown to be more effective in controlling pain than opioid analgesics alone (11). Radiotherapy is also indicated in the management of lymphadenopathy, nerve compression and genitourinary complications secondary to metastasis (11). The second most common palliative treatment is hormonal or androgen deprivation therapy (11).

Radiotherapy combined with hormonal therapy (n = 3 studies) (1, 2, 5) was the most commonly used palliative intervention across 8 studies. This combination achieved the best survival and mortality rates when compared to patients who received radiotherapy or hormonal therapy alone (Table 1, Figures 2, 3). The survival benefit of these combined palliative interventions may be due to improved efficacy of hormonal therapy due to radio-sensitization from radiotherapy (1). Widmark et al. found that the 10-year cumulative incidence of prostate cancer-specific mortality was significantly lower in patients treated with both hormonal-therapy and radiotherapy versus hormonal-therapy alone (11.9% vs. 23.9%; RR = 0.44, 95% CI 0.30 to 0.66) (1). Furthermore, the difference in 10 year cumulative incidence for overall mortality for the same groups was 9.8% (95% CI 0.8-18.8%) for a relative risk of 0.68 (95% CI, 0.52 to 0.89) (1). Based on these findings, Widmark et al. have recommended hormonal-therapy and radiotherapy as the standard of treatment, especially in patients with locally advanced or high-risk local prostate cancer (1). These findings are also corroborated by Lei at al. (12).

There are several limitations of our review, including the limited number of included studies, underreporting of data, and variability in study characteristics, patient characteristics, and type of palliative intervention. Several studies did not report key information regarding time to follow-up, duration of overall survival, Gleason score, Karnofsky Performance Status, and proportion of stage III and IV cancer patients. Among studies that reported the proportion of patients in each clinical stage (1, 2), there was a disproportionate number of stage III patients compared to stage IV patients. Furthermore, many studies had limited follow-up. As a result, nearly half of included studies were excluded from our analysis of five-year overall mortality due to insufficient follow-up periods.

To our knowledge this is the first review performed to determine if palliative care in advanced prostate cancer offers any survival benefits. The two most important findings were that palliative treatments in advanced prostate cancer may have short-term survival benefits and that survival was the greatest in patients who received radiotherapy. Palliative care may only confer a short-term survival benefit due to lack of long-term palliative care administration and follow-up in the eight studies (1-8). For instance, palliative treatments were administered for less than five years in four included studies (3-6, 8). In contrast, median follow-up in studies examining long-term survival was 93 months and median duration of treatment was 25.6 months (13-16). The lack of long-term survival benefits could also be due to an under-reporting of data and patient characteristics in all three studies (1-2, 5) associated with first-line palliative radiotherapy.

Our meta-analysis shows that palliative interventions significantly improve one-year mortality but do not significantly improve five-year mortality when compared to controls. These findings suggest that palliative intervention offers short-term benefits among patients with advanced prostate cancer. However, due to the relatively short time frame of follow-up, wide-range of palliative treatments, and under-reporting of data in studies examining palliative care for advanced prostate cancer, more studies with longer-follow-up comparing long-term palliative care options are needed fully assess the long-term survival impact of palliative interventions.

ACKNOWLEDGMENTS

We thank the generous support of the Bratty Family Fund, Michael and Karyn Goldstein Cancer Research Fund, Joey and Mary Furfari Cancer Research Fund, Pulenzas Cancer Research Fund, Joseph and Silvana Melara Cancer Research Fund and Ofelia Cancer Research Fund.

REFERENCES

[1] Widmark A, Klepp O, Solberg A, Damber J, Angelsen A, Fransson P, et al. Endocrine treatment, with or without radiotherapy, in locally advanced prostate cancer (SPCG-7/SFUO-3): an open randomised phase III trial. Lancet 2009; 373(9660): 301-8.

[2] Warde P, Mason M, Ding K, Kirkbride P, Brundage M, Cowan R, et al. Combined androgen deprivation therapy and radiation therapy for locally advanced prostate cancer: a randomised, phase 3 trial. Lancet 2011; 378(9809): 2104-11.

[3] Mulders P, Molina A, Marberger M, Saad F, Higano C, Chi K, et al. Efficacy and safety of abiraterone acetate in an elderly patient subgroup (aged 75 and Older) with metastatic castration-resistant prostate cancer after docetaxel-based chemotherapy. Eur Urol 2014; 65(5): 875-83.

[4] Dearnaley D. A double-blind, placebo-controlled, randomized trial of oral sodium clodronate for metastatic prostate cancer (MRC PR05 Trial). J Natl Cancer I 2003; 95(17): 1300-11.

[5] Granfors T, Modig H, Damber J, Tomic R. Long-term follow-up of a randomized study of locally advanced prostate cancer treated with combined orchiectomy and external radiotherapy versus radiotherapy alone. J Urol 2006; 176(2): 544-7.

[6] Parker C, Nilsson S, Heinrich D, Helle S, O'Sullivan J, Fosså S, et al. Alpha emitter radium-223 and survival in metastatic prostate cancer. New Engl J Med 2013; 369(3): 213-23.

[7] Nilsson S, Franzén L, Parker C, Tyrrell C, Blom R, Tennvall J, et al. Two-year survival follow-up of the randomized, double-blind, placebo-controlled phase II study of radium-223 chloride in patients with castration-resistant prostate cancer and bone metastases. Clin Genitourin Canc 2013; 11(1): 20-6.

[8] Mitsiades C, Bogdanos J, Karamanolakis D, Milathianakis C, Dimopoulous T, Koutsileris M. Randomized controlled clinical trial of a combination of somatostatin analog and dexamethasone plus zoledronate vs. zoledronate in patients with androgen ablation-refractory prostate cancer. Eur Urol Suppl 2006; 5(2):93.

[9] Novara G, Ficarra V, Mocellin S, Ahlering T, Carroll P, Graefen M, et al. Systematic review and meta-analysis of studies reporting oncologic outcome after robot-assisted radical prostatectomy. Eur Urol 2012; 62(3): 382-404.

[10] Brawley O. Trends in prostate cancer in the United States. J Natl Cancer Inst Mono 2012; 45:152-6.

[11] Iscoe N, Bruera E, Choo R. Prostate cancer: 10. Palliative care. Can Med Assoc J 1999; 160(3): 365.

[12] Lei J, Liu L, Wei Q, Yan S, Song T, Lin F, et al. Systematic review and meta-analysis of the survival outcomes of first-line treatment options in high-risk prostate cancer. Sci Rep 2015; 5: 7713.

[13] Hashine K. Long-term outcomes of 60 Gy conventional radiotherapy combined with androgen deprivation for localized or locally advanced prostate cancer. Jpn J Urol 2005; 35(11): 655-9.

[14] Tewari A, Johnson C, Divine G, Crawford E, Gamito E, Demers R et al. Long-term survival probability in men with clinically localized prostate cancer: a case-control, propensity modeling study stratified by race, age, treatment and comorbidities. J Urol 2004; 171(4): 1513-9.

[15] Walz J, Chun F, Klein E, Reuther A, Saad F, Graefen M et al. Nomogram predicting the probability of early recurrence after radical prostatectomy for prostate cancer. J Urol 2009; 181(2): 601-8.

[16] Berthelet E, Pickles T, Lee K, Liu M, Truong P. Long-term androgen deprivation therapy improves survival in prostate cancer patients presenting with prostate-specific antigen levels >20 ng/mL. Int J Radiat Oncol 2005; 63(3): 781-7.

In: Pain Management Yearbook 2015
Editor: Joav Merrick

ISBN: 978-1-63484-515-1

Chapter 34

ADVANCES IN MANAGEMENT OF NASOPHARYNGEAL CANCER

Tracy CY Shum*, MBBS, Tracy TS Lau, MBBS and Ashley CK Cheng, MBBS
Department of Oncology, Princess Margaret Hospital, Hong Kong

Nasopharyngeal cancer (NPC) tends to metastasize to lymph nodes early and often presents as locally advanced disease. Radical radiotherapy using intensity-modulated radiotherapy (IMRT), with or without chemotherapy, is the current standard treatment for non-metastatic NPC. Radical resection is reserved as salvage treatment. IMRT requires accurate target volume delineation. Co-registering information from MRI and PET-CT improves disease staging and treatment planning. EBV DNA is an increasingly recognized biomarker for detection, prognostication and monitoring of the disease, with ongoing studies being undertaken to extend its clinical utilization in assisting treatment decision. The use of adaptive radiotherapy, taking account of anatomical changes during treatment course, minimizes unintended normal tissue toxicity and maintains tumor coverage, which may translate into improved treatment outcome. Concurrent chemotherapy is recommended for stage II to IVA disease, while induction and adjuvant chemotherapy is given on individual basis. Distant metastasis, being the current dominant pattern of failure, calls for further advances in systemic therapy.

Keywords: nasopharyngeal carcinoma, intensity-modulated radiation therapy, chemotherapy, Epstein-Barr virus DNA

INTRODUCTION

Nasopharyngeal cancer exhibits distinct endemic distribution. While it is rare in most parts of the world, age-adjusted incidence rates among men range from 0.6/100,000 in the United States and Japan, to 11.0 in Singapore, 17.2 among Eskimos, and up to 26.9 in Hong Kong

* Corresponding author: Dr. Tracy Shum MBBS, FRCR, FHKAM (Radiology), Department of Oncology, Princess Margaret Hospital, Hong Kong. Email: scy409@ha.org.hk.

and Guangdong province in Southern China (1). This discriminative geographic distribution is likely due to multifactorial etiology related to EBV infectivity rate, dietary and genetic factors.

In endemic areas, non-keratinizing carcinoma, particularly the undifferentiated subtype, accounts for over 90% of cases; whereas in populations with low incidence, keratinizing squamous cell carcinoma, the less common subtype, may be seen in up to 25% (2).

Non-keratinizing carcinoma subtypes tend to metastasize to lymph nodes early and present as locally advanced disease, but are more radio- and chemosensitive. Radiotherapy, with or without chemotherapy, is therefore the primary treatment. Radical resection, which may be technically demanding and associated with morbidities, is often reserved as salvage treatment. This article will summarize the current standard of care for nasopharyngeal cancer and highlight advances in management of this disease including investigation strategies, radiation techniques and systemic therapy.

Methods

Radiotherapy using intensity-modulated radiotherapy (IMRT) is the backbone of treatment in non-metastatic nasopharyngeal cancer today. IMRT requires highly precise delineation of gross tumor volume (GTV) and clinical target volume (CTV). While computed tomography (CT) is essential for detailed examination of local disease extent, magnetic resonance imaging (MRI) provides added value in better soft tissue contrast resolution and multi-planar capacity. It is also free of bony artifacts and radiation hazards. Studies have shown that MRI provides more accurate definition of invasion into oropharynx, prevertebral muscles and parapharyngeal space, differentiation between primary tumor and retropharyngeal lymph nodes, and refined assessment of skull base, paranasal sinus, and intracranial invasion. Liao et al. (3) demonstrated that MRI resulted in changes T stage in 50% of cases, N stage in 10% of cases and clinical stage in 40% cases compared with CT. Post-radiotherapy fibrosis can also be distinguished from recurrent or residual tumor on MRI.

With these merits, MRI co-registration with CT in treatment planning for radiotherapy improves the accuracy of target delineation, leading to remarkably better PTV coverage and reduced normal tissue complications (4). Nowadays, MRI scanners could be incorporated in treatment planning process directly (5). Large-bore MRI is now commercially available, with provision of immobilization devices, positioning systems (lasers, 4D tracking systems etc.,) and fiducial markers, modified couch tabletop and particularly acquisition sequences suitable for radiotherapy treatment planning. Another development is the accessibility of radiotherapy-dedicated MRI simulator. MRI simulation for head and neck cancers may be increasingly utilized for treatment planning in the near future.

Positron emission tomography–computed tomography (PET-CT) is useful for staging work-up, especially in locally advanced disease. PET-CT has been shown to be more accurate in detecting distant metastases than conventional work-up (chest X-ray, abdominal ultrasound and bone scan) in initial diagnosis (6), with high negative predictive value. After completion of treatment, PET-CT could be employed to detect residual disease, loco-regional relapse and distant metastases. Systematic review performed by Liu et al. (7) reported that FDG-PET had higher sensitivity and specificity than CT and MRI for diagnosis of local residual and recurrent disease. Moreover, the addition of FDG-PET information to CT-based radiotherapy planning could potentially avoid a geographical miss of disease and reduce the target volume size (8). Different methods for defining the borders of PET-CT based GTV are used: I) threshold methods using a fixed SUV or a certain percentage of maximum SUV as the threshold, II) manual method, in which the physician determines the tumor outline on the basis of visual perception of tumor border and III) gradient-based method using the maximum spatial gradient to detect boundaries between the lesion and normal tissue. The third method is considered to be more accurate and reproducible (9, 10).

However, FDG-PET alone has its limitations. For instance, FDG-PET is not ideal for assessment of intracranial disease due to its strong background tracer uptake in the brain as well as poorer image resolution (see Figure 1). Using MRI as the reference imaging modality, the overall sensitivity of FDG-PET for detection of intracranial extension of NPC was only 42.9% (11). In addition, FDG-PET does not provide anatomic details and false positive results exist because FDG is accumulated in metabolically active tissue, including inflammation and infection. Therefore, interpretation of FDG-PET with CT or MRI findings and appropriate timing of performing FDG-PET are important.

FDG-PET is suggested to be performed 3 or 4 months after completion of radiotherapy course when post-treatment inflammatory reaction has subsided.

Role of EBV DNA level

Epstein-Barr virus (EBV) is associated with NPC, specifically the non-keratinizing subtypes, irrespective of ethnic or geographic background. The near-constant association of EBV with NPC suggested an oncogenic role of the virus, with ample supportive evidence serologically and pathologically. Some of these were found to have important clinical implications, including (I) raised IgA levels against EBV (commonly viral capsid antigen and early antigen) in NPC patients as compared to normal controls and cancer patients of other types, (II) demonstrable presence of EBV DNA or RNA in NPC tumor cells by in-situ hybridization technique, and (III) correlation of tumor bulk to plasma levels of IgA against EBV and amounts of copies of EBV DNA (12, 13).

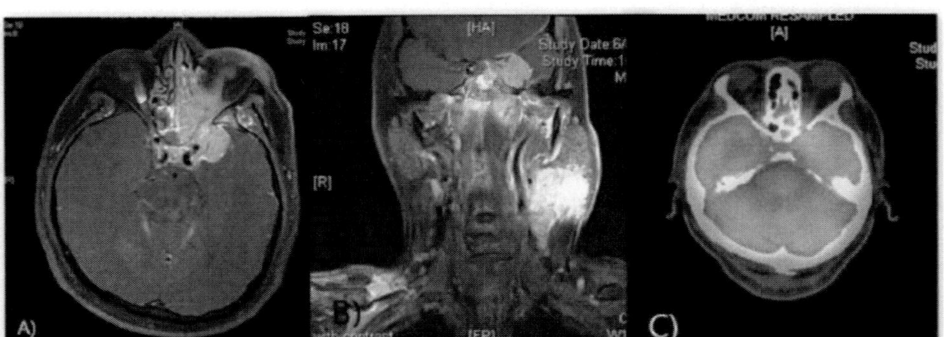

Figure 1. Patient with left intracranial extension detected by MRI (a and b) but not seen in FDG-PET/CT (c).

Circulating plasma EBV DNA, as measured by real-time quantitative polymerase chain reaction (RT-PCR) is therefore increasingly utilized as a useful tool for detection, monitoring and prognostication of NPC.

Diagnosis

A meta-analysis to investigate the diagnostic role of EBV DNA in NPC, overlooking 18 studies conducted in Asia, showed the pooled sensitivity and specificity were 73% and 89% respectively (14). Ongoing studies have been set up to determine if the screening of NPC using plasma EBV DNA analysis would result in the down-staging of NPC cases in asymptomatic individuals (NCT02063399, CUHK).

Prognostication

Plasma/serum EBV DNA concentration is an independent prognostic factor. Pre-treatment EBV DNA correlates with tumor volume (15), recurrence and metastasis within the first year after treatment (16). Patients with early stage disease could be dichotomized by pre-treatment EBV DNA levels (cutoff level of 4000 copies/ mL) into a poor-risk subgroup with survival similar to that of stage III disease, and a good risk subgroup with survival similar to stage I disease (17).

Detectable post-treatment EBV DNA predicts inferior overall survival and relapse-free survival (18) (19). Li et al. (19) reported poorer 2-year overall survival rate (56.3% versus 96.7%, $p < 0.001$) and 2-year relapse-free survival rate (28.6% versus 84.2%, $p < 0.001$) for patients with persistently detectable post-treatment EBV DNA versus those with undetectable post-treatment EBV-DNA.

Some studies further found that levels of post-treatment EBV DNA dominated the effect of pre-treatment EBV DNA for survival endpoints (15)(20). In a study of 170 non-metastatic patients treated with a uniform radiotherapy protocol, Chan et al. (20) reported the relative risk for recurrence was 11.9 for patients with higher post-treatment EBV DNA (> 500 copies/mL) and 2.5 for patients with higher pre-treatment EBV DNA (> 4000 copies/mL). They were then able to divide patients into four subgroups with 1-year progression-free survival rates of 32% (high post-treatment and high pre-treatment EBV DNA), 50% (high post-treatment and low pre-treatment EBV DNA), 84% (low post-treatment and high pre-treatment EBV DNA), and 98% (low post-treatment and low pre-treatment EBV DNA).

In metastatic or recurrent patients undergoing palliative chemotherapy, low pre-treatment plasma EBV DNA level as well as early clearance of plasma EBV DNA after first cycle of chemotherapy were associated with significantly superior survival (21, 22), and the authors suggested that early change of chemotherapy regimen may be considered for patients with slow plasma EBV DNA clearance.

Detection of recurrence

Upon follow-up, regular assessment of EBV DNA levels contributes to earlier detection of tumor recurrence. Significant elevations in EBV DNA could occur up to 6 months before detectable clinical deterioration (23). Wang et al. performed serial monitoring of EBV DNA every 3 to 6 months in 245 treated patients in remission. FDG-PET was arranged when abnormal EBV DNA levels or clinically suspicious signs of recurrence were noted. Plasma EBV DNA levels predicted all NPC recurrences and PET showed high capacity in localizing potential lesion sites (24).

Advances in radiotherapy

Conventional 2D radiotherapy (2D-CRT) starts phase I treatment with large lateral opposing faciocervical fields that cover the primary tumor and upper neck lymphatics in one volume, with matching lower anterior cervical field for lower neck lymphatics. Protection of adjacent critical normal tissues while administering a high dose to tumor is difficult for 2D-CRT, especially in patients with locally advanced disease such as skull base infiltration or intracranial extension. As a result, portions of the tumor are often underdosed with the goal of normal tissue protection. 2D-CRT successfully controls T1 and T2 tumors in 75%-90% of cases, and T3 and T4 tumors in only 50-75% of cases. Nodal control was achieved in 90% of N0 and N1 cases, but control rate has dropped to 70% for N2 and N3 cases (25).

Intensity-modulated radiotherapy (IMRT) offers superior dose conformity to tumor targets with relative sparing of surrounding critical organs such as brainstem, spinal cord, pituitary gland, temporal lobes, eyes, middle and inner ears, and parotid glands. With precise treatment planning, this translates into excellent locoregional control and reduction in toxicity, especially in advanced stage disease. In a randomized controlled trial involving 616 patients with non-metastatic stage I to IVB disease, IMRT was shown to be superior in 5-year local control rate (91% vs 84%, $p = 0.046$), 5-year regional control rates (92% vs 84%, $p = 0.049$) and overall survival at 5 years (80% vs 67%, $p = 0.001$). With respect to late complications, the rates of temporal lobe neuropathy, cranial nerve palsy, trismus, neck fibrosis, late xerostomia and hearing loss were all significantly less in the IMRT group.

Many other studies consistently demonstrated excellent 3-year locoregional control rate of over 90% and 3-year disease-free survival rate of over 80% achieved by IMRT (27-34), even among patients with advanced T3 and T4 disease (35). The RTOG phase II multicenter trial 0225 showed that the excellent 2-year locoregional control rate of over 90% could be reproducible in a multi-institutional setting (36).

Emphasis has also been placed on the prevention of long-term radiation-induced complications. Xerostomia, often caused by conventional RT, could substantially compromise patient's quality of life. Dosimetric studies revealed that a mean radiation dose of 26Gy to parotid glands was the threshold for preservation of stimulated saliva flow. IMRT was significantly better than 2D-CRT in terms of sparing of parotid glands and improved quality of life for early stage disease (37, 38). Kam et al. (38) showed that IMRT had lower incidence of observer-rated severe xerostomia than 2D-CRT (40% vs 82%, p = 0.001) at 1 year after treatment for early stage disease. There was also higher stimulated parotid flow rate as well as a higher stimulated whole saliva flow rate in patients who received IMRT. Wang et al. (39) compared the effect of 3D conformal radiotherapy (3D-CRT) and IMRT on middle ear function and found that IMRT could decrease radiation dose to the middle ear cavity and isthmus and preserved middle ear function better than 3D-CRT. IMRT is therefore the current standard of radiotherapy for NPC. Distant metastasis, occurring in up to 30% of patients, is now the dominant form of failure (29, 30). This indicates the need for more effective systemic therapy, which will be discussed below.

Delivering IMRT

The delivery of IMRT requires high-precision immobilization (see Figure 2) and accurate target volume delineation. Different centers have different protocols regarding clinical target volume (CTV) delineation, dose prescription, dose constraints for organs at risk, acceptance criteria and beam arrangement. In our department, modification of RTOG 0225 protocol is used (see Figure 3).

The gross tumor volume (GTV) includes the primary tumor. Enlarged neck nodes greater than 1 cm or nodes with necrotic center are localized as a separate volume, GTV-N.

The clinical target volume (CTV) includes the subclinical regions at risk of involvement. CTV1 includes entire nasopharynx and covers GTV with 5 mm margin. CTV1 also covers grossly involved nodes with 5 to 10 mm margin, and a greater margin is used for bulky nodes with suspicion of extracapsular spread. CTV2 includes CTV1 with 5 mm margin and potential areas of disease spread, including inferior sphenoid sinus, skull base (including petrous tip, foramen ovale and foramen spinosum), clivus, posterior third of nasal cavity and maxillary antrum, pterygopalatine fossa, parapharyngeal spaces and prevertebral muscles. CTV2 also covers high risk regional lymphatics in the neck, including bilateral retropharyngeal group, posterior level IB, levels II, III and upper half of level V. For cases with involved level II lymph node, the retrostyloid group is also included; whereas for node-negative disease, submandibular glands (posterior level IB) can be spared. CTV3 includes level IV and lower half of level V unless there is gross involvement of levels III and/or IVA. In areas adjacent to critical structures such as brainstem or optic chiasm, the CTV margins could be reduced down to 1 mm. To account for organ motion and daily treatment set-up uncertainties, planning target volume (PTV) is obtained with an additional 3 mm margin beyond CTV.

The organs at risk (OAR) to be localized include eyeballs, lens, optic nerves, optic chiasm, temporal lobes, pituitary gland, brainstem, spinal cord, parotid glands, cochlea, brachial plexus and temporomandibular joints.

The prescribed dose to PTV1, PTV2 and PTV3 is 70 Gy, 60 Gy and 54 Gy respectively to at least 95% volume of targets in 35 fractions over 7 weeks. Radiotherapy is delivered by using a simultaneous integrated boost technique. Nine to eleven coplanar fields are used (Figure 4).

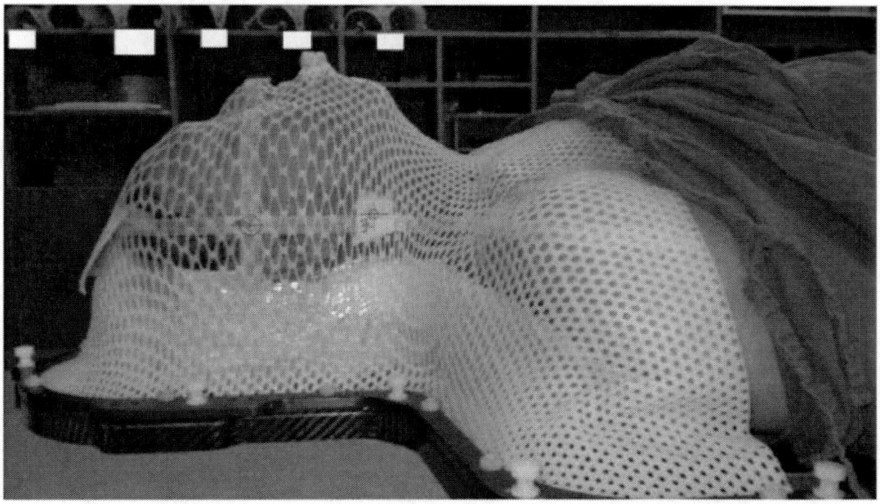

Figure 2. Patient set-up: extended neck, thermoplastic shell, bite block.

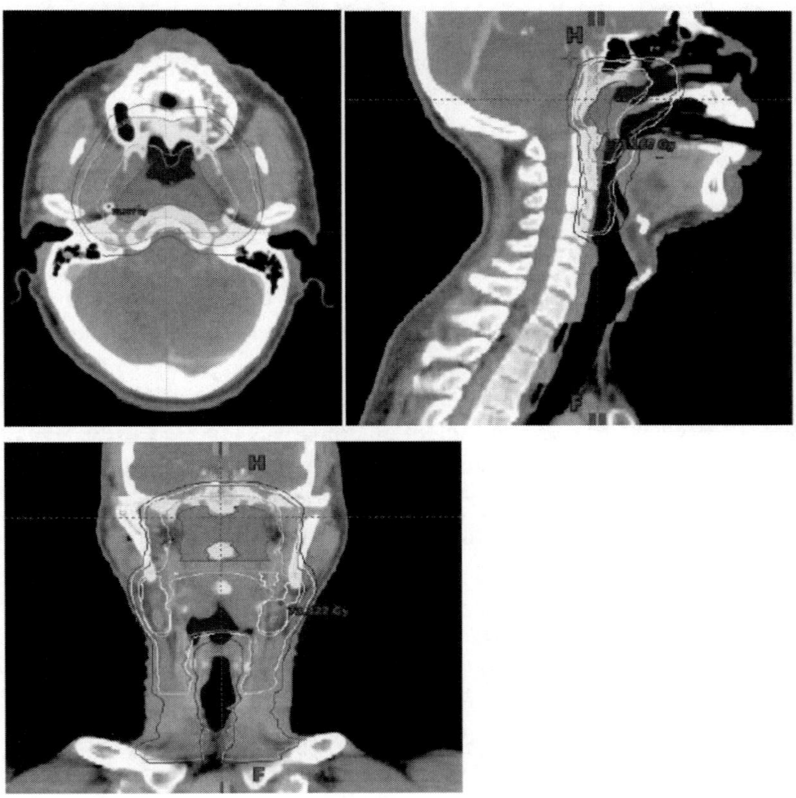

Figure 3. Axial, sagittal and coronal views of dose regions in a NPC RT plan. Red contour: GTV, orange contour: GTV-N, pink and yellow contour: CTV-1, magenta contour: CTV-2, green contour: CTV-3; and their respective coverage by isodose lines.

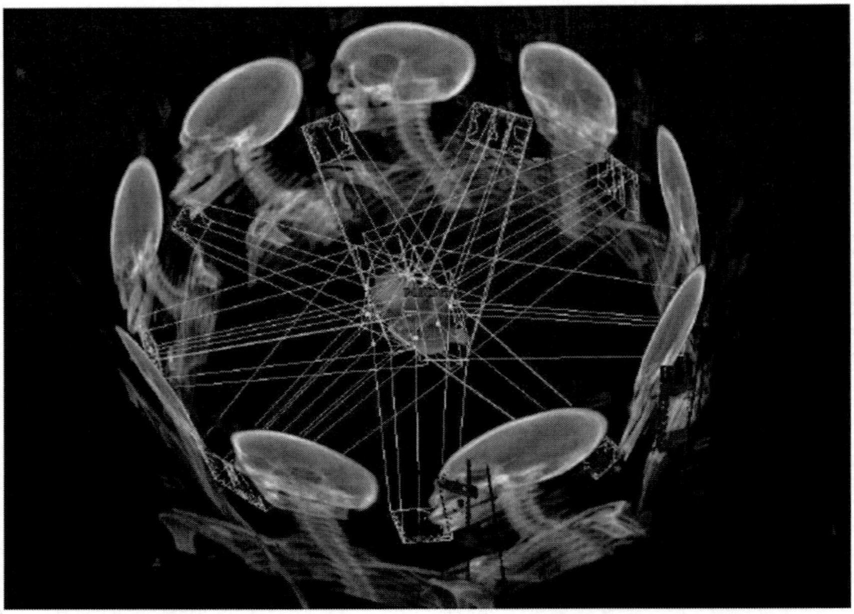

Figure 4. Nine-field IMRT.

Reduced-volume IMRT

While the survival rate of NPC patients has been improved by IMRT and chemotherapy, there has been growing concern regarding late toxicity induced by radiotherapy. As a result, reduced-volume IMRT (RV-IMRT) is being investigated in various studies. Lin et al. (40) reported the use of reduced-volume CTV2 as compared to those defined in the RTOG 0225 and 0615 protocols for 414 patients with non-metastatic NPC. CTV2 covered only maxillary sinus (limited to 5mm anterior to posterior nasal aperture and maxillary mucosa) and anterior third of clivus and cervical vertebrae. Excellent outcome was reported, with 5-year estimated overall survival, local control and regional relapse-free survival being 80%, 95% and 97% respectively. However, 30% of patients (123 patients) received boost treatment after IMRT due to residual disease, including 86 patients in the primary site and 37 patients in cervical lymphatics.

Different strategies of implementing reduced-volume IMRT have been reported. Lin et al. (41) carried out a retrospective analysis of reduced-volume IMRT by reducing the GTV-CTV1 margin (from 7 mm to 0 mm) and CTV1-PTV1 margin (from 7 mm to 5 mm). For the reduced-volume group, the high local relapse-free survival (83.5%), regional relapse-free survival (92.6%) and overall survival (91.0%) rates were in agreement with previous studies. Reduced-volume IMRT also lessens late xerostomia events.

Reducing irradiation volume to the neck had also been explored. As lymph node metastasis in NPC follows an orderly pattern, the probability of skip metastasis in the cervical nodal areas ranges only between 0.2% and 7.9%; and high dose irradiation to the neck may cause side effects such as soft tissue fibrosis and nerve palsy. Gao et al. (42) retrospectively analyzed 410 patients with lymph node-negative (N0) NPC who received radiotherapy to nasopharynx, skull base and upper neck drainage areas, including levels II, III and VA. The elective irradiation to lower neck lymph node levels, including level IV, inferior part of level V and supraclavicular regions was omitted. 4 patients developed neck recurrence and only 1 patient (0.2%) experienced relapse outside the irradiation fields. It was suggested that elective levels II, III, and VA irradiation is adequate for lymph node-negative patients.

Dose escalation

Various strategies have been sought to improve local control of NPC. On the basis of a dose-response relationship between tumor control and radiation dose (43), one strategy is to escalate the radiation dose to the tumor. This dose escalation can be achieved by giving a boost after external irradiation with intracavitary brachytherapy, conformal radiation boost or stereotactic radiosurgery or radiotherapy.

Leung et al. demonstrated that dose escalation with brachytherapy boost 10-12 Gy in 2 weekly fractions after completion of 2D external radiotherapy 66 Gy improved 5-year local control by 8% (96% vs 88%) and overall survival by 11% (91% vs 80%) in patients with T1 to 2a and possibly non-bulky T2b disease (44). However, the addition of brachytherapy boost given by either LDR (11Gy) or HDR (3 Gy per fractions for 3 fractions) technique did not improve local control and overall survival in stage III or non-metastatic stage IV disease (45).

Dose escalation using 3D conformal boost was also reported. Yeh et al. reported that dose escalation to 81Gy failed to show benefits on local control rate for patients with locally advanced NPC treated with radiotherapy alone. Higher radiation doses contribute to a higher incidence of radiation-related complications including xerostomia, hearing impairment and temporal lobe radionecrosis. Dose escalation with IMRT to 76 Gy resulted in 2-year locoregional control rate of 96% in T3 to T4 NPC (35). However, 4% of patients developed severe, life-threatening complication of internal carotid artery aneurysm in the skull base and 42% had moderate to severe hearing loss after treatment.

Fractionated stereotactic body radiation therapy boost was also used for dose escalation and resulted in excellent 3 to 5-year local control rate of over 90% and regional control rate of over 80% (46, 47). However, late toxicities could be severe with radiation-related retinopathy in 4%, carotid aneurysm in 1% and radiographic temporal lobe necrosis in 12% (47).

In summary, studies on dose escalation in improving local control demonstrated inconsistent results with possibility of severe complications.

Accelerated fractionation

Another method to enhance local control is to increase the biologic dose to tumor by accelerated fractionation to counteract the effect of tumor repopulation during treatment. In NPC 99-02 trial (48), Lee et al. demonstrated that concurrent-adjuvant chemotherapy combined with accelerated fractionation (2Gy/ fraction, 6 fractions/ week) significantly reduced failure and cancer-specific deaths, compared with conventional-adjuvant chemotherapy with conventional fractionation. The accelerated fractionation arm with chemotherapy achieved very remarkable 5-year locoregional failure-free survival of 90% and distant failure-free survival of 95% of patients with T3-4N0-1 disease. The combined treatment did not incur excessive acute or late toxicities.

However, the benefit of accelerated fractionation could not be demonstrated in other 3 published randomized trials that evaluated altered fractionation. The trial by Teo et al. on 159 patients (29% with T3-4 tumors) showed that comparing with 60Gy/24fractions/30days, experimental schedule of 71.2Gy/40fractions/30 days did not significantly improve tumor control but incurred excessive neurological toxicities (49% vs 23%) (49). The trial by Daoud et al. on 154 patients (45% with T3-4 tumors) showed that comparing with 70 Gy/35 fractions/7 weeks, experimental schedule of 70.4 Gy/44 fractions/6 weeks did not improve tumor control but incurred more acute mucositis and late skin fibrosis (50). In recent randomized controlled trial NPC-0501, changing the fractionation from conventional to accelerated (6 fractions/week) schedule did not achieve any benefit in progression-free survival but incurred higher toxicities including mucositis and dehydration (51). Based on current evidence, accelerated fractionation is not recommended for patients with locoregionally advanced NPC who receive chemoradiotherapy.

Adaptive radiotherapy

IMRT plans are typically based on a pre-treatment CT simulation that provides a snapshot of patient's anatomy. Nevertheless, during a typical 7-week treatment course, interfractional variations exist due to set-up errors and modification of patient's anatomy. While set-up errors may be reduced by vigorous treatment verification strategy such as the use of daily on-board cone beam CT/ IGRT and online corrections; anatomic changes, which can be a decrease in tumor and nodal volumes, parotid shrinkage, weight loss, alteration in muscle mass and fat distribution, and fluid shift within the body, are often difficult to be corrected by simple couch shifting. Studies have shown that these variations could lead to violation of the original treatment plan and result in poor target coverage and overdosing of organs-at-risk (OARs) in head and neck cancer patients (52, 53).

Adaptive radiotherapy (ART) consists of "the explicit inclusion of the temporal changes in anatomy during the imaging, planning, and delivery of radiotherapy" (54). It usually refers to the modification of treatment plan based on tumor response and normal tissue anatomic changes, and has the potential to counteract the effects of these variations.

Studies on re-planning showed the major dose discrepancies lie in various OARs such as brainstem and parotids, but not in the CTV regions (55-57). In the contrary, Chitapanarux et al. (58) studied 17 stage II to IVB NPC patients treated with IMRT using a two-phase adaptive radiotherapy protocol. Their results showed that the adapted re-plan provided a higher dose to the target volumes with better homogeneity, and a lower dose to the OARs. The D_{min} of all PTVs was increased; the D_{max} of the spinal cord and brainstem were decreased in 94% of patients (by 1.6–5.9 Gy and 2.1–9.9 Gy respectively), and the D_{mean} of the contralateral parotid was decreased in 70% of patients (by 0.2–4.4 Gy).

Fung et al. (59) developed a recommendation on ART strategy by quantifying the anatomic changes of the posterolateral wall of nasopharynx (P-NP), neck region and parotid glands in NPC patients during their RT course. Recruited 30 patients in their study, they showed that P-NP, parotid gland and neck volumes significantly regressed over time, with mean loss rates being 0.99, 1.35 and 0.39%/ day respectively. The parotid gland shifted medially and superiorly by a mean of 0.34 and 0.24 cm respectively. The neck region showed non-rigid posterior displacement, which increased from upper to lower neck. Their analysis proposed three re-plans scheduled at 9th, 19th and 29th fractions.

Nonetheless, there is still limited evidence whether these dosimetric advantages of ART would translate into improved patient outcomes. Zhao et al. (60) carried out a retrospective analysis on 33 patients with re-planning done and case-matched them with 66 control patients without re-planning. They showed that re-planning improved 3-year local progression-free survival for patients who had locally advanced primary (T3/4) and decreased the late effects for patient staged N2/3.

Another challenge is the interpretation of dose distribution on treatment plans as the configurations of tumors and surrounding tissues change over time. Leung et al. (61) extended the use of non-linear image registration of CT sets to the radiation dose. Since CT and dose were inherently in-register, the entire dose distribution could be deformed using the same deformation field derived from the CTs. Normal tissue complication probability could then be computed for various critical organs.

Practically, ART could heavily increase the department workloads and operative cost, as CT scanning, contouring and plan optimization would need to be repeated regularly. Automation of the different processes involved and development of an optimal strategy are required. At the moment, there is still considerable potential for further improvement in near real-time processes involving 3D CT image acquisition, automated segmentation, deformable registration, and modification of IMRT parameters, possibly including re-planning, to be performed just before the delivery of each fraction (54). Owing to such technical challenges and cost-effectiveness issue, prospective studies with larger sample sizes will have to be conducted to address the safety and clinical outcomes of ART, before it becomes a widely adopted approach.

ADVANCES IN CHEMOTHERAPY

As advance in radiotherapy achieves good local and regional control, distant metastasis becomes the main pattern of recurrence, especially in those with loco-regionally advanced disease. Many clinical studies investigated the benefit of chemotherapy for NPC.

Role of concurrent chemotherapy

Intergroup-0099 study (62) was the first phase III trial that achieved a significant survival benefit using cisplatin (100 mg/m^2) on D1, 22 and 43 concurrent with radiotherapy at conventional fractionation 70 Gy in 35-39 fractions, followed by combination of cisplatin (80 mg/m^2) and fluorouracil (1000 mg/m^2 for 4 days) every 4 weeks for 3 cycles. The addition of chemotherapy resulted in both superior 3-year progression-free survival rate (69% vs 24%, $p < 0.001$) and 3-year survival rate (78% vs 47%, $p = 0.005$). This regimen becomes the standard of care in locoregionally advanced NPC.

Three Asian studies with a similar design of Intergroup-0099 study were performed in Hong Kong, Singapore and China. In the Hong Kong NPC 9901 study (63), patients were treated with a chemotherapy schedule that was identical to that of Intergroup-0099 study. The chemoradiotherapy arm (CRT) had significantly higher 3-year failure-free survival (72% vs 62%, p = 0.027), mostly as a result of an improvement in locoregional control (92% vs 82%, p=0.005). However, there was no improvement in distant control and overall survival. On the other hand, the Singapore and China studies employed varied dosing of cisplatin from the Intergroup 0099 regimens, and showed significant improvement in both distant control, disease-free and overall survival with CRT. In the Singapore SQNP01 study (64)(65), patients on CRT received concurrent cisplatin (25mg/m^2 D1-4) on weeks 1, 4 and 7 of RT and adjuvant cisplatin (20mg/m^2 on D1-4) and fluorouracil (1000mg/m^2 on D1-4) every 4 weeks for 3 cycles. With a median follow-up of 4.9 years, the CRT arms showed superior 5-year disease-free survival (55% vs 45%) and overall survival (65% vs 46%) rates. The hazard ratios for disease-free survival and overall survival were 0.67 (p = 0.04) and 0.58 (p = 0.01) respectively. In the study performed in China (66), the CRT arm used concurrent cisplatin (40mg/m^2 on D1) weekly during RT, followed by cisplatin (80mg/m^2 on D1) and fluorouracil (800mg/m^2 on D1-5) every 4 weeks for 3 cycles after completion of RT. With a median follow-up of 29 months, the 2-year overall survival, failure-free survival, distant failure-free survival, and locoregional failure-free survival rates for the combined treatment arm and RT-alone arm were 90% vs 80% (p = 0.003), 85% vs 73% (p = 0.001), 87% vs 79% (p = 0.024) and 98% vs 92% (p = 0.007), respectively.

Three studies have compared concurrent chemotherapy with radiotherapy (without adjuvant chemotherapy) vs radiotherapy alone. In the trial performed by Chan et al. (67), 350 patients with stage II to IV NPC were randomized to receive either weekly cisplatin (40mg/m2/week) with RT or RT alone. After a median follow-up of 66 months, a borderline significant 11% improvement in overall survival from 59% (RT group) to 70% (CRT group) (p = 0.065) and a trend for improvement in disease-free survival (6% improvement, p = 0.16) were shown. In the trial performed by Li et al. (68), 115 patients were randomized to either radiotherapy alone or CRT with weekly oxaliplatin 70mg/m2 for six doses. After a median follow-up of 24 months, there was a significant difference in 2-year overall survival (100% vs 77%), relapse-free survival (96% vs 83%), and metastasis-free survival (92% vs 80%) in favor of the CRT arm. Lin et al. (69) compared concurrent chemoradiotherapy with cisplatin and fluorouracil versus radiotherapy alone for patients with stage III to IV NPC. CRT arm had statistically significant better 5-year overall survival (72% vs 54%) and 5-year progression-free survival (72% vs 53%).

The meta-analysis by Baujat et al. (70), based on 1753 patients from 8 randomized trials, confirmed that the use of chemotherapy offered an absolute survival benefit of 6% at 5 years, improving it from 56% to 62%. The risk reduction seemed to be greatest for concurrent chemotherapy at approximately 40%, suggesting that chemotherapy may act as a radiosensitizer. No evidence of an overall survival benefit was observed with induction and adjuvant chemotherapy.

The meta-analysis performed by Zhang et al. (71) included seven phase III randomized controlled trials (total 1608 patients) done in endemic areas focusing on the impact of concurrent chemoradiotherapy comparing with RT alone on patients with locally advanced NPC. Risk ratios of 0.63 (95% CI, 0.50 to 0.80), 0.76 (95% CI, 0.61 to 0.93) and 0.74 (95% CI, 0.62 to 0.89) were observed for 2-, 3- and 5-year overall survival respectively in favor of the concurrent chemoradiotherapy group.

The current evidence indicates that concurrent chemoradiotherapy is the most effective treatment modality for improvement of overall survival for locally advanced nasopharyngeal cancer.

Role of adjuvant chemotherapy

One major discussion regarding the design of Intergroup 0099 is the contribution of an adjuvant phase. Two phase 3 trials of pure adjuvant chemotherapy trials did not show a positive effect on overall survival or relapse-free survival (72, 73). A recent phase 3 trial by Chen et al. (74) evaluated the contribution of adjuvant chemotherapy to concurrent chemoradiotherapy. 508 patients with non-metastatic stage III or IV (except T3-4N0) NPC were randomly assigned to receive concurrent chemoradiotherapy plus adjuvant chemotherapy or concurrent chemoradiotherapy alone. Adjuvant cisplatin and fluorouracil chemotherapy did not significantly improve failure-free survival in locoregionally advanced disease. The 2-year failure-free survival rate was 86% in the concurrent chemoradiotherapy plus adjuvant chemotherapy group and 84% in concurrent chemoradiotherapy only group (HR 0.74, p = 0.13). However, 18% of patients did not receive any adjuvant chemotherapy and 19% of patients discontinued adjuvant chemotherapy after starting treatment in this trial. The improvement in survival benefit may be hampered by poor compliance to adjuvant chemotherapy.

In the meta-analysis by Baujat et al. (70), no evidence of an overall survival benefit and an event free-survival benefit was observed with adjuvant chemotherapy. The meta-analysis performed by Zhang et al. (71) attempted to identify the additional benefit of adjuvant chemotherapy (AC) for patients receiving concurrent chemoradiotherapy (CCRT). Subgroup analyses showed that both loco-regional recurrences (RR 0.65, 95% CI 0.45 to 0.95) and distant failure (RR 0.71, 95% CI 0.54 to 0.92) were improved in CCRT+AC arms compared with RT alone. However, the RR of death with CCRT+AC was not significant (p = 0.18). This lack of demonstrable survival difference might be due to increased mortality related to chemotherapy toxicities, and possibly successful salvage after relapse.

The meta-analysis project done by the MAC-NPC collaborative group, released its latest update in 2015 (75). The analyzed data from 19 trials and 4806 patients, with a median follow-up of 7.7 years, confirmed that the addition of chemotherapy to radiotherapy significantly improved overall survival (HR 0.79, absolute benefit at 5 years 6.3%), and the benefit was consistent across all analyzed endpoints (including PFS, locoregional and distant control, cancer mortality). This meta-analysis also examined the effect of concomitant chemotherapy with or without adjuvant chemotherapy as distinct groups. The interaction between benefit of chemotherapy on overall survival and the timing of chemotherapy was statistically significant, in favor of concomitant plus adjuvant chemotherapy (HR 0.65, 0.56-0.76) and concomitant without adjuvant chemotherapy (HR 0.80, 0.70-0.93), but not adjuvant chemotherapy alone or induction chemotherapy alone. However, despite the seemingly greatest benefit gained by the CCRT+AC, the difference on overall survival gain between CCRT alone and CCRT+AC is not statistically significant, and the authors have agreed that these two schedules are very close in terms of benefit.

Given the limited patient compliance to adjuvant chemotherapy after concomitant chemoradiotherapy and the uncertain benefit but actual risks of adjuvant treatment, patient selection is important. Large-scale trials are exploring the utilization of post-treatment EBV DNA level to select out the right patients for adjuvant chemotherapy (NCT00370890 and NCT02135042). In summary, the exact contribution of adjuvant chemotherapy remains to be addressed in further studies.

Role of induction chemotherapy

One strategy for further therapeutic benefit is to use induction-concurrent chemotherapy. Chemotherapy tolerance was better in induction phase than in adjuvant phase. Studies showed that 95% patients could tolerate 3 cycles of induction chemotherapy (76), comparing to only 50-75% of the patients who received the three planned adjuvant chemotherapy cycles in the MAC-NPC analysis (75). Induction chemotherapy has two potential benefits: more effective eradication of micro-metastases and shrinkage of primary tumor to allow a wider margin for irradiation, especially in locally advanced cases with intracranial involvement. Lee et al. reported induction chemotherapy achieved significant down-staging of T-category in 35% of patients and reduction of gross tumor volume by 61% on average (76). Hui et al. reported significant improvement of 3-year overall survival from 67.7% to 94.1% using 2 cycles of induction chemotherapy docetaxel and cisplatin, compared with concurrent chemoradiotherapy alone for patients with stage III to IVB NPC (77). In the meta-analysis by Baujat et al. though no evidence of an overall survival benefit was observed, a benefit of event-free survival with risk reduction of 18% was demonstrated in the subset of trials using induction chemotherapy (70).

Conclusion of chemotherapy

The addition of chemotherapy to standard radiotherapy provides a 6% survival benefit at 5 years in patients with NPC. The benefit of concurrent chemotherapy has been confirmed by multiple trials and meta-analyses. Induction chemotherapy can downstage the tumor and has benefit in event-free survival. Adjuvant chemotherapy potentially furthers survival benefit but appropriate patient selection is the key. The risk of distant metastases remains significant. Intensification of chemotherapy regime, incorporation of newer cytotoxic drugs or development of novel agents to improve efficacy should be explored in future trials.

CONCLUSION

Radical radiotherapy using IMRT is the current standard of management for NPC. Concurrent chemoradiotherapy with cisplatin, with or without induction or adjuvant chemotherapy with cisplatin and fluorouracil, is used in locoregionally advanced disease. MRI and PET-CT improve accuracy of target delineation in radiotherapy planning, as well as detection of residual disease and recurrence. Pre- and post-treatment EBV DNA levels are of prognostic value and may be useful in guiding treatment. Distant metastasis, being the dominant pattern of failure, calls for further advances in systemic therapy.

REFERENCES

[1] Curado M, Edwards B, Shin H, Storm H, Ferlay J, Heanue M, et al. Cancer incidence in five continents. Lyon, France: IARC Scientific Publications, 2007.

[2] Barnes L, Eveson JW, Reichart P, Sidransky D. Pathology and genetics of head and neck tumours. WHO Classif Tumour 2005; (9): 163–75.

[3] Liao XB, Mao YP, Liu LZ, Tang LL, Sun Y, Wang Y, et al. How does magnetic resonance imaging influence staging according to AJCC staging system for nasopharyngeal carcinoma compared with computed tomography. Int J Radiat Oncol Biol Phys 2008; 72(5): 1368-77.

[4] Emami B, Sethi A, Petruzzelli GJ. Influence of MRI on target volume delineation and IMRT planning in nasopharyngeal carcinoma. Int J Radiat Oncol Biol Phys 2003; 57(2): 481-8.

[5] Devic S. MRI simulation for radiotherapy treatment planning. Med Phys 2012; 39(11): 6701.

[6] Ng SH, Chan SC, Yen TC, Rung CC, Liao CT, Ko SF, et al. Staging of untreated nasopharyngeal carcinoma with PET/CT: comparison with conventional imaging workup. Eur J Nucl Med Mol Imaging 2009; 36: 12-22.

[7] Liu T, Xu W, Yan WL, Ye M, Bai YR, Huang G. FDG-PET, CT, MRI for diagnosis of local residual or recurrent nasopharyngeal carcinoma, which one is the best: A systematic review. Radiother Oncol 2007; 85(3): 327-35.

[8] Zheng XK, Chen LH, Wang QS, Wu HB, Wang HM, Chen YQ, et al. Influence of FDG-PET on computed tomography-based radiotherapy planning for locally recurrent nasopharyngeal carcinoma. Int J Radiat Oncol Biol Phys 2007; 69(5): 1381-8.

[9] Werner-Wasik M, Nelson AD, Choi W, Arai Y, Faulhaber PF, Kang P, et al. What is the best way to contour lung tumors on PET scans? Multiobserver validation of a gradient-based method using a NSCLC digital PET phantom. Int J Radiat Oncol Biol Phys 2012; 82(3): 1164-1171

[10] Zhang G, Han D, Ma C, Lu J, Sun T, Liu T, et al. Gradient-based delineation of the primary GTV on FLT PET in squamous cell cancer of the thoracic esophagus and impact on radiotherapy planning. Radiat Oncol 2015; 10(1): 11.

[11] Lim TC, Chua ML, Chia GS, Ng DC, Ong SC, Wee JT, et al. Comparison of MRI, CT and 18 F-FDG-PET / CT for the detection of intracranial disease extension in nasopharyngeal carcinoma. Head Neck Oncol 2012; 4(2): 1-8.

[12] Lo YMD, Chan LYS, Lo K, Leung S, Zhang J, Chan ATC, et al. Quantitative analysis of cell-free Epstein-Barr virus DNA in plasma of patients with nasopharyngeal carcinoma advances in brief quantitative analysis of cell-free Epstein-Barr Virus DNA in plasma of patients with nasopharyngeal carcinoma 1999; 1: 1188–91.

[13] Ma BBY, King A, Lo YMD, Yau YY, Zee B, Hui EP, et al. Relationship between pretreatment level of plasma Epstein-Barr virus DNA, tumor burden, and metabolic activity in advanced nasopharyngeal carcinoma. Int J Radiat Oncol Biol Phys 2006; 66(3): 714-20.

[14] Han BL, Xu XY, Zhang CZ, Wu JJ, Han CF, Wang H, et al. Systematic review on Epstein-Barr virus (EBV) DNA in diagnosis of nasopharyngeal carcinoma in asian populations. Asian Pacific J Cancer Prev 2012; 13(6): 2577-81.

[15] Hou X, Zhao C, Guo Y, Han F, Lu LX, Wu SX, et al. Different clinical significance of pre- and post-treatment plasma Epstein-Barr virus DNA load in nasopharyngeal carcinoma treated with radiotherapy. Clin Oncol 2011; 23(2): 128-33.

[16] Lo YM, Chan a T, Chan LY, Leung SF, Lam CW, Huang DP, et al. Molecular prognostication of nasopharyngeal carcinoma by quantitative analysis of circulating Epstein-Barr virus DNA. Cancer Res 2000; 60(24): 6878-81.

[17] Leung SF, Zee B, Ma BB, Hui EP, Mo F, Lai M, et al. Plasma Epstein-Barr viral deoxyribonucleic acid quantitation complements tumor-node-metastasis staging prognostication in nasopharyngeal carcinoma. J Clin Oncol 2006; 24(34): 5414-8.

[18] Lin J-C, Wang W-Y, Liang W-M, Chou H-Y, Jan J-S, Jiang R-S, et al. Long-term prognostic effects of plasma epstein-barr virus DNA by minor groove binder-probe real-time quantitative PCR on nasopharyngeal carcinoma patients receiving concurrent chemoradiotherapy. Int J Radiat Oncol Biol Phys 2007; 68(5): 1342-8.

[19] Lin J-C, Wang W-Y, Chen KY, Wei Y-H, Liang W-M, Jan J-S, et al. Quantification of plasma Epstein-Barr virus DNA in patients with advanced nasopharyngeal carcinoma. N Engl J Med 2004; 350(24): 2461-70.

[20] Chan ATC, Lo YMD, Zee B, Chan LYS, Ma BBY, Leung S-F, et al. Plasma Epstein-Barr virus DNA and residual disease after radiotherapy for undifferentiated nasopharyngeal carcinoma. J Natl Cancer Inst 2002; 94(21): 1614-9.

[21] An X, Wang FH, Ding PR, Deng L, Jiang WQ, Zhang L, et al. Plasma Epstein-Barr virus DNA level strongly predicts survival in metastatic/recurrent nasopharyngeal carcinoma treated with palliative chemotherapy. Cancer 2011; 117(16): 3750-7.

[22] Wang WY, Twu CW, Chen HH, Jan JS, Jiang RS, Chao JYC, et al. Plasma EBV DNA clearance rate as a novel prognostic marker for metastatic/recurrent nasopharyngeal carcinoma. Clin Cancer Res 2010; 16(3): 1016-24.

[23] Lo YMD, Chan LYS, Chan ATC, Leung S, Lo K, Zhang J, et al. Quantitative and temporal correlation between circulating cell-free Epstein-Barr virus DNA and tumor recurrence in nasopharyngeal carcinoma advances in brief virus DNA and tumor recurrence in nasopharyngeal carcinoma. Cancer Res1999; 59: 5452–5.

[24] Wang WY, Twu CW, Lin WY, Jiang RS, Liang KL, Chen KW, et al. Plasma Epstein-Barr virus DNA screening followed by by cell-free Epstein-Barr Virus DNA and tumor recurrence in nasopharyngeal carcinoma advances in brief virus DNA and tumor. Cancer 2011; 117(19): 4452-9.

[25] Lee AW, Poon Y, Foo W, Law SC, Cheung FK, Chan DK, et al. Retrospective analysis of 5037 patients with nasopharyngeal carcinoma treated during 1976–1985: Overall survival and patterns of failure. Int J Radiat Oncol 1992; 23(2): 261–70.

[26] Peng G, Wang T, Yang KY, Zhang S, Zhang T, Li Q, et al. A prospective, randomized study comparing outcomes and toxicities of intensity-modulated radiotherapy vs. conventional two-dimensional radiotherapy for the treatment of nasopharyngeal carcinoma. Radiother Oncol 2012; 104(3): 286-93.

[27] Ng WT, Lee MCH, Hung WM, Choi CW, Lee KC, Chan OSH, et al. Clinical outcomes and patterns of failure after intensity-modulated radiotherapy for nasopharyngeal carcinoma. Int J Radiat Oncol Biol Phys 2011; 79(2): 420-8.

[28] Bakst RL, Lee N, Pfister DG, Zelefsky MJ, Hunt M, Kraus DH, et al. Hypofractionated dose-painting intensity modulated radiation therapy with chemotherapy for nasopharyngeal carcinoma: A prospective trial. Int J Radiat Oncol Biol Phys 2011; 80(1): 148-53.

[29] Wolden SL, Chen WC, Pfister DG, Kraus DH, Berry SL, Zelefsky MJ. Intensity-modulated radiation therapy (IMRT) for nasopharynx cancer: Update of the Memorial Sloan-Kettering experience. Int J Radiat Oncol Biol Phys 2006; 64(1): 57-62.

[30] Lee N, Xia P, Quivey JM, Sultanem K, Poon I, Akazawa C, et al. Intensity-modulated radiotherapy in the treatment of nasopharyngeal carcinoma: An update of the UCSF experience. Int J Radiat Oncol Biol Phys 2002; 53(1): 12-22.

[31] Lin S, Pan J, Han L, Zhang X, Liao X, Lu JJ. Nasopharyngeal carcinoma treated with reduced-volume intensity-modulated radiation therapy: Report on the 3-year outcome of a prospective series. Int J Radiat Oncol Biol Phys 2009; 75(4): 1071-8.

[32] Kam MKM, Teo PML, Chau RMC, Cheung KY, Choi PHK, Kwan WH, et al. Treatment of nasopharyngeal carcinoma with intensity-modulated radiotherapy: The Hong Kong experience. Int J Radiat Oncol Biol Phy. 2004; 60(5): 1440-50.

[33] Tham IWK, Hee SW, Yeo RMC, Salleh PB, Lee J, Tan TWK, et al. Treatment of nasopharyngeal carcinoma using intensity-modulated radiotherapy: The national cancer centre Singapore experience. Int J Radiat Oncol Biol Phys 2009; 75(5): 1481-6.

[34] Wong FCS, Ng AWY, Lee VHF, Lui CMM, Yuen K-K, Sze W-K, et al. Whole-field simultaneous integrated-boost intensity-modulated radiotherapy for patients with nasopharyngeal carcinoma. Int J Radiat Oncol Biol Phys 2010; 76(1): 138-45.

[35] Kwong DLW, Sham JST, Leung LHT, Cheng ACK, Ng WM, Kwong PWK, et al. Preliminary results of radiation dose escalation for locally advanced nasopharyngeal carcinoma. Int J Radiat Oncol Biol Phys 2006; 64(2): 374-81.

[36] Lee N, Harris J, Garden AS, Straube W, Glisson B, Xia P, et al. Intensity-modulated radiation therapy with or without chemotherapy for nasopharyngeal carcinoma: Radiation therapy oncology group phase II trial 0225. J Clin Oncol 2009; 27(22): 3684-90.

[37] Pow EHN, Kwong DLW, McMillan AS, Wong MCM, Sham JST, Leung LHT, et al. Xerostomia and quality of life after intensity-modulated radiotherapy vs. conventional radiotherapy for early-stage nasopharyngeal carcinoma: Initial report on a randomized controlled clinical trial. Int J Radiat Oncol Biol Phys 2006; 66(4): 981-91.

[38] Kam MKM, Leung S-F, Zee B, Chau RMC, Suen JJS, Mo F, et al. Prospective randomized study of intensity-modulated radiotherapy on salivary gland function in early-stage nasopharyngeal carcinoma patients. J Clin Oncol 2007; 25(31): 4873-9.

[39] Wang SZ, Li J, Miyamoto CT, Chen F, Zhou LF, Zhang HY, et al. A study of middle ear function in the treatment of nasopharyngeal carcinoma with IMRT technique. Radiother Oncol 2009;93(3):530-3.

[40] Lin S, Pan J, Han L, Guo Q, Hu C, Zong J, et al. Update report of nasopharyngeal carcinoma treated with reduced-volume intensity-modulated radiation therapy and hypothesis of the optimal margin. Radiother Oncol 2014; 110(3): 385-9.

[41] Lin Y-W, Chen C-C, Lin L-C, Lee SP. The impact of reduced-volume, intensity-modulated radiation therapy on disease control in nasopharyngeal carcinoma. PLoS One 2015; 10(4): e0125283.

[42] Gao Y, Zhu G, Lu J, Ying H, Kong L, Wu Y, et al. Is elective irradiation to the lower neck necessary for N0 nasopharyngeal carcinoma? Int J Radiat Oncol Biol Phys 2010; 77(5): 1397-402.

[43] Teo PML, Leung SF, Tung SY, Zee B, Sham JST, Lee AWM, et al. Dose-response relationship of nasopharyngeal carcinoma above conventional tumoricidal level: a study by the Hong Kong nasopharyngeal carcinoma study group (HKNPCSG). Radiother Oncol 2006; 79(1): 27-33.

[44] Leung TW, Wong VYW, Sze WK, Lui CMM, Tung SY. High-dose-rate intracavitary brachytherapy boost for early T stage nasopharyngeal carcinoma. Int J Radiat Oncol Biol Phys 2008; 70(2): 361-7.

[45] Rosenblatt E, El-Gantiry M, Elattar I, Afiane M, Benjafaar N, Abubaker S, et al. Brachytherapy boost in loco-regionally advanced nasopharyngeal carcinoma: A prospective randomized trial of the international atomic energy agency. Int J Radiat Oncol 2011; 81(2): S4-5.

[46] Chen HHW, Tsai S-T, Wang M-S, Wu Y-H, Hsueh W-T, Yang M-W, et al. Experience in fractionated stereotactic body radiation therapy boost for newly diagnosed nasopharyngeal carcinoma. Int J Radiat Oncol Biol Phys 2006; 66(5): 1408-14.

[47] Hara W, Loo BW, Goffinet DR, Chang SD, Adler JR, Pinto H, et al. Excellent local control with stereotactic radiotherapy boost after external beam radiotherapy in patients with nasopharyngeal carcinoma. Int J Radiat Oncol Biol Phys 2008; 71(2): 393-400.

[48] Lee AWM, Tung SY, Chan ATC, Chappell R, Fu YT, Lu TX, et al. A randomized trial on addition of concurrent-adjuvant chemotherapy and/or accelerated fractionation for locally-advanced nasopharyngeal carcinoma. Radiother Oncol 2011; 98(1): 15-22.

[49] Teo PML, Leung SF, Chan ATC, Leung TWT, Choi PHK, Kwan WH, et al. Final report of a randomized trial on altered-fractionated radiotherapy in nasopharyngeal carcinoma prematurely terminated by significant increase in neurologic complications. Int J Radiat Oncol Biol Phys 2000; 48(5): 1311-22.

[50] Daoud J, Toumi N, Siala W, Ghorbel A, Drira MM, Frikha M. Results of a prospective randomised trial comparing conventional radiotherapy to split course bifractionated radiation therapy in patients with nasopharyngeal carcinoma. Radiother Oncol 2007; 85(1): 17-23.

[51] Lee AWM, Ngan RKC, Tung SY, Cheng A, Kwong DLW, Lu T-X, et al. Preliminary results of trial NPC-0501 evaluating the therapeutic gain by changing from concurrent-adjuvant to induction-concurrent chemoradiotherapy, changing from fluorouracil to capecitabine, and changing from conventional to accelerated radiotherapy. Cancer 2015; 121(8): 1328-38.

[52] O'Daniel JC, Garden AS, Schwartz DL, Wang H, Ang KK, Ahamad A, et al. Parotid gland dose in head-and-neck intensity-modulated radiotherapy: is what you plan what you get? Int J Radiat Oncol Biol Phys 2007; 69(4): 1290–6.

[53] Hansen EK, Bucci MK, Quivey JM, Weinberg V, Xia P. Repeat CT imaging and replanning during the course of IMRT for head-and-neck cancer. Int J Radiat Oncol Biol Phys 2006;64(2):355–62.

[54] Castadot P, Lee J, Geets X, Gr, GrX, V. Adaptive radiotherapy of head and neck cancer. Semin Radiat Oncol 2010; 20(2): 84-93.
[55] Wang X, Lu J, Xiong X, Zhu G, Ying H, He S, et al. Anatomic and dosimetric changes during the treatment course of intensity-modulated radiotherapy for locally advanced nasopharyngeal carcinoma. Med Dosim 2010; 35(2): 151–7.
[56] Zhang X, Li M, Cao J, Luo JW, Xu GZ, Gao L, et al. Dosimetric variations of target volumes and organs at risk in nasopharyngeal carcinoma intensity-modulated radiotherapy. Br J Radiol 2012; 85(1016): 506–13.
[57] Jin X, Han C, Zhou Y, Yi J, Yan H, Xie C. A modified VMAT adaptive radiotherapy for nasopharyngeal cancer patients based on CT-CT image fusion. Radiat Oncol 2013; 8(1): 277.
[58] Chitapanarux I, Chomprasert K, Nobnaop W, Wanwilairat S, Tharavichitkul E, Jakrabhandu S, et al. A dosimetric comparison of two-phase adaptive intensity-modulated radiotherapy for locally advanced nasopharyngeal cancer. J Radiat Res 2015; 56(3): 529-38.
[59] Fung WWK, Wu VWC, Teo PML. Developing an adaptive radiation therapy strategy for nasopharyngeal carcinoma. J Radiat Res 2014; 55(2): 293-304.
[60] Zhao L, Wan Q, Zhou Y, Deng X, Xie C, Wu S. The role of replanning in fractionated intensity modulated radiotherapy for nasopharyngeal carcinoma. Radiother Oncol 2011; 98(1): 23-7.
[61] Leung LHT, Wong WKH, Cheng ACK, Kan MWK, Cheung JYC, Lam NKH, et al. A new approach to computing normal tissue complication probability of an intensity-modulated radiotherapy treatment with stereotactic radiotherapy boost of nasopharyngeal carcinoma: a case study. Med Dosim 2011; 36(2): 138-44.
[62] Al-Sarraf M, LeBlanc M, Giri PG, Fu KK, Cooper J, Vuong T, et al. Chemoradiotherapy versus radiotherapy in patients with advanced nasopharyngeal cancer: Phase III randomized Intergroup study 0099. J Clin Oncol 1998; 16: 1310-1317.
[63] Lee AWM, Lau WH, Tung SY, Chua DTT, Chappell R, Xu L, et al. Preliminary results of a randomized study on therapeutic gain by concurrent chemotherapy for regionally-advanced nasopharyngeal carcinoma: NPC-9901 trial by the Hong Kong Nasopharyngeal Cancer Study Group. J Clin Oncol 2005; 23(28): 6966-75.
[64] Wee J, Tan EH, Tai BC, Wong HB, Leong SS, Tan T, et al. Randomized trial of radiotherapy versus concurrent chemoradiotherapy followed by adjuvant chemotherapy in patients with American Joint Committee on Cancer/International Union Against Cancer stage III and IV nasopharyngeal cancer of the endemic variety. J Clin Oncol 2005; 23(27): 6730-8.
[65] Wee J, Tan EH, Tai BC, Wong HB, Leong SS, Tan T, et al. Final Report of SQNP01 - A phase III randomized trial comparing RT with chemo-RT for locally advanced nasopharyngeal cancer. Int J Radiat Oncol 2006; 66(3): S16.
[66] Chen Y, Liu M-Z, Liang S-B, Zong J-F, Mao Y-P, Tang L-L, et al. Preliminary results of a prospective randomized trial comparing concurrent chemoradiotherapy plus adjuvant chemotherapy with radiotherapy alone in patients with locoregionally advanced nasopharyngeal carcinoma in endemic regions of china. Int J Radiat Oncol Biol Phys 2008; 71(5): 1356-64.
[67] Ngan RKC, Teo PML, Mok TSK, Johnson PJ, Peter HK, Zee BCY. Overall survival after concurrent cisplatin – radiotherapy compared with radiotherapy alone in locoregionally advanced nasopharyngeal carcinoma. J Natl Cancer Inst 2005; 97(7): 536–9.
[68] Zhang L, Zhao C, Peng PJ, Lu LX, Huang PY, Han F, et al. Phase III study comparing standard radiotherapy with or without weekly oxaliplatin in treatment of locoregionally advanced nasopharyngeal carcinoma: Preliminary results. J Clin Oncol 2005; 23(33): 8461–8.
[69] Lin J-C, Jan J-S, Hsu C-Y, Liang W-M, Jiang R-S, Wang W-Y. Phase III study of concurrent chemoradiotherapy versus radiotherapy alone for advanced nasopharyngeal carcinoma: positive effect on overall and progression-free survival. J Clin Oncol 2003; 21(4): 631–7.
[70] Baujat B, Audry H, Bourhis J, Chan ATC, Onat H, Chua DTT, et al. Chemotherapy in locally advanced nasopharyngeal carcinoma: An individual patient data meta-analysis of eight randomized trials and 1753 patients. Int J Radiat Oncol Biol Phys 2006; 64(1): 47-56.
[71] Zhang L, Zhao C, Ghimire B, Hong M-H, Liu Q, Zhang Y, et al. The role of concurrent chemoradiotherapy in the treatment of locoregionally advanced nasopharyngeal carcinoma among

endemic population: a meta-analysis of the phase III randomized trials. BMC Cancer 2010; 10(1): 558.

[72] Chi K-H, Chang Y-C, Guo W-Y, Leung M-J, Shiau C-Y, Chen S-Y, et al. A phase III study of adjuvant chemotherapy in advanced nasopharyngeal carcinoma patients. Int J Radiat Oncol Biol Phys 2002; 52(5): 1238-44.

[73] Kwong DLW, Sham JST, Au GKH, Chua DTT, Kwong PWK, Cheng ACK, et al. Concurrent and adjuvant chemotherapy for nasopharyngeal carcinoma: A factorial study. J Clin Oncol 2004; 22(13): 2643-53.

[74] Chen L, Hu C-S, Chen X-Z, Hu G-Q, Cheng Z-B, Sun Y, et al. Concurrent chemoradiotherapy plus adjuvant chemotherapy versus concurrent chemoradiotherapy alone in patients with locoregionally advanced nasopharyngeal carcinoma: a phase 3 multicentre randomised controlled trial. Lancet Oncol 2012; 13(2): 163-71.

[75] Blanchard P, Lee A, Marguet S, Leclercq J, Ng WT, Ma J, et al. Chemotherapy and radiotherapy in nasopharyngeal carcinoma: an update of the MAC-NPC meta-analysis. Lancet Oncol 2015; 16(6): 645-55.

[76] Lee AWM, Lau KY, Hung WM, Ng WT, Lee MCH, Choi CW, et al. Potential improvement of tumor control probability by induction chemotherapy for advanced nasopharyngeal carcinoma. Radiother Oncol 2008; 87(2): 204-10.

[77] Hui EP, Ma BB, Leung SF, King AD, Mo F, Kam MK, et al. Randomized phase II trial of concurrent cisplatin-radiotherapy with or without neoadjuvant docetaxel and cisplatin in advanced nasopharyngeal carcinoma. J Clin Oncol 2009; 27(2): 242-9.

In: Pain Management Yearbook 2015
Editor: Joav Merrick

ISBN: 978-1-63484-515-1

Chapter 35

INTERSTITIAL BRACHYTHERAPY IN GYNECOLOGICAL MALIGNANCIES: IMPROVING PATIENT OUTCOMES

Laura D'Alimonte, MRT(T), MHSc and Eric Leung[*], MD, MSc, FRCPC
Odette Cancer Centre, Sunnybrook Health Sciences Centre,
Toronto, Ontario, Canada

Radiation therapy has become a well-established treatment for the management of advanced gynecological cancers. Standard of care can include external beam radiation therapy with concurrent chemotherapy and internal intracavitary brachytherapy. Brachytherapy plays an important role in the management of cervical cancer, endometrial cancer and vaginal cancer, as it allows very high ablative doses of radiation to be delivered directly to the tumour with a sharp dose drop-off allowing for surrounding normal tissue to be spared. Interstitial brachytherapy is an effective treatment option for patients with locally advanced or recurrent gynecological cancer. It involves a complex procedure with detailed radiation planning and physics.

Keywords: brachytherapy, gynecological cancer, oncology

INTRODUCTION

In Canada, gynecological malignancies account for approximately 12% of all new malignancies in women (1). Although the incidence and mortality are on the decline in western societies, there remains a significant proportion of patients who suffer from uncontrollable or incurable disease. Gynecological cancer patients who present with low risk, early stage disease are routinely managed with local treatment such as surgery. For those who

[*] Corresponding author: Eric Leung MD, MSc, FRCPC, Sunnybrook Odette Cancer Centre, 2075 Bayview Ave, Toronto, ON, Canada. E-mail: Eric.Leung@sunnybrook.ca.

present with locally advanced disease, management is more challenging and often requires a multi-modality approach.

Radiation therapy has become a well-established treatment for the management of advanced gynecological cancers. Standard of care can include external beam radiation therapy with concurrent chemotherapy and internal intracavitary brachytherapy which involves the insertion of radioactive seeds into an organ cavity via a brachytherapy applicator (2). Brachytherapy plays an important role in the management of cervical cancer, endometrial cancer and vaginal cancer, as it allows very high ablative doses of radiation to be delivered directly to the tumour with a sharp dose drop off allowing for surrounding normal tissue to be spared (2). With the adoption and integration of 3D imaging techniques, 3 year local control rates in cervix cancer have improved with many of the leading Groupe Europeen de Curietherapie and the European Society for Radiotherapy and Oncology (GEC-ESTRO) institutions reporting 85%-100% local control rates depending on disease stage (3-7). However, in some instances such as extensive disease or distortion of anatomy (8), standard intracavitary brachytherapy is inadequate to achieve these results and the use of interstitial needles has been recommended (9, 10).

Interstitial brachytherapy has been shown to be an effective treatment for disease that would be inadequately managed with traditional brachytherapy (8, 11-13). With this technique, needles are inserted directly through tissue and into the tumour allowing for very high doses of radiation to be delivered to the target volume, while minimizing or sparing radiation dose to the surrounding normal tissue (8, 11-15). The utilization of interstitial needles in the management of gynecological malignancies has been growing in popularity worldwide. This technique allows for a tailored treatment approach by creating an individualized radiation treatment plan through the implantation of interstitial needles directly into the tumour volume (8).

Historically, interstitial implantations were performed using low dose rate (LDR) brachytherapy techniques (12). However, high dose rate (HDR) brachytherapy techniques offers several advantages over LDR techniques including; reduced occupational exposure, and the ability to optimize treatment plans (12). With the increasing availability of 3D imaging options for treatment planning, in particular, MRI imaging, radiation doses can be fully optimized to optimally deliver ablative radiation doses to the tumour volume in an effort to improve patient outcomes (8). This article will explore the interstitial brachytherapy technique including, indications for this treatment, the various techniques currently used to deliver these very high radiation doses, the technical aspects associated with this technique and an overview of the current outcomes associated with this treatment.

ROLE OF INTERSTITIAL BRACHYTHERAPY FOR GYNECOLOGICAL MALIGNANCIES

When a tumour cannot be optimally encompassed by standard intracavitary brachytherapy technique, interstitial brachytherapy is recommended to achieve an optimal dose distribution to the target volume (13). Both the American Brachytherapy Society (ABS) and GEC-ESTRO define several different clinical scenarios that warrant the use of interstitial brachytherapy over standard (intracavitary) techniques (16-18).

Scenario 1

The use of interstitial needles is recommended in patients who present with extensive cervical cancer including large tumours that extend into the parametrium which would result in an inadequate target volume coverage if a standard intracavitary technique was used. Cases with extensive disease in the cervix, obliteration of the cervical os, narrow fornices, extension of disease into the lower vagina or infiltration laterally into the parametria are all indications for the use of interstitial brachytherapy as the use of standard intracavitary applicators are associated with high local failures and increased risk of organs at risk complications (19).

Scenario 2

For women who present with a recurrence inside an area previously irradiated restricting the use of further external beam irradiation, the use of interstitial brachytherapy is a viable treatment option. In these cases, highly conformal radiation doses are required to ablate the recurrence and are safely deliverable via interstitial brachytherapy.

Scenario 3

The use of interstitial needles is recommended for women who present with a primary vaginal malignancy when the target volume cannot be adequately encompassed with standard intracavitary brachytherapy techniques.

Scenario 4

Patients with vaginal recurrences especially from endometrial cancer have been recognized as good candidates for interstitial brachytherapy techniques with potential sparing of the bladder and rectum. These techniques have been shown to improve dose distribution particularly deeply infiltrating tumours.

Scenario 5

There are some instances where there is an anatomical distortion that doesn't allow for the use of standard brachytherapy techniques. In these instances, interstitial brachytherapy is recommended.

TECHNIQUE

The development of interstitial brachytherapy for the management of gynecological cancers was first reported in the 1950's using a free-hand placement of radioactive needles (radium

226 or cobalt 60) (16). Modern day techniques include the use of a transperineal or transvaginal template which has resulted in improved needle placement for better tumour volume coverage (15). Transvaginal templates are well-described in the literature (16) with transperineal templates more widely used clinically.

There are two main types of transperineal templates used clinically; the Martinez Universal Perineal Interstitial Template (MUPIT) (20) and the Syed-Neblett Template (21). The MUPIT was designed to treat not only gynecological malignancies but also prostatic, anorectal and perineal tumours where the Syed-Neblett template is strictly used for gynecological malignancies (16). There are several similarities between the two templates. Both templates are designed with evenly-spaced holes allowing for the insertion of needles through the perineum (Figure 1). A central hole within the template allows for the housing of a vaginal cylinder which can also be loaded with needles to be placed for vaginal dosing and anchoring. The vaginal cylinder is designed to be hollow in the middle to allow for the use of a uterine tandem for cases that may require it (Figure 1).

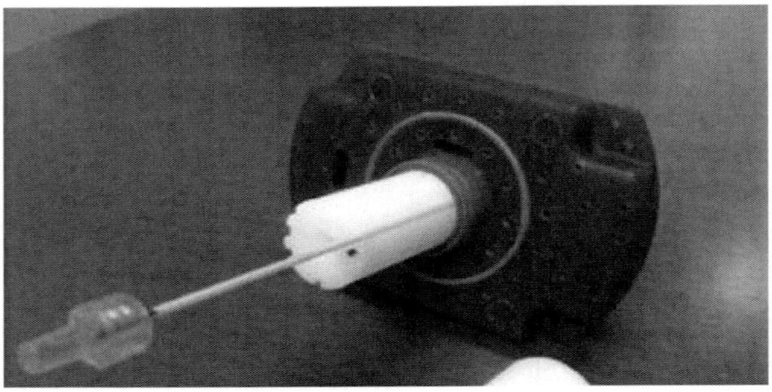

Figure 1. Syed-Neblett transperineal template (Part #790, Best Medical International).

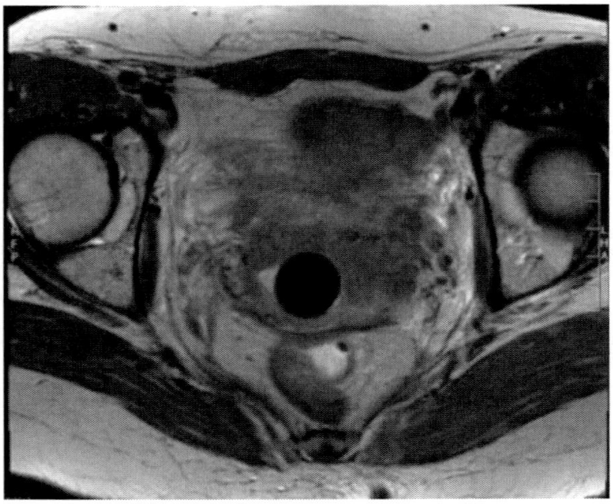

Figure 2. Pre-brachytherapy MRI images with dummy cylinder.

TREATMENT PROCESS: THE ODETTE CANCER CENTRE EXPERIENCE

Pre-brachytherapy imaging

The gynecological interstitial program at the Odette Cancer Centre (OCC), Sunnybrook Health Sciences Centre was established in 2014. Identified interstitial brachytherapy candidates undergo a pre-treatment MRI with a vaginal cylinder in place. These images provide sufficient information about tumour/target extent in relation to the treatment applicator prior to treatment (see Figure 2).

Implantation

The implantation procedure is performed with the patient under general anesthetic in the lithotomy position. In cervical cancer cases, the uterine tandem is inserted under transabdominal ultrasound for positioning (Figure 3).

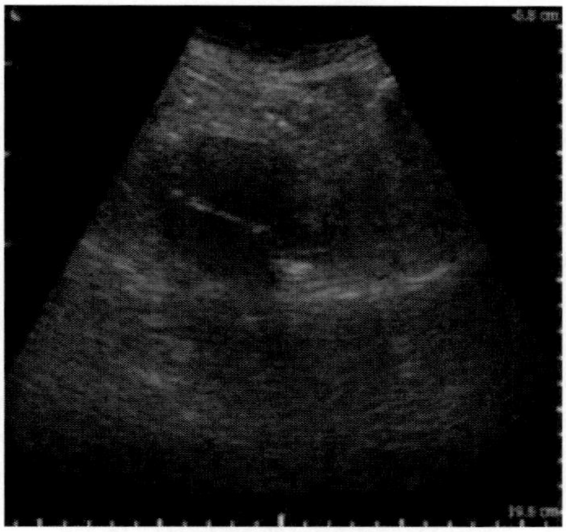

Figure 3. Transabdominal ultrasound image with tandem in uterus.

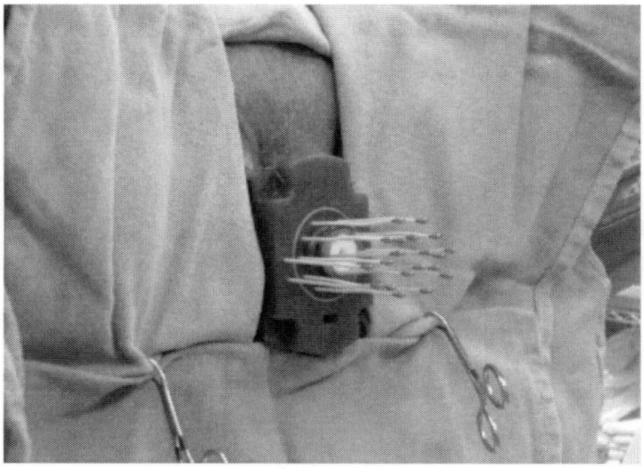

Figure 4. Transperineal template with needles affixed to patient.

After, the vaginal cylinder is inserted; the template is then affixed to the vaginal cylinder. Needles are then inserted into the hole positions that correspond to the location of the tumour. The number and position of needles is dependent on the size and shape of disease on pre-brachytherapy imaging and upon clinical examination. Typically, 15 to 25 needles are inserted through the holes of the template. Once all needles are in place, they are advanced to a final depth to cover the superior aspect of the disease which is based on the pre-brachytherapy MR imaging. All needles are then secured to the template. Finally the template is sutured to the perineum (see Figure 4). Patients' legs are brought down from lithotomy and wedges are placed under their knees to tilt the pelvis slightly upwards. They are then sent to recovery until they are ready to be planned.

Planning and treatment

With the availability of three dimensional (3D) imaging increasing worldwide over the last several decades, the use of 3D imaging for brachytherapy treatment planning has been increasing (13). At present, all OCC interstitial patients are CT-planned with a strict bladder-filling protocol with contrast to aid in defining the bladder wall contours. In addition, rectal tubes are inserted to minimize or eliminate gas from the rectum. A planning CT scan of the whole pelvis is obtained with a slice thickness of 1.5 mm. For image acquisition, the stainless steel obturators located in the plastic needles are replaced with CT dummy marker lines to allow for optimized catheter digitization during planning (see Figure 5).

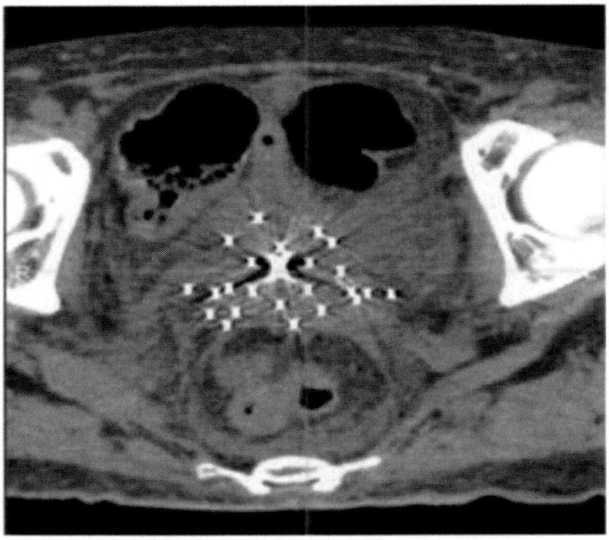

Figure 5. Axial pelvic CT with markers in place.

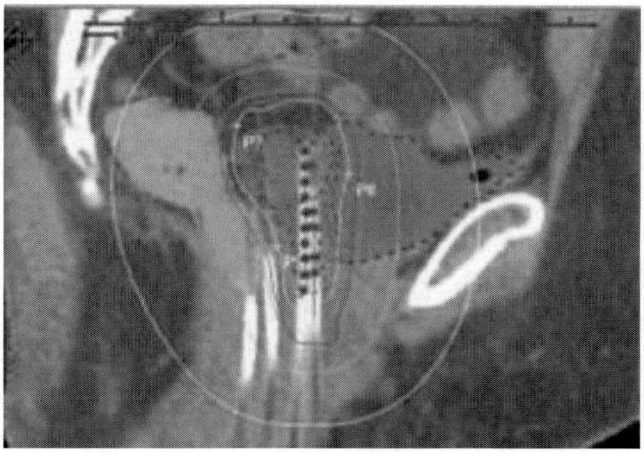

Figure 6. Sagittal view of pelvis with target and OARs contoured.

Once complete, the CT scan is imported into brachytherapy planning software. The CT images are fused with the pre-brachytherapy MRI imaging sequences. After, target volumes and organs at risk (bladder, rectum, sigmoid and small bowel) are contoured. With the adoption of 3D imaging for better visualization of target volumes and organs at risk, the GEC-ESTRO working group have successfully introduced adaptive target concepts for brachytherapy in locally advanced cervical cancer (22, 23). The key target concepts are image based definitions of a high risk clinical target volume (HRCTV) and an intermediate risk clinical target volume (IRCTV) defined at the time of brachytherapy (22). These brachytherapy target concepts are applied not only for cervical cancer but have also been adopted for other gynecological malignancies such as vagina or recurrent endometrium. The gross target volume (GTV) is defined utilizing the pre-treatment imaging, the clinic examination at diagnosis and the clinical examination under anesthesia at the time of implantation (see Figure 6).

Prescribed dose, dose constraints

The optimal dose and fractionation schedule to be delivered with this technique has yet to be defined (8). However, the increasing availability of 3D imaging for treatment planning and the transition from low dose rate (LDR) to high dose rate (HDR) treatments, has led to the investigation of several dose fractionation schemas. There is variability of high dose rate gynecologic ISBT practice in published institutional series and guidelines, and questions remain regarding adequate total dose, the optimal number of implants, and the number of fractions per implant (8). Nonetheless, currently used dose targets and constraints are based on the GEC-ESTRO guidelines (22) with the primary goal of treatment to achieve an HRCTV D90 over the prescription dose and the V100 over 90%, D2cc < 490 cGy per fraction for the rectum, sigmoid, small bowel and D2cc < 630 cGy per fraction for the bladder.

Patients receive between 3 to 4 HDR treatments by remote afterloading techniques. Implantation and first treatment are completed on Day 1. The minimum separation between fractions is 6 hours. Before each treatment delivery, the positions of the catheters are checked by measuring the catheter free length in relation the perineal template. After the last fraction, the implant is removed and the patient is discharged home once medically stabilized.

OUTCOMES

Interstitial brachytherapy is a radiotherapy treatment that allows for an individualized radiation therapy treatment plan to be planned and delivered through directly implanting needles into a tumour/target volume allowing for high doses of radiation to be deposited directly into the tumour while minimizing dose delivered to the surrounding normal tissue (8).

There is a growing body of evidence that report the outcomes of HDR interstitial brachytherapy for gynecological malignancies that would otherwise be treated inadequately with standard treatments. However, the criticisms of these works are that they are single institutional experiences, generally retrospective in nature, low patient numbers, heterogeneous groups of patients with relatively short follow up. In addition, there is significant variation between the reported series in terms of dose per fraction and total dose prescribed (13). Despite these drawbacks, there is compelling evidence to support further investigation of interstitial brachytherapy techniques. Selected results are reported in Table 1.

The earliest reported HDR interstitial brachytherapy series was in 1999, Demanes et al. (19). They performed three interstitial implants each one week apart delivering two HDR fractions of either 5.5 Gy or 6 Gy for a total of 6 fractions over 3 weeks utilizing 2D radiographs to develop patient treatment plans (19). They report an overall local control (LC) rate of 81% with a disease free survival (DFS) rate of 6.5% (19).

With the increased availability and use of 3D volumetric imaging, subsequent series altered the dose fractionation in an effort to minimize the total treatment duration. Thibault et al. (12) reported their experience using CT-based interstitial brachytherapy for the treatment of both primary gynecological disease (n = 34) and recurrent gynecological disease (n = 9). They report poorer outcomes associated with recurrent disease compared to patients with primary disease with reported LC rates at 2 years was 45% versus 87% respectively. Reported overall survival rates at 2 years were 86% for primary cancer, 16.7% for recurrent cancers. Similar results are reported by Lee et al. (2013). In total, 68 women (34 with recurrent disease) underwent CT-based volumetric planning with a reported 86% local control rate at 2 years and a 64% overall survival rate at 2 years post treatment (26). In a recent single institution study conducted by D'Souza et al. (2014), 64 women (primary and recurrent disease) were treated with a CT based volumetric planned interstitial HDR brachytherapy. In their series, they report a local control rate of 68% at 3 years and an overall survival rate of 73% at 3 years (9). The variability in outcomes is likely due to differences in patient population (primary site of disease, primary vs. recurrent disease).

Table 1. HDR-ISBT literature

Authors (Ref)	Patient population	No. pts	Total dose (Gy)	Fractions	Median follow-up (Mths)	Local control (%)	Survival (%)	Late toxicity (%)
Demanes et al. (19)	Cervix	62	33-36	6	40	81%	DFS @ 5yrs = 48%	6.5%
Beriwal et al. (11)	Cervix, vagina	16	18.75	5	22	@ 5yrs 63% (cervix), 100% (vagina)	CSS @ 5yrs = 64%	7%
Kannen et al. (24)	Cervix	47	18.25-25	5	14.6	61%	DFS @ 2yrs = 43% OS @ 2yrs = 59%	10%
Sharma et al. (25)	Cervix	42	20	2	23	62%	RFS @ 3yrs = 47%	9%
Lee et al. (26)	cervix, endometrium vagina, ovarian, vulva	68	12.5-48	2-9	17	86%	OS @2yrs = 64% PFS@2yrs = 60%	13%
Pinn-Bingham et al. (27)	Cervix	116	36 + hyperthermia	2	35	85.3	DFS@3yrs = 68% OS@3yrs = 58%	13%
D'Souza et al. (9)	Cervix, vagina, vulva, endometrium	47	12-24	2-4	34.8	@3yrs 68%	RFS@3yrs = 65% OS@3yrs = 73%	29%
Thibault et al. (12)	Cervix, vagina, vulva, endometrium	43	18-35	3-7	19.3	Primary=87% Recurrent=45%	OS@ 2yrs Primary = 86% Recurrent = 16.7%	28%

DFS = disease free survival.
CSS = cause specific survival.
OS = overall survival.
RFS = recurrence free survival.
PFS = progression free survival.

The incidence of severe (grade 3+) complications post interstitial HDR brachytherapy ranges from 7% to 29% (9, 11, 12, 24-27). Potential complications that have been reported in the literature include; vaginal necrosis, proctitis, small bowel obstruction, fistula, bleeding. Variability in toxicity rates can be related to treatment factors such as total radiation dose, dose per fraction, proximity of target volumes to OARs, the use of multimodality therapy (external beam radiation therapy, chemotherapy, surgery) or patient factors (9).

Conclusion

Interstitial brachytherapy is an effective treatment option for patients with locally advanced or recurrent gynecological cancer. It involves a complex procedure with detailed radiation planning and physics. With the increased availability of volumetric imaging for both the planning of brachytherapy treatment and guidance of needles during the procedure will continue to improve outcomes for patients.

References

[1] Navaneelan T. Trends in the incidence and mortality of female reproductive system cancers. Statistics Canada. Accessed 2015 July 31. URL: http://www.statcan.gc.ca/pub/82-624-x/2015001/article/14095-eng.htm.

[2] Viswananthan AN, Beriwal S, De Los Santos JF, Demanes DJ, Gaffney D, et al. American Brachytherapy Society consensus guidelines for locally advanced carcinoma of the cervix. Part II: High-dose-rate brachytherapy. Brachytherapy 2011; 11: 47-52.

[3] Potter R, Georg P, Dimopoulous JC, Grimm M, Berger D, Nesvacil N, et al. Clinical outcomes of protocol based image (MRI) guided adaptive brachytherapy combined with 3D conformal radiotherapy with or without chemotherapy in patients with locally advanced cervical cancer. Radiother Oncol 2011; 100(1): 116-23

[4] Tanderup K, Nielsen SK, Nyvang GB, Pedersen EM, Rohl L, Aagaard T, et al. From point A to the sculpted pear: MR image guidance significantly improves tumour dose and sparing of organs at risk in brachytherapy of cervical cancer. Radiother Oncol 2010; 94(2): 173-80.

[5] Nomden CN, de Leeuw AA, Roesink JM, Tersteeg RJ, Moerland MA, Witteveen PO, et al. Clinical outcome and dosimetric parameters of chemo radiation including MRI guided adaptive brachytehrapy with tandem ovoid applicators for cervical cancer patients: a single institution experience. Radiother Oncol 2013; 107(1): 69-74.

[6] Lindegaard JC, Tanderup K, Nielsen SK, Haack S, Gelineck J. MRI-guided 3D optimization significantly improves DVH parameters of pulsed dose rate brachytherapy in locally advanced cervical cancer. Int J Radiat Oncol Biol Phys 2008; 71(3): 756-64.

[7] Rijkmans EC, Nout RA, Rutten IHHM, Ketelaars M, Neelis KJ, Laman MS, et al. Improved survival of patients with cervical cancer treated with image guided brachytherapy compared with conventional brachytherapy. Gynecol Oncol 2014; 135: 231-8.

[8] D'Souza D, Wiebe E, Patil N, Sugimoto A, Prefontaine M, Aulakh S, et al. CT-based interstitial brachytherapy in advanced gynaecologic malignancies: Outcomes from a single institution experience. Brachytherapy 2014: 13: 225-32.

[9] Dimopoulos JC, Kirisits C, Petric P, Georg P, Lang S, Berger D, et al. The Vienna applicator for combined intracavitary and interstitial brachytherapy of cervical cancer: clinical feasibility and preliminary results. Int J Radiat Oncol Biol Phys 2006; 66(1): 83-90.

[10] Nomden CN, De Leeuw AA, Moerland MA, Roesink JM, Tersteeg RJ, Jurgenliemk-Shulz IM. Clinical use of the Ultrecht applicator for combined intracavitary/interstitial brachytherapy treatment in locally advanced cervical cancer. Int J Radiat Oncol Biol Phys 2012; 82(4): 1424-30.

[11] Agrawal PP, Singhal SS, Neema JP, Vyas RK, Rathi AK, Bahadur AK. The role of interstitial brachytehrapy using template in locally advanced gynecolgical malignancies. Gynecol Oncol 2005; 99: 169-75.

[12] Beriwal S, Bhatnagar A, Heron DE, Selvaraj R, Mogus R, Kim H, et al. High dose rate interstitial brachytherapy for gynecologic malignancies. Brachytherapy 2006; 5: 218-22.

[13] Thibault I, Lavallee MC, Aubin S, Laflamme N, Vigneault E, et al. Inverse planned gynecologic high dose rate interstitial brachytherapy: Clinical outcomes and dose volume histogram analysis. Brachytherapy 2012; 11: 181-91.

[14] Beriwal S, Heron DE, Mogus R, Edwards RP, Kelley JL, Sukumvanich P. High dose rate brachytehrapy(HDRB) for primary or recurrent cancer in the vagina. Radiat Oncol 2008; 13: 3-7.

[15] Fokdal L, Tanderup K, Nielsen SK, Christensen HK, Rohl L, Pedersen EM, et al. Image and laparscopic guided interstitial brachytherapy for locally advanced primary or recurrent gynaecological cancer using the adaptive GEC-ESTRO target concept. Radiother Oncol 2011; 100: 473-9.

[16] Haie-Meder C, Gerbaulet A, Potter R. The GEC-ESTRO handbook of brachytherapy, ESTRO, Brussels: ESTRO, 2002.

[17] Viswanathan AN, Thomadsen B. American Brachytherapy Society consensus guidelines for locally advanced carcinoma of the cervix. Brachytherapy 2012; 11: 33-46.

[18] Beriwal S, Demanes JD, Erickson B, Jones E, De Los Santos JF, Cormack RA, et al. American Brachytherapy Society consensus guidelines for interstitial brachytherapy for vaginal cancer. Brachytherapy 2012; 11: 68-75.

[19] Demanes JD, Rodriguez RR, Bendre DD, Ewing TL. High dose rate transperineal interstitial brachytherapy for cervical cancer: High pelvic control and low complication rates. Int J Radiat Oncol Biol Phys 1999; 45(1): 105-12.

[20] Martinez A, Cox RS, Edmunson GK. A multiple-site perineal applicator (MUPIT) for treatment of prostatic, anorectal and gynecological malignancies. Int J Radiat Oncol Biol Phys 1984; 10: 297-305.

[21] Syed AMN, Puthawala AA, Neblett D. Transperineal interstitial-intracavitary "Syed-Neblett" applicator in the treatment of carcinoma of the uterine cervix. Endocurie Hypertherm Oncol 1986; 2: 1-13.

[22] Haie-Meder C, Potter R, Van Limbergen E, Barillot I, De Brabandere M, Dimopoulos J, et al. Recommendations from gynecological (GYN) GEC-ESTRO working group (I): concepts and terms in 3D image based 3D treatment planning in cervix cancer brachytherapy with emphasis on MRI assessment of GTV and CTV. Radiother Oncol 2005; 74: 235-45.

[23] Potter R, Haie-Meder C, Van Limbergen E, Barillot I, De Brabandere M,Dimopoulos J, et al. Recommendations from gynecological (GYN) GEC-ESTRO working group (II): concepts and terms in 3D image based treatment planning in cervix cancer brachytherpay-3D dose volume parameters and aspects of 3D image-based anatomy, radiation physics, radiobiology. Radiother Oncol 2006; 78: 67-77.

[24] Kannan N, Beriwal S, Kim H, Houser C, Mogus R, Sukumvanich P, et al. High dose rate interstitial computed tomography-based brachytherapy for the treatment of cervical cancer: Early results. Brachytherapy 2012; 11: 408-12.

[25] Sharma DN, Rath GK, Thulkar S, Kumar S, Subramani V, Julka PK. High dose rate interstitial brachytherapy using two weekly sessions of 10 Gy each for patients with locally advanced cervical carcinoma. Brachytherapy 2011; 10: 242-8.

[26] Lee LJ, Damato AL, Viswananthan AN. Clinical outcomes of high dose rate interstitial gynecologic brachytherapy using real time CT guidance. Brachytherapy 2013; 12: 303-10.

[27] Pinn-Bingham M, Puthawala AA, Syed N, Sharma A, DiSaia P, Berman M, et al. Outcomes of high dose rate interstitial brachytherapy in the treatment of locally advanced cervical cancer: Long term results. Int J Radiat Oncol Biol Phys 2012; 85(3): 714-20.

In: Pain Management Yearbook 2015
Editor: Joav Merrick

ISBN: 978-1-63484-515-1

Chapter 36

SOCIAL WORK IN END-OF-LIFE CARE: A REVIEW OF THE MOST HIGHLY CITED PAPERS

Blair Henry**, *Michael Lam, Ronald Chow,
Leonard Chiu, Selina Chow, Edward Chow,
Henry Lam, Natalie Pulenzas and Breanne Lechner
Sunnybrook Health Sciences Centre, Toronto, Ontario, Canada

Background: This study provides a bibliography on the topic of social work in end-of-life (EOL) care, based on the 50 most highly cited papers in this field as presented in the Scopus database.

Method: A search was conducted in Scopus to determine the most frequently cited papers in the area of social work in EOL care. To limit the results to references highly relevant to social work, the phrases 'social work' and 'social worker' were searched as both subject and title keywords. The results were then combined with the subject keywords 'end of life', 'palliative care', 'hospice care', and 'terminal care'.

Results: A total of 193 references dating between 1987 and 2011 were found on social work in EOL care.

Discussion: Literature on this topic is limited. A majority (68%) of the top 50 cited articles were published in a 6 year period between 2000 and 2006. A total of 14 journals were involved, with the Journal of Social Work in end-of-life and Palliative Care publishing the most articles on the list. The top articles were further reviewed with 15 key topics identified.

Keywords: social work, social worker, end of life, palliative care, hospice care, terminal care, bibliography

---

* Corresponding author: Blair Henry, Sunnybrook Health Sciences Centre, 2075 Bayview Avenue, Toronto, ON, Canada. E-mail: Blair.Henry@sunnybrook.ca.

INTRODUCTION

The provision of high quality end-of-life (EOL) care depends on the involvement and contributions made by social workers. This is particularly relevant for addressing the complex psychosocial needs of both patients and families (1). The field of EOL care is changing and evolving, and with the expected increase in demands for these services due to our aging population, the profession of social work will need to be able to keep up with both the demand and skills necessary to meet these demographic changes.

The changes in EOL care have also called for an evidence-based approach to the provision of hospice and palliative care that is supported by both research and scholarship. It will also be a requirement for social work to provide skilled clinical interventions that are backed by strong evidence (2).

To this end, a strategic review of the literature can provide a profession such as social work with the opportunity to examine how the historical factors of the past have shaped the direction of scholarship, and by doing so can identify where gaps in knowledge generation exists. However, when undertaking a review of the literature it is understood that a vast majority of published articles are never referenced even once, and so those that are cited often are arguably assumed to have impacted the field and patient care (3).

Noted as far back as the NASW Standards (2004), "the role of social work—a profession steeped in the same basic principles and values that characterize palliative and end-of-life care—is on a similar trajectory." Social workers have an incredible opportunity to influence this field, and given the demographic changes occurring in society, the need for trained social workers specialized in EOL will undoubtedly increase. The purpose of this review is to provide social workers and social work students with a bibliography of highly cited articles in the social work and EOL.

METHODS

A search was conducted in Scopus to determine the most frequently cited papers in the area of social work in EOL care. Scopus by Elsevier is one of the largest abstract and citation database of peer-reviewed literature and it was chosen for this project because it offers 20% more coverage than Web of Science for citation analysis purpose while providing more consistent accuracy than Google Scholar (4).

Given our interest in works which are highly relevant to the field of social work, we excluded papers which only touched upon social work as an aside or those only marginally related to the field. Our search criteria required that the phrases 'social work' or 'social worker' had to appear in both the subject keyword field and the article title field of Scopus in order to qualify. We then combined the resulting set of references with another search criteria of subject keywords 'end of life', 'palliative care', 'hospice care' or 'terminal care'. The top fifty cited articles in the field of EOL and social work were identified.

RESULTS

The overall results of our literature search are presented in Figure 1 as a Venn diagram, showing the results of three groups of keyword search terms and the resulting overlap using the Boolean operator "AND". As evidenced in the Venn diagram we extended our search to also include 'ethics' as a third category, in an attempt to identify how involved the literature on social work in EOL care related to ethical dilemmas and issues.

DISCUSSION

The Scopus search for social work in EOL care identified a surprisingly low number of references. Only 193 publications met our search criteria. The small number of reported publications is partly due to the strict search criteria used for encompassing social work, but is also reflective of the relative scarcity of literature highly relevant to social work in EOL care.

The full bibliographic listing of the top 50 cited articles that dealt with social work in EOL care is presented in Table 1. The papers span a publication period of 26 years, with the first article published in 1987 and the last in 2011. However, 58% of the articles appeared in print over the 7 year period between 2000 and 2006.

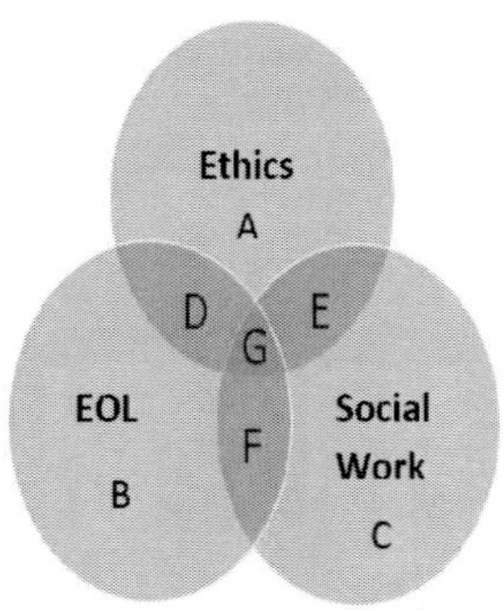

Item	Description	Number of papers
A	ETHICS	175 986
B	EOL	67 447
C	SOCIAL WORK*	6 616
D	ETHICS AND EOL	6 508
E	ETHICS AND SOCIAL WORK	300
F	EOL AND SOCIAL WORK	193
G	EOL AND ETHICS AND SOCIAL WORK	16

* Rigorous search criteria with requirement in both keyword and title field.

Figure 1. Overall Search Results.

Table 1. Top 50 Most Highly Cited Papers on Social Work and End-of-Life Care

Rank	Paper	Times Cited
1	Ganzini L, Harvath TA, Jackson A et al. (2002) Experiences of Oregon nurses and social workers with hospice patients who requested assistance with suicide. N Engl J Med 347(8):582-8	92
2	Christ GH, Sormanti M et al. (2000) Advancing social work practice in end-of-life care. Soc Work Health Care 30(2):81-99	78
3	Gwyther LP, Altilio T, Blacker S, et al. (2005) Social work competencies in palliative and end-of-life care. Journal of social work in end-of-life and palliative care. 1(1):87-120	43

Table 1. (Continued).

Rank	Paper	Times Cited
4	Kramer BJ, Christ GH, Bern-Klug M et al. (2005) A national agenda for social work research in palliative and end-of-life care. Journal of Palliative Medicine. 8(2):418-431	39
5	Csikai EL, Raymer M (2005) Social workers' educational needs in end-of-life care. Social Work in Health Care. 41(1):53-72	34
6	Csikai EL, Bass K (2000) Health care social workers' views of ethical issues, practice, and policy in end-of-life care. Social Work in Health Care. 32(2):1-22	33
7	Kovacs PJ, Bronstein LR (1999) Preparation for oncology settings: What hospice social workers say they need. Health and Social Work. 24(1):57-64	31
8	Reese DJ, Brown DR (1997) Psychosocial and spiritual care in hospice: differences between nursing, social work, and clergy. The Hospice Journal. 12(1):29-41	31
9	Ross E (1993) Preventing burnout among social workers employed in the field of AIDS/HIV. Social Work in Health Care. 18(2):91-108	28
10	Davidson KW, Foster Z (1995) Social work with dying and bereaved clients: Helping the workers. Social Work in Health Care. 21(4):1-16	26
11	Csikai EL (2004) Social workers' participation in the resolution of ethical dilemmas in hospice care. Health and Social Work. 29(1):67-76	25
12	Kovacs PJ, Bellin MH, Fauri DP (2006) Family-centered care: A resource for social work in end-of-life and palliative care. Journal of Social Work in End-of-Life and Palliative Care. 2(1):13-27	23
13	Miller PJ, Hedlund SC, Murphy KA (1998) Social work assessment at end of life: Practice guidelines for suicide and the terminally ill. Social Work in Health Care. 26(4):23-36	22
14	Miller LL, Harvath TA, Ganzini L et al. (2004) Attitudes and experiences of Oregon hospice nurses and social workers regarding assisted suicide. Palliative Medicine. 18(8):685-691	21
15	Sheldon FM (2000) Dimensions of the role of the social worker in palliative care. Palliative Medicine. 14(6):491-498	21
16	Beresford P, Croft S, Adshead L (2008) 'We don't see her as a social worker': A service user case study of the importance of the social worker's relationship and humanity. British Journal of Social Work. 38(7):1388-1407	20
17	Luptak M (2004) Social work and end-of-life care for older people: A historical perspective. Health and Social Work. 29(1):7-15	20
18	Bosma H, Johnston M, Cadell S et al. (2010) Creating social work competencies for practice in hospice palliative care. Palliative Medicine. 24(1):79-87	19
19	MacDonald D (1991) Hospice social work: a search for identity. Health and Social Work. 16(4):274-280	18
20	Kulys R, Davis MA (1987) Nurses and social workers: rivals in the provision of social services?. Health and Social Work. 12(2):101-112	18
21	Jones BL (2006) Companionship, control, and compassion: A social work perspective on the needs of children with cancer and their families at the end of life. Journal of Palliative Medicine. 9(3):774-788	17
22	Walsh-Burke K, Csikai EL (2005) Professional social work education in end-of-life care: contributions of the Project on Death in America's Social Work Leadership Development program. Journal of Social Work in End-of-Life and Palliative Care. 1(2):11-26	16
23	Wesley C, Tunney K, Duncan E (2004) Educational needs of hospice social workers: Spiritual assessment and interventions with diverse populations. American Journal of Hospice and Palliative Medicine. 21(1):40-46	16

Rank	Paper	Times Cited
24	Babler JE (1997) A comparison of spiritual care provided by hospice social workers, nurses, and spiritual care professionals. The Hospice Journal.. 12(4):15-27	16
25	Huff MB, Weisenfluh S, Murphy M et al. (2006) End-of-life care and social work education: What do students need to know?. Journal of Gerontological Social Work. 48(2):219-231	13
26	Christ GH, Blacker S (2005) Setting an agenda for social work in end-of-life and palliative care: an overview of leadership and organizational initiatives. Journal of Social Work in End-of-Life and Palliative Care. 1(1):9-22	13
27	Bern-Klug M, Kramer BJ, Linder JF (2005) All aboard: advancing the social work research agenda in end-of-life and palliative care. Jounral of Social Work in End-of-Life and Palliative Care. 1(2):71-86	13
28	Baker ME (2000) Knowledge and attitudes of health care social workers regarding advance directives. Social Work in Health Care. 32(2):61-74.	13
29	Meier DE, Beresford L (2008) Social workers advocate for a seat at palliative care table. Journal of Palliative Medicine. 11(1):10-14	12
30	Mccormick AJ, Engelberg R, Curtis JR (2007) Social workers in palliative care: Assessing activities and barriers in the intensive care unit. Journal of Palliative Medicine. 10(4):929-937	12
31	Heyman JC, Gutheil IA (2006) Social work involvement in end of life planning. Journal of Gerontological Social Work. 47(4):47-61	12
32	Sharp JW, Blum D, Aviv L (1993) Elderly men with cancer: Social work interventions in prostate cancer. Social Work in Health Care. 19(1):91-107	12
33	McCormick AJ, Curtis JR, Stowell-Weiss P et al. (2010) Improving social work in intensive care unit palliative care: Results of a quality improvement intervention *. Journal of Palliative Medicine. 13(3):297-304	11
34	Sanders S, Swails P (2009) Caring for individuals with end-stage dementia at the end of life: A specific focus on hospice social workers *. Dementia. 8(1):117-138	11
35	Black K (2007) Advance care planning throughout the end-of-life: Focusing the lens for social work practice. Journal of Social Work in End-of-Life and Palliative Care. 3(2):39-58	11
36	Arnold EM, Artin KA, Griffith D et al. (2007) Unmet needs at the end of life: Perceptions of hospice social workers. Journal of Social Work in End-of-Life and Palliative Care. 2(4):61-83	11
37	Brandsen CK (2005) Social work and end-of-life care: reviewing the past and moving forward. Journal of Social Work in End-of-Life and Palliative Care. 1(2):45-70	11
38	Mackelprang RW, Mackelprang RD (2005) Historical and contemporary issues in end-of-life decisions: Implications for social work. Social work. 50(4):315-324	11
39	Clausen H, Kendall M, Murray S et al. (2005) Would palliative care patients benefit from social workers' retaining the traditional 'casework' role rather than working as care managers? A prospective serial qualitative interview study. British Journal of Social Work. 35(2):277-285	11
40	Csikai EL (1999) Euthanasia and assisted suicide: issues for social work practice. Journal of Gerontological. Social Work. 31(4):49-63	11
41	Bomba PA, Morrissey MB, Leven DC (2011) Key role of social work in effective communication and conflict resolution process: Medical Orders for Life-Sustaining Treatment (MOLST) program in New York and shared medical decision making at the end of life. Journal of Social Work in End-of-Life and Palliative Care. 7(1):56-82	10
42	Agnew A, Duffy J (2010) Innovative approaches to involving service users in palliative care social work education. Social Work Education. 29(7):744-759	10

Table 1. (Continued).

Rank	Paper	Times Cited
43	Lacey D (2005) Nursing home social worker skills and end-of-life planning. Social Work in Health Care. 40(4):19-40	10
44	Black RB (1989) Challenges for social work as a core profession in cancer services. Social Work in Health Care. 14(1):1-14	10
45	Rose SL, Shelton W (2006) The role of social work in the ICU: Reducing family distress and facilitating end-of-life decision-making. Journal of Social Work in End-of-Life and Palliative Care. 2(2):3-23	9
46	Reese DJ, Raymer M, Orloff SF (2006) The Social Work Assessment Tool (SWAT). Journal of Social Work in End-of-Life and Palliative Care. 2(2):65-95	9
47	Jones BL (2006) Pediatric palliative and end-of-life care: The role of social work in pediatric oncology. Journal of Social Work in End-of-Life and Palliative Care. 1(4):35-62	9
48	Werner P, Carmel S, Ziedenberg H (2004) Nurses' and social workers' attitudes and beliefs about and involvement in life-sustaining treatment decisions. Health and Social Work. 29(1):27-35	9
49	Becker JE (2004) Oncology social workers' attitudes toward hospice care and referral behavior. Health and Social Work. 29(1):36-45	9
50	Manetta AA, Wells JG (2001) Ethical issues in the social worker's role in physician-assisted suicide. Health and Social Work. 26(3):160-166	9

The bibliographic listing was sorted and ranked by the number of citations received. The most highly cited paper in this group (Rank 1 in Table 1) received a total of 92 cites (5). By comparison a search for a related topic of EOL and ethics resulted in a top paper which received 455 cites (2). When looking at the top 50 articles for social work and EOL 66% obtained less than 20 cites. We decided to present the top 50 articles only since the total cites received drop below 10 after the 44th ranked paper on the list.

Our analysis identified that 42 out of the top 50 cited articles came out of the US (84%), 4 from the UK (8%), and one each from Canada (2%), Israel and South Africa. The author with the most (1) publications is Ellen L Csikai of the School of Social Work, at the University of Alabama. Another institution with the most affiliations (5) within this group of articles is the School of Social Work at Columbia University (8). In addition 33 out of the 50 articles describe results from a mix of qualitative and quantitative research, of which the most popular was the standard survey methodology (n=20). Only two studies involved chart reviews and three employed a review of the literature. No interventional studies were noted in the review of these articles.

An analysis of the top 50 papers showed that articles were published in a total of 14 separate academic journals (Table 2). Sixty percent of them were printed in only three journals: Journal of Social Work in end-of-life and Palliative care; Social Work in Health Care; and, Health and Social Work.

Of particular interest are the topics represented in this group of papers (Table 3). Interestingly 14 (28%) of the publication involved a review of the evolving role of social work in EOL care and 8 articles focused on the education and professional development.

As previously discussed, we undertook a separate search in Scopus to identify the printed articles involving social work, EOL care and ethics. Table 4 presents the 16 articles retrieved, ranked in order of citations received.

Though the number of times an article is referenced is typically an indication of its impact on the academic community, several limitations exist with a study of this nature. Firstly the number of citations an article receives is not a definitive indication of the quality of the work, and that several other factors can be at play in this manifestation (7).

Table 2. Number of papers by Journal

Journal	Number
Journal of Social Work in End-of-Life and Palliative Care	12
Social Work in Health Care	10
Health and Social Work	8
Journal of Palliative Medicine	5
Palliative Medicine	3
Journal of Gerontological Social Work	3
The Hospice journal	2
Dementia	1
Social Work	1
British Journal of Social Work	1
Social Work Education	1
British Journal of Social Work	1
New England Journal of Medicine	1
American Journal of Hospice and Palliative Medicine	1

Table 3. Primary Topics of the Top 50 Papers

Topic	No. of Papers
Role of SW in EOL care	14
Educational Needs/ Professional Development	8
Advance Care Planning	5
Physician Assisted Dying/Euthanasia	5
Ethical Issues	3
Practice standards and guidelines	3
Working with older adults	3
SW Research Agenda EOL	2
Occupational Stress and burn out	2
SW Assessment Tools	2
Working with children and Cancer	2
SW Leadership in EOL Care	2
EOL in ICU	2
Working with dementia	1
Unmet needs at EOL	1

Additionally, the relatively low number of total articles identified to date is indicative of a field that may need further empirical research, and that a top 50 list may be too premature to name as having a significant impact of this field. Our search did not look at the grey literature on this subject matter which will bias the results of our article.

Table 4. Papers on Social Work, Ethics, and End-of-Life Care

Rank	Papers	Times Cited
1	Csikai EL, Raymer M (2005). Social workers' educational needs in end-of-life care. Social Work in Health Care. 41(1):53-72	34
2	Csikai EL, Bass K (2000). Health care social workers' views of ethical issues, practice, and policy in end-of-life care. Social Work in Health Care. 32(2):1-22	33
3	Csikai EL (2004). Social workers' participation in the resolution of ethical dilemmas in hospice care. Health and Social Work. 29(1):67-76	25
4	Luptak M (2004). Social work and end-of-life care for older people: A historical perspective. Health and Social Work. 29(1):7-15	20
5	Bomba PA, Morrissey MB, Leven DC (2011). Key role of social work in effective communication and conflict resolution process: Medical Orders for Life-Sustaining Treatment (MOLST) program in New York and shared medical decision making at the end of life. Journal of Social Work in End-of-Life and Palliative Care. 7(1):56-82	10
6	Manetta AA, Wells JG (2001). Ethical issues in the social worker's role in physician-assisted suicide. Health and Social Work. 26(3):160-166	9
7	Stein GL, Sherman PA (2005). Promoting effective social work policy in end-of-life and palliative care. Journal of Palliative Medicine. 8(6):1271-1281	5
8	Csikai EL, Roth S, Moore C (2004). Ethical problems in end-of-life care decision making faced by oncology social workers and the need for practice guidelines. Journal of Psychosocial Oncology. 22(1)1:18	5
9	Miller PJ, Mesler MA, Eggman ST (2002). Take some time to look inside their hearts: Hospice social workers contemplate physician assisted suicide. Social Work in Health Care. 35(3):53-64	4
10	Holloway M (2009). Dying old in the 21st century: A neglected issue for social work. International Social Work. 52(6):713-725	3
11	Roff S (2001). Analyzing end-of-life care legislation: A social work perspective. Social Work in Health Care. 33(1):51-68	3
12	Holmes KA (1980). Euthanasia: a social work perspective. Health and Social Work. 5(4):5-12	3
13	Sanders S, Bullock K, Broussard C (2012). Exploring Professional Boundaries in End-of-Life Care: Considerations for Hospice Social Workers and Other Members of the Team. Journal of Social Work in End-of-Life and Palliative Care. 8(1):10-28	1
14	Altilio T, Otis-Green S (2006). "Res ipsa loquitur" . . . It speaks for itself . . . Social work-values, pain, and palliative care. Journal of Social Work in End-of-Life and Palliative Care. 1(4):3-6	0
15	Dennis MK, Washington KT, Koenig TL (2014). Ethical dilemmas faced by hospice social workers. Social Work in Health Care. 53(9):950-968	0
16	Kwon SA, Kolomer S, Alper J (2014). The Attitudes of Social Work Students Toward End-of-Life Care Planning. Journal of Social Work in End-of-Life and Palliative Care. 10(3):240-256	0

To our understanding, this is the first report to identify the top cited papers covering the field of social work in EOL care. Limitations aside it does stand as a point of reference for social workers and social work students interested in EOL care, and perhaps even a clarion call for social workers to undertake a rigorous and evidenced- based research agenda forward to better represent their important contribution to the evolving field of EOL care.

ACKNOWLEDGMENTS

We thank the generous support of the Bratty Family Fund, Michael and Karyn Goldstein Cancer Research Fund, Joey and Mary Furfari Cancer Research Fund, Pulenzas Cancer Research Fund, Joseph and Silvana Melara Cancer Research Fund, and Ofelia Cancer Research Fund.

REFERENCES

[1] National Association of Social Workers. NASW standards on palliative and end of life care. Washington, DC: National Association of Social Workers, 2004.

[2] Sprung CL, Cohen SL, Sjokvist P, Baras M, Bulow H, Hovilehto S, et al. End-of-life practices in European intensive care units: The Ethicus study. JAMA 2003; 290(6): 790-7.

[3] Bhandari M, Busse J, Devereaux PJ, Montori VM, Swiontkowski M, Tornetta Iii P, et al. Factors associated with citation rates in the orthopedic literature. Can J Surg 2007; 50: 119-23.

[4] Falagas ME, Pitsouni, EI, Malietzis, GA, Pappas G. Comparison of PubMed, Scopus, Web of Science, and Google Scholar: strengths and weaknesses. FASEB J 2008; 22(2): 338-42.

[5] Ganzini L, Harvath TA, Jackson A, Goy ER, Miller L, Delorit M. Experiences of Oregon nurses and social workers with hospice patients who requested assistance with suicide. N Engl J Med 2002; 347(8): 582-8.

[6] Altillo T, Gardia G, Otis-Green S. Social work practice in palliative and end-of-life care: a report from the summit. J Soc *Work End Life* Palliat Care 2007; 3(4): 68-86.

[7] Weale AR, Bailey M, Lear PA. The level of noncitation of articles within a journal as a measure of quality: a comparison to the impact factor. BMC Med Res Methodol 2004; 4: 14.

[8] Christ GH, Blacker S. Setting an agenda for social work in end-of-life and palliative care: an overview of leadership and organizational initiatives. J Soc *Work End Life* Palliat Care 2005; 1(1): 9-22.

SECTION FIVE: ACKNOWLEDGMENTS

In: Pain Management Yearbook 2015
Editor: Joav Merrick
ISBN: 978-1-63484-515-1

Chapter 38

ABOUT THE EDITOR

Joav Merrick, MD, MMedSci, DMSc, born and educated in Denmark is professor of pediatrics, child health and human development, Division of Pediatrics, Hadassah Hebrew University Medical Center, Mt Scopus Campus, Jerusalem, Israel and Kentucky Children's Hospital, University of Kentucky, Lexington, Kentucky United States and professor of public health at the Center for Healthy Development, School of Public Health, Georgia State University, Atlanta, United States, the medical director of the Health Services, Division for Intellectual and Developmental Disabilities, Ministry of Social Affairs and Social Services, Jerusalem, the founder and director of the National Institute of Child Health and Human Development in Israel. Numerous publications in the field of pediatrics, child health and human development, rehabilitation, intellectual disability, disability, health, welfare, abuse, advocacy, quality of life and prevention. Received the Peter Sabroe Child Award for outstanding work on behalf of Danish Children in 1985 and the International LEGO-Prize ("The Children's Nobel Prize") for an extraordinary contribution towards improvement in child welfare and well-being in 1987.

Contact:

Office of the Medical Director, Health Services, Division for Intellectual and Developmental Disabilities, Ministry of Social Affairs and Social Services, POBox 1260, IL-91012 Jerusalem, Israel. E-mail: jmerrick@zahav.net.il

In: Pain Management Yearbook 2015
Editor: Joav Merrick

ISBN: 978-1-63484-515-1

Chapter 39

About the National Institute of Child Health and Human Development in Israel

The National Institute of Child Health and Human Development (NICHD) in Israel were established in 1998 as a virtual institute under the auspices of the Medical Director, Ministry of Social Affairs and Social Services in order to function as the research arm for the Office of the Medical Director. In 1998 the National Council for Child Health and Pediatrics, Ministry of Health and in 1999 the Director General and Deputy Director General of the Ministry of Health endorsed the establishment of the NICHD.

Mission

The mission of a National Institute for Child Health and Human Development in Israel is to provide an academic focal point for the scholarly interdisciplinary study of child life, health, public health, welfare, disability, rehabilitation, intellectual disability and related aspects of human development. This mission includes research, teaching, clinical work, information and public service activities in the field of child health and human development.

Service and academic activities

Over the years many activities became focused in the south of Israel due to collaboration with various professionals at the Faculty of Health Sciences (FOHS) at the Ben Gurion University of the Negev (BGU). Since 2000 an affiliation with the Zusman Child Development Center at the Pediatric Division of Soroka University Medical Center has resulted in collaboration around the establishment of the Down Syndrome Clinic at that center. In 2002 a full course on "Disability" was established at the Recanati School for Allied Professions in the Community, FOHS, BGU and in 2005 collaboration was started with the Primary Care Unit of the faculty and disability became part of the master of public health course on "Children and society". In the academic year 2005-2006 a one semester course on "Aging with disability" was started as part of the master of science program in gerontology in our collaboration with the Center for Multidisciplinary Research in Aging. In 2010 collaborations with the Division of Pediatrics, Hadassah Hebrew University Medical Center, Jerusalem, Israel around the National Down Syndrome Center and teaching students and residents about intellectual and developmental disabilities as part of their training at this campus.

Research activities

The affiliated staff have over the years published work from projects and research activities in this national and international collaboration. In the year 2000 the International Journal of Adolescent Medicine and Health and in 2005 the International Journal on Disability and Human Development of De Gruyter Publishing House (Berlin and New York) were affiliated with the National Institute of Child Health and Human Development. From 2008 also the International Journal of Child Health and Human Development (Nova Science, New York), the International Journal of Child and Adolescent Health (Nova Science) and the Journal of Pain Management (Nova Science) affiliated and from 2009 the International Public Health Journal (Nova Science) and Journal of Alternative Medicine Research (Nova Science). All peer-reviewed international journals.

National collaborations

Nationally the NICHD works in collaboration with the Faculty of Health Sciences, Ben Gurion University of the Negev; Department of Physical Therapy, Sackler School of Medicine, Tel Aviv University; Autism Center, Assaf HaRofeh Medical Center; National Rett and PKU Centers at Chaim Sheba Medical Center, Tel HaShomer; Department of Physiotherapy, Haifa University; Department of Education, Bar Ilan University, Ramat Gan, Faculty of Social Sciences and Health Sciences; College of Judea and Samaria in Ariel and in 2011 affiliation with Center for Pediatric Chronic Diseases and National Center for Down Syndrome, Department of Pediatrics, Hadassah Hebrew University Medical Center, Mount Scopus Campus, Jerusalem.

International collaborations

Internationally with the Department of Disability and Human Development, College of Applied Health Sciences, University of Illinois at Chicago; Strong Center for Developmental Disabilities, Golisano Children's Hospital at Strong, University of Rochester School of Medicine and Dentistry, New York; Centre on Intellectual Disabilities, University of Albany, New York; Centre for Chronic Disease Prevention and Control, Health Canada, Ottawa; Chandler Medical Center and Children's Hospital, Kentucky Children's Hospital, Section of Adolescent Medicine, University of Kentucky, Lexington; Chronic Disease Prevention and Control Research Center, Baylor College of Medicine, Houston, Texas; Division of Neuroscience, Department of Psychiatry, Columbia University, New York; Institute for the Study of Disadvantage and Disability, Atlanta; Center for Autism and Related Disorders, Department Psychiatry, Children's Hospital Boston, Boston; Department of Paediatrics, Child Health and Adolescent Medicine, Children's Hospital at Westmead, Westmead, Australia;

International Centre for the Study of Occupational and Mental Health, Düsseldorf, Germany; Centre for Advanced Studies in Nursing, Department of General Practice and Primary Care, University of Aberdeen, Aberdeen, United Kingdom; Quality of Life Research Center, Copenhagen, Denmark; Nordic School of Public Health, Gottenburg, Sweden, Scandinavian Institute of Quality of Working Life, Oslo, Norway; The Department of Applied Social Sciences (APSS) of The Hong Kong Polytechnic University Hong Kong.

Targets

Our focus is on research, international collaborations, clinical work, teaching and policy in health, disability and human development and to establish the NICHD as a permanent institute at one of the residential care centers for persons with intellectual disability in Israel in order to conduct model research and together with the four university schools of public health/medicine in Israel establish a national master and doctoral program in disability and human development at the institute to secure the next generation of professionals working in this often non-prestigious/low-status field of work.

Contact

Professor Joav Merrick, MD, MMedSci, DMSc
Medical Director, Health Services, Division for Intellectual and Developmental Disabilities, Ministry of Social Affairs and Social Services, POB 1260, IL-91012 Jerusalem, Israel.
E-mail: jmerrick@zahav.net.il

SECTION SIX: INDEX

INDEX

C

D

E

F

G

J

K

L

M

N

O

P

Q

R

S

T

U

V

W

X

Z